NURSING SHIFTS IN SICHUAN

NURSING SHIFTS IN SICHUAN

CANADIAN MISSIONS AND
WARTIME CHINA, 1937–51

Sonya Grypma

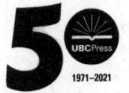

30 29 28 27 26 25 24 23 22 21   5 4 3 2 1

Printed in Canada on FSC-certified ancient-forest-free paper (100% post-consumer recycled) that is processed chlorine- and acid-free.

LIBRARY AND ARCHIVES CANADA CATALOGUING IN PUBLICATION

Title: Nursing shifts in Sichuan : Canadian missions and wartime China, 1937-51 / Sonya Grypma.
Names: Grypma, Sonya, 1965- author.
Description: Includes bibliographical references and index.
Identifiers: Canadiana (print) 20210291079 | Canadiana (ebook) 20210291591 | ISBN 9780774865715 (hardcover) | ISBN 9780774865722 (paperback) | ISBN 9780774865739 (PDF) | ISBN 9780774865746 (EPUB)
Subjects: LCSH: Peking Union Medical College—History. | LCSH: Hua xi xie he da xue—History. | LCSH: United Church of Canada. West China Mission—History. | LCSH: Nursing—Study and teaching—China—History—20th century. | LCSH: Nursing—China—History—20th century. | LCSH: Missions, Medical—China— Sichuan Sheng—History—20th century. | LCSH: Sino-Japanese War, 1937-1945— Refugees—China.
Classification: LCC RT81.C6 G79 2021 | DDC 610.73071/151—dc23

Canadä

UBC Press gratefully acknowledges the financial support for our publishing program of the Government of Canada (through the Canada Book Fund) and the British Columbia Arts Council.

This book has been published with the help of a grant from the Canadian Federation for the Humanities and Social Sciences, through the Awards to Scholarly Publications Program, using funds provided by the Social Sciences and Humanities Research Council of Canada.

UBC Press
The University of British Columbia
2029 West Mall
Vancouver, BC V6T 1Z2
www.ubcpress.ca

to Sylvia Ann (Visser) Slagter (1963–2018)

Contents

Illustrations and Tables

Tables

Abbreviations

AJN	*American Journal of Nursing*
CMB	China Medical Board
FAU	Friends Ambulance Unit
FMB	Foreign Mission Board
ICN	International Council of Nurses
IHD	International Health Division of the Rockefeller Foundation
LMS	London Missionary Society
MEM	Mass Education Movement
NAC	Nurses Association of China
NCM	North China Mission
PUMC	Peking Union Medical College (*Beijing Xiehe*)
PUMC-SNA	PUMC School of Nursing Archives
RF	Rockefeller Foundation
SCM	South China Mission
UMASC	University of Manitoba Archives and Special Collections
UNRRA	United Nations Rehabilitation and Relief Administration
WCM	United Church of Canada West China Mission
WCUU	West China Union University (*Huaxi Xiehe*)
WHO	World Health Organization
WMS	Woman's Missionary Society
YMCA	Young Men's Christian Association

Historical Highlights

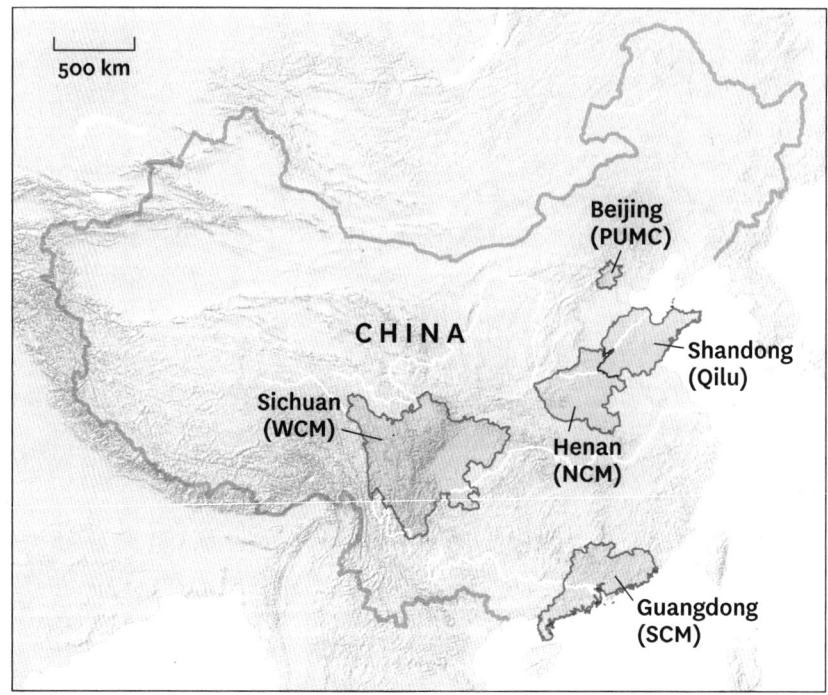

FIGURE 0.1 Location of Canadian missions and key northern medical universities in China. | Map by Eric Leinberger.

Political events	West China Mission events	Nursing events
1860: Second Opium War ends	1865: Adeline (Galliland) Hart is first Canadian missionary sent to China	1884: First missionary nurse
	1875: Canadian doctor Leonora Howard King to China under American Methodist Mission	1888: First Canadian missionary nurse
	1888: Canadian Presbyterian missionaries to North China (NCM)	
	1891: Dr. and Mrs. Hart, Dr. Omar, and Mrs. Kilborn among 9 Canadian Methodist missionaries to depart for West China (Sichuan)	
	1892: First dispensary opened at WCM	
	1894: Men's Hospital started in Chengdu (FMB)	
	1895: Women's Hospital started in Chengdu (WMS); Jennie Ford, first nurse at WCM	
1900: Boxer Uprising	1902: Presbyterian missionaries to Guangdong (SCM)	1907: Cora Simpson arrives in China
1908: Empress Dowager dies	1906: Nurse Caroline Wellwood sails for China	1909: NAC established, with Caroline Hart as president
	1909: Wellwood trains 2 Chinese women to dispense medicine	

1865–99

1900–09

Political events	WCM events	PUMC events	Nursing events
1910: Manchurian plague	1910: Canadian Methodists join 4 other denominations to found WCUU	1914: Rockefeller Foundation establishes China Medical Board	1911: China Medical Commission examines state of missionary hospitals
1911: Overthrow of Qing Dynasty	1911: Missionaries evacuate Chengdu	1915: CMB purchases Union Medical College from LMS, opens PUMC on site	1912: Missionaries hold NAC meeting during exile; Nina Gage becomes NAC president
1912: Republic of China established	1913: WCM opens men's nursing school	1917: Premedical school opens to men	1914: 5th NAC Conference; nursing named *Hushi*
1916: President Yuan Skikai dies	1914: WCUU Medical College opens	1918: Ruth Ingram becomes dean of nursing	
1919: May Fourth Movement	1915: WCM opens women's nursing school		

1910–19

Political events	WCM events	PUMC events	Nursing events
	1918: First nurse graduate of WCM 1919: Women's School of Nursing registers with NAC	1919: Premedical school opens to women; medical college opens; RF sponsors Committee for Study of Nursing Education in United States	1919: Anna Wolf appointed dean and superintendent of nursing at PUMC
1926: Chiang Kai-shek leads Northern Expedition 1928: Nanjing declared national capital	1920: Men's School of Nursing registers with NAC 1921: Leslie Kilborn to WCM 1922: WCUU incorporated 1925: Canadian Methodists and Presbyterians join as United Church of Canada 1926: Cora Kilborn to China as missionary nurse 1927: Great missionary exodus	1920: PUMC School of Nursing admits first students 1922: Two nursing programs: diploma and degree 1923: Vera Nieh admitted to PUMC 1925: Beijing Health Station opens	1920: *Nursing Journal of China* starts 1922: NAC joins ICN; Cora Simpson is NAC executive secretary 1923: *Goldmark Report* published in USA 1928 Lillian Wu first Chinese NAC president
1931: Japan annexes Manchuria 1932: Japan bombs Shanghai 1937: Marco Polo Bridge Incident; Japan occupies Beijing 1938: Mass migration of millions to Free China 1939: 47 institutions have migrated to West China and 21 to Shanghai; first major bombing of Chongqing	1936: Renji hires first Chinese principal and first Chinese head nurse 1937: Qilu Medical School, National Central University migrate to West China, hosted at WCUU 1938: Men's and Women's Hospital combined into United Hospital; only women students now accepted at WCM (United Hospital) 1939: WCUU is hosting 5 evacuated universities	1930: Gertrude Hodgman becomes dean 1934: Vera Nieh first secretary of Central Board of Nursing Education 1937: Hodgman agrees to step down as dean but wartime interrupts departure 1938: Chou Meiyu turns down dean position	1931: Chou Meiyu leaves PUMC for MEM 1934: Ministry of Education organizes Central Board of Nursing Education; replaces some of NAC functions 1937: NAC Headquarters open in Nanjing; some staff relocate to West China

1910–19

1920–29

1930–39

1940: Chongqing designated China's wartime capital

1941: Pearl Harbor; US declares war on Japan

1945: US drops atomic bombs on Hiroshima/Nagasaki; Japan surrenders

1945: Civil war between Nationalists, Communists

1949: Mao Zedong declares victory, establishes People's Republic of China

1940: WCM Hospital destroyed by fire; NCM Clara Preston, Dorothy Boyd, Margaret Gay, and Ernest Struthers relocate to WCM; Cora Kilborn to Canada

1941: Dorothy Boyd, Clara Preston, Margaret Gay depart China

1942: Caroline Wellwood returns to Canada

1943: New University Hospital opens

1944: Cora Kilborn returns to China

1946: WCUU starts baccalaureate program

1949: Chengdu surrenders to Communist army

1940: Vera Nieh becomes first Chinese dean of nursing; Henry Houghton to West China to gather info about PUMC evacuees

1941: Japanese occupy PUMC; 14 Western staff and families arrested/interned

1942: Classes discontinue at PUMC

1943: Claude Forkner signs agreement with WCUU; Refugee PUMC admits in first nursing class

1946: PUMC school returns to Beijing

1941: Japanese takeover of PUMC School of Nursing; enemy aliens placed under house arrest

1943: PUMC nurses arrive at WCUU; Chou Meiyu opens first Army Nursing School

1949: ICN recognizes Republic of China in Taiwan as China's government; Peoples Republic of China removed from ICN membership

1950: People's Republic of China enters Korean War

1950: Cora Kilborn resigns

1951: Canada closes all China missions

1952: Remaining 6 missionaries depart Chengdu

1951: Communist government takes over PUMC; Vera Nieh replaced by Communist Party member

1951: University-level education for nurses in China ends

Key People

Name	Alternate name	Main affiliation	Main position
Balfour, Marshall C.	M.C. Balfour	RF, IHD	Director
Beard, Mary		RF, IHD	Associate director
Best, Allan E.		WCM	Hospital director/ superintendent
Boyd, Dorothy		WCM	Missionary nurse
Chang, Stephen		PUMC	Professor of medicine
Chen, C.C.		PUMC	Board of trustees
Chou Meiyu	Zhou Meiyu	PUMC	Nurse
Chu Chen, Bernice	Chu Phi-hui; Zhu Bihui	PUMC	Nurse
Crawley, Mary		WCM	Missionary nurse
Eggleston, Margery		CMB	Secretary
Ferguson, Mary		PUMC	Secretary
Forkner, Claude		CMB	Director
Fox, Dorothy		WCM	Missionary nurse
Gay, Margaret		WCM	Missionary nurse
Grant, John B.		PUMC	Head, public health
Greene, Roger		PUMC	Acting director
Gunn, Selskar M.		RF	Vice-president
Harrison, Adelaide		WCM	WMS secretary-treasurer
Harris, Winifred		WCM	WMS secretary treasurer
Hodgman, Gertrude		PUMC	Dean of nursing
Houghton, Harry	Houghton, Henry S.	PUMC	Acting director
Hsu Ai-Chu	Xu Ai-chu	PUMC	Nurse
Ingram, Ruth		PUMC	Acting superintendent

Name	Alternate name	Main affiliation	Main position
Kilborn, Cora		WCM	Nursing principal, Renji
Kilborn, Leslie		WCM	Dean of medicine, WCUU
Lee, Margaret		WCM	Missionary nurse
Lin, Evelyn	Lin Sz-sing	PUMC	Nurse
Lobenstine, Edwin		CMB	Director?
McCabe, Anne		PUMC	Chief, health visiting
McIntosh, Janet M.		WCM	Missionary nurse
Miller, Isabelle		WCM	Missionary nurse
Nieh, Vera	Nieh Yuchan	PUMC	Dean of nursing
Pao Ai-Ching	Pao, Gertrude	PUMC	Nurse
Preston, Clara		WCM	Missionary nurse
Tallman, Anna		WCM	Missionary nurse
Taylor, Lillian		WCM	Missionary nurse
Taylor, Mrs. Hugh		UCC	WMS executive secretary
Tennant, Mary		RF, IHD	Assistant director, nursing consultant
Wang, Hilda	Wang Ia fang	PUMC	Nurse
Wang Hsui-ying	Wang Shuiying/ Wang Xiuying	PUMC	Assistant dean of nursing
Whiteside, Faye		PUMC	Acting dean of nursing
Wu, Lillian	Wu Zheying	PUMC	Nurse, NAC president

Foreword

For Mainland Chinese, the mention of Canada's historical medical connection to China automatically brings to mind Dr. Norman Bethune. Bethune's ongoing fame in China can be attributed to Chairman Mao Zedong's article "Learn from Bethune," published in December 1939. This article commemorated Bethune as "a Canadian Communist Party member who, in order to aid China's Resistance to the Japan Invasion, was sent by the Canadian and American Communist Parties, travelling from ten thousand miles away to China, where he consecrated his life." In China, Bethune's image is so recognizable as a heroic icon of a selfless Western doctor that his fame has overshadowed the considerable medical efforts of other Canadians, especially missionaries. But this is changing.

In *Nursing Shifts in Sichuan: Canadian Missions and Wartime China, 1937–51*, Sonya Grypma, a Canadian historian of nursing and past dean of a Canadian school of nursing, continues her groundbreaking work on Canadian missionaries and their footprint in China. Her previous books (*Healing Henan: Canadian Nurses at the North China Mission, 1888–1947* and *China Interrupted: Japanese Internment and the Reshaping of a Missionary Community*) focused on Canadian missionaries at the North China Mission. In this third book, Grypma expands her lens to include Canadians in West China as well as Chinese nursing leaders from the Peking Union Medical College (PUMC, considered "the darling child of the Rockefeller Foundation"). The title of this book invites readers to consider how such disparate groups connected with each other during the War of Resistance against Japan. As Grypma reveals, it was the wartime migration of millions to West China that brought these contrasting groups together on the campus of the West China Union University for three years. Here they discovered a common purpose: to support, equip, and sustain the Chinese during a brutal war.

In this book, Sonya Grypma captures and contextualizes a very important period in the history of nursing in China. For thousands of years before missionaries from the West introduced modern Western medicine into China, the Chinese had used their own medicine to heal illness and preserve health. However, caring for the sick had always been done by lay people and was seen as the responsibility of family members. Missionaries opened up hospitals and brought to Chinese society the idea of caring for illness outside of the family. Since caring for patients in hospitals necessitates nurses, in the late nineteenth century medical missionaries also introduced modern nursing in China. At that time, both hospitals and missionaries were foreign to Chinese society, and theirs was an arduous existence.

As Sonya Grypma notes in this volume, nursing history in China has played out against a tumultuous and unsettled backdrop. It is a history interwoven with wars, political uncertainty, and changes in regimes. The first Western nurse, Elizabeth McKetchnie, arrived in China in 1884. At that time, China was undergoing the collapse of the (anti-Christian) Qing Dynasty. In order to address the severe shortage of nurses, medical missionaries set up schools to train Chinese nurse assistants, mostly males from poor families. During the Boxer Rebellion in 1900, missionaries and their approach to medicine were relentlessly attacked. In 1908, at the peak of the anti-missionary movement, missionary nurses established the Nurses Association of China (NAC, now the Chinese Nurses Association). Three years later, Dr. Sun Yat-sen led a revolution to overthrow the Qing Dynasty and establish the Republic of China. It was during the Republican Era (1911–49) that Western medicine became central to China's new scheme for modernity, and modern nursing development accelerated.

The establishment of a school of nursing and a public health nursing program at the PUMC in 1920 was a significant milestone in nursing history. Although foreign nurses still dominated and led nursing education and practice in China during this period, Chinese female nurses became increasingly visible professionally. In 1928, Lillian Wu became the first

Chinese president of the NAC, marking the beginning of the transition in nursing leadership from foreigners to Chinese. In 1927, after a series of wars between warlords, Chiang Kai-shek united most of China under his leadership. For ten years, China enjoyed a period of cherished peace. During this decade, the country established a national public health care administration system through which the Ministry of Education and National Health Administration began to pay more attention to nursing education. The government nationalized nursing education and practice standards and took over nursing registration and qualification examinations from the NAC. When the War of Resistance against Japan broke out in 1937, nursing in China experienced further dramatic changes: the number of Chinese nurses grew, foreign nurses were replaced, military and public health nursing was established, and nursing education became even more deeply established.

In the years leading up to the War of Resistance, the relationship between nursing and Christianity in China had grown increasingly tenuous. The PUMC School of Nursing exemplified a growing commitment to science and to university-level education rather than the apprenticeship training common to missionary nursing schools. The PUMC was also unique in holding nursing education to be valuable as, and not subservient to, medical education. The PUMC, with its high standards, produced a cohort of Chinese nursing leaders well prepared for the increasingly nationalized educational and public health systems.

In *Nursing Shifts in Sichuan*, Grypma examines two distinct groups of nurses: Canadian missionaries and the Chinese nurses of the PUMC. The parallel footprints of these groups crossed and eventually merged into one path in "Free China" – the interior territories in West China that remained unoccupied by the Japanese throughout the war. At the end of her book, Grypma describes the termination of both the Canadian missionary undertaking in West China and the PUMC after the eruption of the Korea War, when all the Westerners, including the last Canadian missionaries, were forced to leave China. China closed all of its collegiate nursing programs, including the PUMC, in 1951, marking the end of an era in China's nursing history.

I have known Sonya Grypma since 2012. She was one of the contributors to the book *Medical Transitions in Twentieth-Century China,* written as part of the China Medical Board Centennial Series, coauthoring the chapter on nursing history in China. I was impressed by her knowledge of and research into China's nursing history, since nursing history has been poorly studied in China. In that chapter, she divided China's history of nursing before 1949 into three distinct periods: nursing as Christian service, as a profession, and as a patriotic service, and she gave the study of the nursing history a new and insightful angle. In this new book, Sonya discusses issues of race, class, and gender as she recounts the stories of both Canadian and Chinese nurses. It builds on her previous books on Canadian missionary nursing in China, extending beyond accounts of relatively isolated evangelical Canadian missionaries to include the widely influential, scientifically educated cohort of PUMC nurses. In so doing, this book encompasses overlapping narratives that include the fate of missionary nurses and the experiences of "heroic" Chinese nursing leaders, all of whom faced the hardship, chaos, and life-threatening risk during wartime.

Sonya's books are based on extensive archival research. She has made research trips to the Rockefeller Archive Center in New York as well as to archives in Canada and China. We've met up in Beijing whenever she's made research trips to the PUMC Archives here, and have had good conversations about our shared interest in nursing history. In addition to our friendship, I have benefited from and been inspired by her academic advice, her zest for research, her vigor as a nursing leader, and her knowledge about China and the nursing profession.

Today, nursing has become an indispensable part of the health care system in China. However, nurses lack the strong voice needed for them to secure a more respectable status and to be acknowledged for their important role. In reading *Nursing Shifts in Sichuan* and Sonya's detailed and vivid description of the courage, persistence, and fortitude of the PUMC nursing leaders in rebuilding the School of Nursing in West China, I cannot help but see a parallel to China's current fight against the outbreak of COVID-19. As I write this, more than 28,000 nurses from different parts of China have been sent to the epicenter of the epidemic – in Wuhan and surrounding areas – as frontline workers in high-risk settings fighting against a very contagious disease. Nurses now in the fight against COVID-19 are connected to the heritage of the achievements of their predecessors during wartime seventy years ago.

Yuhong Jiang, PhD
School of Humanities and Social Sciences,
Peking Union Medical College
Beijing, China, February 2020

Preface

One need look no further than the outbreak of COVID-19 to recognize the swiftness with which a health crisis can change the trajectory of world history – and nursing history within it. The World Health Organization's (WHO) declaration of a global pandemic on 11 March 2020 occurred less than two weeks after UBC Press approved publication of this book. Avenues to archives so critical to my research are now indefinitely closed. When the WHO designated 2020 as the Year of the Nurse and the Midwife in honour of Florence Nightingale's birth 200 years ago, little did they know how fitting that designation would become. Tributes to nurses and other health care workers have been ubiquitous, including noisy neighbourhood acknowledgments nightly at 7 p.m., the hour of shift changes. Nurse volunteers – including graduates from my own institution – have travelled to the frontlines of the pandemic in northern Italy and New York City to volunteer in makeshift hospitals set up to contain the surge of patients. In China, nursing leaders – including colleagues who have supported me in the research for this book – left their homes and families for two months to work at the frontlines in Wuhan. Cao Yingjuan, professor and director of nursing at the Qilu Hospital of Shandong University in Jinan, emailed me in February from Hubei, where she had travelled with 130 colleagues from her institution to support the fight against COVID-19. They were surprised and delighted to meet up with a Huaxi (Guiyang) team at the airport in Wuhan, and subsequently worked together at the same hospital in Hubei. It had been eighty-three years, she told me, since nurses from those institutions had worked together; the last time was during the War of Resistance against Japan.

As I write this (July 2020), the story of COVID-19 is still unfolding. My home province of British Columbia has just entered Phase 3 of its Restart Plans, having successfully flattened the COVID-19 curve through stringent public health measures led by an extraordinary public health officer, Dr. Bonnie Henry. In the meantime, the United States is experiencing a worrisome surge in COVID-19 cases, prompting Canada to extend its closure of our shared 9,000-kilometre border yet again. With one eye warily on daily case counts, the Canadian Association for Schools of Nursing has advocated for nursing education in Canada to be deemed an essential service. Nursing leaders across Canada are working through ways to ensure that nursing education is both safe and not delayed. Behind the scenes, nurses who work in leadership positions in universities — including in provosts' and presidents' offices — are helping their institutions make safe decisions regarding the reopening of campuses. We are, in short, living through a global disruption whose impact, though still unknown, will be historic. For future historians, then, seeking to examine how COVID-19 reshaped the health care landscape regionally and globally (as it will inevitably do), here is my advice: Follow the nurses.

A NOTE ON SPELLINGS AND TERMINOLOGY

Wherever possible, Pinyin spellings are used in this book for names of places. This is to help readers situate places on a present-day map of China. Wade-Giles spelling is used in cases where Pinyin could not be ascertained. (Places frequently referenced in this book appear in the list below, which provides both the Pinyin spellings and their Wade-Giles equivalent.) In contrast, for people's names, I generally use the Wade-Giles spellings that are found in the records, unless the Pinyin name is well known (for example, "Mao Zedong" rather than "Mao Tsetung"). Where a person has both an English and a Chinese given name, the English name is generally used, with the surname following the given name.

Finally, I have chosen to use present-day educational terminology in situations where archival terms conflict or might be confusing. For

Pinyin/ Contemporary	Wade-Giles/ Common	Pinyin/ Contemporary	Wade-Giles/ Common
Anyang/Zhangde	Changte	Luzhou	Luchow/Jiangyang
Beijing	Peking/Peiping	Pengxian	Penghsien
Beidaihe	Peitaiho	Pudong	Pootung
Baoji/Paoki	Pao-chi	Qingdao	Tsintao/Tsingtao
Chengdu	Chengtu	Qilu	Cheeloo
Chongqing	Chungking	Renshou	Jenshow
Dingxian	Ting Hsien	Rongxian	Junghsien
Fuzhou	Foochow/Fowchow	Sanqui	Kweiteh/Shangkiu
Fujian	Fukien	Shaanxi	Shensi
Gansu	Kansu	Shandong	Shantung
Guangdong	Kuangtung	Sichuan	Szechwan
Guangzhou	Canton/Kwangchow	Suzhou	Soochow
Guiyang	Kweiyang	Taiwan	Formosa
Nanjing	Nanking	Tianjin	Teintsien
Guizhou	Kweichou/Kweichow	Weihui	Weihwei
Guilin	Kweilin/Kueilin	Weixian	Weihsien
Guomindong	Kuomintang/KMT	Wuhan/Hankou	Wuhan/Hankow
Hangzhou	Hanchow	Xian	Sian
Hebei	Hopei	Yenching	Yanjing
Henan	Honan	Zhengzhou	Chengchow
Huaiqing	Hwaiking	Zhejiang	Chekiang
Jinan	Tsinan	Zhongzhou	Chungcho
Lanzhou	Lanchow	Ziliujing/Zigong	Tzeliutsin
Leshan	Kiating/Jiading		

example, I use the term "program" rather than "course" when referring to a series of courses leading to a diploma or degree. I also favour the terms "university-level" or "baccalaureate" over "collegiate" or "high-grade," although I use all of these. I use the terms "Western nursing" and "modern nursing" interchangeably, both referring to scientific and hospital-based nursing, which is aligned with Western medicine and science. Also, I generally use the term "School of Nursing" for educational institutions for nurses at both hospitals and universities. Finally, I use the terms "West China" and "Free China" interchangeably. While both terms generally refer to the province of Sichuan, Free China included all unoccupied regions in China's southwest.

NURSING SHIFTS IN SICHUAN

Introduction

Nursing, Shifted

What [Peking Union Medical College Dean of Nursing] Miss [Vera] Nieh and her faculty have achieved during the war has shown the finest quality of Chinese professional women. We all are very proud of them.

— *I.C. Yuan (China Medical Board), 1946*

In July 1943, nurses at the United Church of Canada West China Mission (WCM) in Chengdu, Sichuan, waited with nervous anticipation for the arrival of a new group of academic refugees at the campus of the West China Union University (WCUU), a Christian university run by four Protestant missions.[1] The WCUU was already hosting four evacuated universities from Japanese-occupied areas of China. For the previous three years, WCM nurses had been working out of two makeshift hospitals in Chengdu after the WCM Women's Hospital was destroyed by fire, likely arson, in 1940.[2] Plans had been made to build a new university hospital on the WCUU campus to replace the Women's Hospital, now in ruins, but these plans were hampered by wartime conditions. Although Chengdu, in its isolation, had thus far not been occupied by the Japanese, it had experienced the full impact of the Sino-Japanese War through six years of air raids, displacement, and war-related trauma. A combination of extreme inflation and restricted transportation was causing a critical shortage of food, medical equipment, and supplies. There was also a shortage of nurses. Prior to the war, as many as sixteen Canadian missionary nurses were working in West China at any given time. In 1943, there were only four. Nor were there enough Chinese nurses at the mission; graduates of the Canadian nursing schools were quickly seconded by the government to help with the war effort.[3]

The wartime nursing shortage impacted not only patient care and staff morale, but also the training of physicians. Since opening in 1914, the WCUU Medical College had always relied on the Canadian mission hospitals for the clinical training of medical students. That is, despite the "union" nature of the WCUU, the medical, hospital, and nursing services in Chengdu were, in fact, almost entirely a Canadian enterprise, primarily overseen and staffed by WCM missionaries. The WCM had ten mission stations in Sichuan, five of which had hospitals with small nurses' training schools. The main training school, called Renji, was closely affiliated with the WCUU in Chengdu, and had been run primarily out of the WCM Women's Hospital. Canadian missionary nurses supervised the nursing services of the WCM hospitals and ran the associated nursing schools, while Chinese nursing students provided much of the day-to-day patient care under the watchful eye of graduated ("graduate") nurses. In other words, the WCUU Medical School was (indirectly but fully) reliant on Chinese nursing students; WCUU medical students obtained their clinical (hands-on) training in hospitals that were staffed mainly by nursing students and their instructors. The shortage of nurses and medical training schools translated into a shortage of medical training. In brief, the WCUU was keen to see its nursing educational programs flourish.

Up until this period, the WCM nursing schools, including Renji, offered "low-grade" nursing programs – an approach to nursing education common in China at the time. In "low-grade" schools, nursing students were junior middle school graduates who received three years of apprenticeship-style training in the hospitals. In contrast, the Peking Union Medical College (PUMC) in Beijing, which was sponsored by the Rockefeller Foundation, offered China's only "high-grade" (collegiate) nursing program.[4] At the PUMC, nursing students were senior high school graduates who had to meet university entrance requirements and complete a year of university-level prerequisites before entering nursing school. Whereas WCM graduates received a nursing diploma, PUMC graduates received both a diploma and a baccalaureate degree. The PUMC approach to nursing education was trailblazing. It reflected the Rockefeller Foundation's aim to prepare nursing *leaders*, not simply rank-and-file nurses. Given this context, it is not surprising that, in July 1943, the Woman's Missionary Society (WMS) and WCUU in Chengdu were so eagerly awaiting the arrival of what would be its fifth refugee academic institution. It would now host the elite PUMC School of Nursing.

One of the "most astonishing phenomena" in the War of Resistance against Japan was the mass migration involving thousands of students and hundreds of professors to West ("Free") China.[5] Although the migration started immediately after Japan invaded China in 1937, the PUMC remained in place in Beijing. In December 1941, the Japanese army used the pretext of America's declaration of war after Pearl Harbor to take over the PUMC. Within months, its faculty and students were scattered around China, with many migrating to the safety of Free China, a dangerous journey of 1,500 miles. The PUMC dean of nursing, Vera Nieh, and her brother set out for Free China in March 1943. Tragically, he was killed by Chinese soldiers along the way.[6] After connecting with PUMC staff and alumnae in Chongqing, Vera Nieh agreed to take up the task to open the "refugee PUMC" School of Nursing on the WCUU campus.

Nursing Shifts in Sichuan examines how wartime unsettled dominant Western views and missionary approaches to nursing education, specifically through the evacuation of the PUMC from Beijing to the Canadian WCM. The refugee PUMC was hosted for three years by what it considered a "backwater" institution, during a time when most Canadians and Americans had either evacuated wartime China or were interned under the Japanese. This book details the story of the last sustained period of transnational relationships (and knowledge flows) between China, Canada, and the United States, as the Rockefellers, through the PUMC, aimed to develop a Chinese nursing elite. They succeeded to the point where PUMC alumnae held virtually all of the most important nursing positions in China during wartime, and even transformed Western nursing at the Canadian WCM, only to see all modern nursing programs in China shut down in 1951. That it would be thirty-five years before these same alumnae brought modern nursing back to China, in the 1980s, is both a cautionary tale of the transient nature of transnational relations and a treatise on the resilience of educated women.

Today, at a time of exponential (and some would say, unchecked and uncritical) increase in demands for transnational educational exchanges between China and Canada,[7] *Nursing Shifts in Sichuan* provides a timely, instructive, and fresh perspective on modern nursing as one of the most consequential additions to the Chinese health care landscape in the early twentieth century, and a liberating movement for Chinese women. Although it is well-recognized that Protestant missionaries introduced modern nursing to China, and that the PUMC had an enduring effect on Chinese nursing leadership, scholarly emphasis has been on a one-way flow of knowledge: from West to East – from Americans and Canadians to the Chinese. *Nursing Shifts in Sichuan* charts a new path in Chinese nursing history, one that draws and examines linkages between nursing education at two distinct but influential institutions, the PUMC and the WCUU. Seeking to understand the transition of modern nursing as Chinese actors replaced Canadian and American ones at these two institutions, this book traces multi-directional knowledge flows by following the geographic movements of and documented conversations by and about key individuals at these educational institutions. It takes special note of interpersonal conflicts as markers of differing – and shifting – values, beliefs, and assumptions, especially about nursing practice and education. As a social history, *Nursing Shifts in Sichuan* offers insight into how class, religion, gender, and nationality influenced interactions between nurses and physicians, staff and administrators, missionaries and civil servants, and Americans, Canadians, and Chinese. And it provides a transnational frame that grants historical agency to both Western *and* Chinese nurses, examining, importantly, how Chinese nursing faculty at the PUMC influenced Canadian nursing by inspiring the development of the first baccalaureate program for nurses at the WCUU in 1946. Finally, it underscores how modern nursing, so ubiquitous across the globe today (and still a primary avenue for women to access higher education), is a social construct with beginnings, evolutions, and endings.

The History of Modern Nursing in China

Missionaries are widely credited with introducing modern nursing to China. The missionary era (1935–52) was a time of unprecedented change in China. Characterized by war, political upheaval, and the introduction of modern medicine in the country, this period reformulated the health care and educational landscape and the nature of women's work in China.[8] One of the most visible changes was the establishment of modern hospitals, centres of science, hygiene, and efficiency whose mandate for round-the-clock nursing care eventually became the raison d'être for nurses' training schools in hospitals across China – and for foreign-trained nurses who could teach Florence Nightingale's methods.[9] The term "modern nursing," as used here, was a systematic, hospital-based system of care of the sick that encompassed nurses' training and nursing practice under the same roof. Fashioned after the three-year apprenticeship training program for women developed by Nightingale in the late nineteenth century, modern nursing valued science and medical knowledge (even if it was unevenly applied). Modern nursing was closely associated with Western medicine. Until the understanding of nursing expanded in the 1920s to include public health, modern nursing was a result of, and dependent upon, the practice of Western medicine and the construction of Western hospitals, where most nursing education took place.[10]

In this book, the term "medical missions" refers to the domain of medical doctors, whereas "missionary nursing" refers to the domain of nurses. This distinction is to ensure that the work of nurses is not inadvertently subsumed into, or rendered invisible by, the work of physicians. The history of nursing in China during the missionary era can be divided roughly into four stages: introduction, professionalization, nationalization, and fragmentation (see the summary in Table I.1).[11] The first stage, from 1884 to 1914, was characterized by the arrival of missionary nurses, whose primary aim was to assist missionary physicians in their work. The first American missionary nurse, Elizabeth McKetchnie, arrived in Shanghai in 1884. The first Canadian missionary nurse, Harriet Sutherland, arrived in Zhifu, Shandong, in 1888. Both came to China to support the work of missionary physicians – McKetchnie to help Dr. Elizabeth Reifsynder to open the Margaret Williamson Memorial Hospital for Women and Children, Sutherland to help Dr. James Frazer Smith in the medical work being planned by the "Honan Seven" (Canada's first group of missionaries to China, who worked in Henan, a remote, interior province). Nurses who trained in the late nineteenth century were expected to be skilled at ventilating rooms, determining water potability, disinfecting "clothing, rooms and bodily discharges," and sanitizing dwellings.[12] Early missionary physicians were pragmatic in their acknowledgment of the need for missionary nurses, whose practical skills and gender proved useful in China: as Dr. Frazer Smith noted, missionary nurses (all women) could open the door to the care of female patients who would otherwise never consider coming to a dispensary or hospital to be cared for by a male physician.

Although missionary nurses were an advantage to medical missionaries (i.e., physicians) seeking access to female patients, they were limited in the type of hands-on care they could provide themselves; Chinese social mores prevented women from giving physical care to male patients. When missionaries arrived in China, care of the sick was a family responsibility, and care could be performed only by a household member of the same gender as, and of lower status than, the patient.[13] Work that involved caring for sick bodies was considered menial to the extreme, and there was little incentive for Chinese women to enter nursing programs. As C.T. Liu has noted, "it was always difficult for the Chinese to accord professional status to individuals who either performed menial duties, or touched the human body, as nurses invariably did."[14] In these early years, then, young men drawn from poorly educated classes provided physical care to male patients. Over the course of forty years (1888–1928), schools were opened in Fuzhou, Nanjing, Wuhan, Shanghai, Hangzhou, Guangzhou, Tianjin, Anjing, and Beijing.[15] These were preprofessional programs that offered free room and board, and enrolled only a handful of students – mostly men from families favouring the missionary enterprise. Women in China were still uneducated and not expected to work in public places or care for anyone unrelated to them.

The professionalization stage, from 1914 to 1927, included the growth of the Nurses Association of China (NAC) and the development of nursing as a standardized profession. The emphasis was on training Chinese nurses in hospital-based programs headed by missionaries. Two significant events in China in 1911 helped to generate an increased interest in science and Western medicine. First, the Qing Dynasty was overthrown and replaced by the Republic of China, with Dr. Sun Yat-sen as

TABLE I.1 Four stages of nursing history in China, 1884–1951

Stage	Years	Characteristics	Nursing milestones	Key events
Introduction	1884–1914	Missionary nurses assist missionary physicians; pre-professional nursing schools established for Chinese men	1884: Arrival of first missionary nurse (American) 1888: Arrival of first Canadian missionary nurse	1910–11: Manchurian plague 1911: Overthrow of Qing Dynasty; 1912: Establishment of Republic of China
Professionalization	1914–27	Emphasis on training Chinese nurses in hospital-based programs headed by missionaries	1914: First Nurses Association of China conference; nurses have title *hushi* ("caring scholar") 1920: PUMC opens first university-level nursing program 1926: 112 schools have registered with NAC	1927: Great missionary exodus; Nationalist army takeover of China, with government established in Nanjing
Nationalization	1927–37	Chinese nurse leaders step into administrative and teaching roles	1928: Appointment of first Chinese president and secretary of NAC 1930: NAC headquarters moved to Nanjing	1928: Establishment of Ministry of Health, Ministry of Education in Nanjing
Fragmentation	1937–51	Japanese occupation and mass migration of universities and refugees to West ("Free") China; internment of foreign nurses; Western institutions forced to close in 1951	1937: NAC leaders withdraw to wartime capital in Chongqing, Sichuan; PUMC School of Nursing migrates to Sichuan, hosted by the West China Union University in Chengdu	1937: Outbreak of War of Resistance against Japan; wartime capital set up in Sichuan 1945: Outbreak of civil war 1949: Mao Zedong comes to power 1952: Remaining missionaries depart China

president. Second, the Manchurian plague (1910–11) swept through China and received a multinational medical response. That same year, the China Medical Commission (a committee of the Christian Medical Association of China) became interested in the state of the missionary hospitals, and discovered that there were only 140 trained nurses in all of China, and that only half of the hospitals in China had a nurse.[16] Cora E. Simpson, who headed up a nurses' training school in Fuzhou, toured missionary hospitals in China and observed their lack of sufficient staff to care for patients.[17] Urging a more systematic approach to nurses' training in China, Simpson helped to move the NAC, established in 1909, to take a more active role. Holding its first annual meeting in 1914, the NAC introduced the word *hushi* ("caring scholar") to represent the title of nurse and called on all nurses' training schools to register with the NAC and all graduates to hold the title *hushi*. Four missionary hospital schools registered. The curriculum laid out by the NAC recommended a program of study of three years. By 1920, 52 training schools had registered; by 1926 there were 112.[18]

By the time the Peking Union Medical College School of Nursing opened in 1920, nursing had already been established as an acceptable profession for young women in China. As an elite university, however, the PUMC raised the attractiveness of nursing education even further by appealing to families seeking opportunity for their daughters to enhance their social status. Applications were competitive. Prospective PUMC students not only had to meet university entrance standards, but they also had to be proficient in English. While this narrowed the pool of prospective applicants considerably, it also allowed the PUMC to attract students from upper-class families. Unlike schools who attracted students as a way to raise the students' social status, PUMC desired students who *came with* a high social status.

The nationalization stage of modern nursing history in China, from 1927 to 1937, was characterized by Chinese nurse leaders stepping into administrative and teaching roles previously held by missionaries. Although the years 1925 to 1927 were characterized by rising nationalism and related anti-Christian movements (culminating in the great missionary exodus of 1927, during which 8,300 missionaries fled their mission stations), the decade thereafter was a period of relative peace, when the fledgling Nationalist government ruled from Nanjing. The NAC conference in Shanghai in 1930 recorded a Chinese attendance of 2,000, which was tenfold that of Western nurses.[19] During this period, the Ministry of Health became interested in the promotion of public health. By 1935, China reported 217 nursing schools – one national, ten provincial, and 206 private.[20] However, the "curriculum was made up to suit the need and convenience of hospitals, and students were brought in as cheap labor to work in the wards."[21] To redress the situation, the Nationalist government's Commission on Medical Education put together ten six- to nine-month fellowships for teacher training and practical experience at the PUMC School of Nursing. By 1936, the NAC recognized over 6,000 registered nurses, very few of whom were foreign.

The fourth stage, fragmentation (1937–51), which started with the Japanese occupation, was characterized by chaos, wartime trauma, and displacement of both nurses and patients. The nursing profession and higher education suffered severely during the eight-year War of Resistance against Japan. Most of the mission hospitals were in East China and soon found themselves within the Japanese occupied areas.[22] A mass migration of educational institutions to the relative safety of West China did not generally include private schools, most of which lacked the independent means or leadership to withdraw to Free China. As we have seen, even the PUMC School of Nursing did not relocate until 1943. Some of the NAC leadership remained in Nanjing under Japanese surveillance, while others withdrew to Free China's wartime capital of Chongqing, in Sichuan. As John Watt notes, "during this period nursing established itself as not only a woman's calling but an activity requiring professional competence."[23] *Nursing Shifts in Sichuan* takes place during this fourth stage, which ended with the expulsion of Westerners and the closure of collegiate nursing schools, including the PUMC and WCUU, in 1951.

REFUGEE PUMC: COLLIDING CULTURES

The PUMC School of Nursing's period of refuge at the WCUU from 1943 to 1946 was a landmark in Chinese nursing history. These years also mark a pivotal time in the career of Vera Nieh. Celebrated as PUMC's first Chinese dean of nursing, Vera Nieh was a PUMC alumnus and a Rockefeller fellow. She was a model of the type of graduate the Rockefeller Foundation's China Medical Board (CMB) envisioned when it started a nursing program at the PUMC in 1920. Vera Nieh was well educated, having attended the Keen Anglo-Chinese girls mission school in Tianjin, the PUMC in Beijing, the University of Toronto, Columbia University, and the University of Michigan. By the time Vera Nieh took the helm of PUMC in 1940, she had secured a spot in a tightknit, international network of nursing's elite, with a well-trodden path between Chinese and Western circles. Evacuating Beijing in 1943 after the Japanese takeover of the PUMC campus, she came to West China with administrative, educational, and wartime experience. Once there, she was given a clear mandate by the CMB: to reopen the PUMC School of Nursing on the WCUU campus in Chengdu. This meant creating a space for university-level nursing education in a setting established and long occupied by nurses from the Canadian West China Mission (WCM) and their "low-grade" nurses' training.

Vera Nieh wasted no time. The refugee PUMC took in its first class of first-year students in 1943, adding a new cohort of students each year after that. When the PUMC nursing faculty and all of its students followed Nieh back to Beijing in 1946, the WCUU opened its own baccalaureate program for nurses. The program ran under the leadership of Canadian missionary nurse Cora Kilborn until she evacuated to Canada in 1950.

Were it not for the Japanese takeover of the PUMC in 1941, it is highly unlikely that nurses from the Canadian WCM and the PUMC would have crossed paths. Although both groups played significant roles in the establishment of nursing in China, they were separated geographically and by national, ethnic, religious, and class differences that were deeply ingrained, making each group wary of the other. Their coming together was a collision of disparate worlds of nursing, representing differing priorities and practices. The WCM and PUMC nursing schools opened within five years of each other – the WCM in 1915, the PUMC in 1920.[24] A key difference between them was that Canadian missionaries had been in West China for almost three decades before the first nursing school was opened there in 1915. Nursing at the WCM was, and remained, an extension of medical mission priorities: the primary purpose of nurses' training was to staff mission hospitals. In contrast, the PUMC aimed to develop nursing leaders. It emphasized university-level preparation of nursing leaders in administration, education, and public health, and offered a baccalaureate degree. Its incoming students were older than at the WCM (eighteen-year-old university students as opposed to fifteen-year-old junior middle school graduates) and had been taught in English. Furthermore, PUMC alumnae, armed with a degree and English fluency, were well positioned to (and did) pursue master's degrees from leading institutions in the United States. PUMC graduates had opportunities that WCM graduates could only dream of.

Despite the eagerness with which the West China missionaries received the PUMC refugees, it became quickly apparent that the PUMC personnel were less interested in a partnership than in a physical space in which they could re-establish their own programs. Although the WCM (Renji) program was officially an "affiliate" of the PUMC program and shared clinical teaching space at the University Hospital, the two programs ran independently of each other. Vera Nieh had little appetite to adapt or improve the Renji program. Rather, she sought to build the PUMC program on a new foundation, accepting a fresh group of incoming students in 1943. Her vision to recreate the PUMC in West China was met with resistance both within the West China Mission and, perhaps more surprisingly, in the China Medical Board itself. Power struggles became virulent in West China, where, as Nicole Elizabeth Barnes puts it, Nieh experienced a "stunning degree of sexism."[25] Her superiors characterized her as aggressive and psychologically unstable, and schemed for her resignation. They were not successful.

While physicians and others *with* positional power tried to force Vera Nieh from her job as dean in the early 1940s, students and others *without* traditional power tried to force Cora Kilborn from hers a few years later, in 1950. That year, Kilborn, a China-born missionary nurse from a highly respected missionary family, experienced an uprising among her students, who characterized her as inept and controlling. To make matters worse, a PUMC alumnus working at the WCUU slapped Kilborn in the face during a disagreement – something that was unthinkable, and astounds even today. Given her family background and position as a dean of nursing, both Chinese and nursing norms dictated that Kilborn be shown the utmost respect. This slap signalled – and symbolized – the end to Western influence in Chinese nursing at the WCUU. Kilborn departed China shortly afterward, having given twenty-four years of missionary service to Chengdu.

The presence of PUMC nurses in wartime Sichuan helped to unsettle nursing as understood and taught by missionary nurses there. For missionary nurses, nursing was an opportunity to sooth the suffering of strangers – a social imperative rooted in Christ's mandate to his followers to care for the poor and sick. Nursing education emphasized a virtuous character and altruistic service to God and others. While this view aligned well with Florence Nightingale's model, it was slow to catch up to scientific advances and the promise of public health embraced by the founders of the PUMC. For PUMC nurses, nursing was a scientifically based means toward a population-based end: a healthy citizenry. Their view of nursing was inspired by findings from the 1923 *Goldmark Report*, a comprehensive survey of nursing in the United States by the Rockefeller Foundation's Committee for the Study of Nursing Education.[26] The report proved crucial in determining Rockefeller Foundation health priorities and decisions, which, in turn, were taken up by the PUMC. The view of public health as an avenue to strengthen the citizenry became particularly relevant during China's War of Resistance against Japan. It aligned well with an emerging view of nursing in West China as a patriotic – and not simply altruistic – practice. By healing and strengthening the citizenry, Chinese nurses could help liberate China from foreign (most urgently Japanese, but also Western) occupation and influence. In this way, the presence of the PUMC in West China unsettled local notions of what it meant to be nurses. By the time the Japanese occupation ended, Chinese nursing students in Chengdu were no longer satisfied with Western nursing as previously taught and practised. For the first time, nursing students began to voice strong opinions and agitate for change. After sixty years, nursing in West China was coming into its own.

SOURCES: ACCESSING MULTIPLE PERSPECTIVES

Nursing Shifts in Sichuan is based on a wide range of material obtained from personal collections and visits to archives across four countries over an eight-year period. Archives included the Rockefeller Archive Center (New York), the PUMC Archives (Beijing), Bedford College Archives (London, UK), United Church of Canada Archives (Toronto), and University of Manitoba Archives (Winnipeg). The personal collections were primarily from missionary relatives with whom I worked on earlier studies of the United Church of Canada North China Mission in Henan; some of the material overlapped with or was otherwise relevant to this study of United Church of Canada WCM in Sichuan. Sources include institutional committee minutes and correspondence, telegrams, confidential memos, personal letters, photos, self-published memoirs, and unpublished interview transcripts and audio recordings. They also include books written by missionaries and others working and living in China, many of which I have collected via rare book collections and bookstores over the years.

For the past several years, historians of nursing have favoured a critical approach to historical analysis, one that uses constructs of identity (race, gender, class) as a lens through which to understand how power imbalances have shaped nursing work. Analysis has long shifted away from a focus on the "grand dames" of nursing. Instead, nursing history has moved "from an era of heroic biography to an era more interested in the archeology of humbler lives," making work on the ordinary daily lives of subjects more possible and desirable.[27] At first glance, a book like *Nursing Shifts in Sichuan* that foregrounds an elite institution may seem to risk losing historians' calls to focus on ordinary women and the lives of lesser-known figures.[28] However, despite the notoriety of the Rockefellers and the disproportionate privilege held by those associated with the PUMC, it is really the deans of nursing who emerge as the actors with both the most prestige and the most conflicted relations. Gertrude Hodgman (PUMC dean of nursing, 1930–40), Vera Nieh, and Cora Kilborn were constantly embroiled in power struggles, particularly in relation to their relatively low status within their respective organizations – as women (versus men), nurses (versus physicians), and, in the case of Vera Nieh, Chinese (versus Western).

This study focuses on the transition in modern nursing from Canadian and American actors to Chinese ones at two distict institutions, the PUMC and WCUU. Primary sources reviewed include institutional documents from these two institutions, as well as personal correspondence, memoirs, and interview transcripts of nursing educators, students, alumnae, and administrators who worked or studied at either (or both) of them. Although most of the primary sources originate in China, they were almost exclusively written in English. At the PUMC, this could have been because the nursing programs were taught in English and all Chinese students and educators were required to be fluent in English. At the WCUU, nursing programs were taught in Chinese, but correspondence was generally geared to other English-speaking missionaries or family members. In any case, nursing educators and administrators – be they Chinese, Canadian, or American – were expected to be bilingual. Even during the wartime years, when the PUMC was staffed entirely by Chinese, internal records were in English. What this underscores is an understanding of modern nursing in China as a transnational project as much as a national one. *Nursing Shifts in Sichuan,* then, is less a study of Chinese nursing per se than a study of nursing as a global phenomenon. If the use of English in the early years was colonial residue, its persistence during wartime points to its currency for *these particular* Chinese nurses who wished to be, or remain, part of the global nursing community.

As a historian of nursing, I approach this work with an awareness of my own subjectivity. In this, I draw on the work of Pamela Sugiman who, in her study of interned Japanese Canadians in Canada, noted how her own identity as a third-generation Japanese Canadian whose parents were interned in British Columbia in the Second World War influenced her work.[29] Situating herself as a co-constructor of the narrative, Sugiman recognized the need to consider her own motivations and needs alongside those of her subjects. Similarly, I recognize that my own experiences and perspectives as a former dean of nursing at a private, faith-based university necessarily influences my work. I have been writing about nursing history in China for many years now, having started by researching Canadian missionary nurses in Henan,[30] branching out to missionary nurses who were interned under the Japanese in China,[31] and then to broader, co-authored studies of nursing as a whole in China, including at Qilu and the PUMC.[32] In the last few years, however, I have been working as a university administrator, including as a dean of nursing, and my administrative insights inevitably influence my reading of the materials. For example, I am sensitive to, and surprised by, how little has changed in terms of gendered and other power differences in nursing – particularly a view that nursing (still predominantly a female profession) does not require (or deserve) advanced education. As a regular writer and reader of committee minutes, I am also sensitive to evidence of committee members' subversive attempts to circumvent, leverage, or disrupt decisions they disagree with – for nurses, this usually means decisions they believed would be harmful to nursing. And, as the former dean of the only private Christian nursing program in Canada, I am sensitive to ways in which missionaries positioned themselves in relation to the PUMC and vice versa: whereas missionaries viewed themselves as virtuous carriers of Christian culture, PUMC members viewed missionaries as well-intentioned but insulated remnants of a bygone era. Finding myself cheering for the underdogs in this story, I also find it sobering that, in the face of the tidal wave of socio-political change headed their way, nurses in China had little control over the destiny of modern nursing there.

OVERVIEW OF CHAPTERS

This book is divided into two parts, roughly before and after the 1942 closure of the PUMC. Part 1 (Chapters 1–4) examines the contexts of nursing at the WCM and the PUMC that helped shaped the values, beliefs, and identities of nurses at both places. Nurses took up the mantle of their respective institutions, embodying the ideal that advancing nursing was core to a nation's development and progress. Whereas Canadian missionaries were inspired by religious ideals, American nurses were motivated by the idea of a well-funded educational experiment in which to test new ideals. In both cases, wartime interrupted and reshaped the way these ideals were transferred and taken up by their Chinese protégées. Part 2 (Chapters 5–8) explores the nature and impact of bringing two worlds of nursing together as the refugee PUMC entered a space that had been occupied by Canadian missionaries since the 1890s.

The story of nursing in China, like the story of missionaries in China, is one of "repeated disturbances and wars, with repeated withdrawals and returns" of Western nurses.[33] To capture what living on the edge of evacuation meant not only to Westerners, but also to Chinese nurses, this book is organized into eight thematic chapters that overlap somewhat chronologically. Chapter 1 (1914–33) sets the stage. It examines the early influence of missionary nurses on professional nursing development in China, introduces the WCM and its most significant family, the Kilborns. It provides a historical context for the PUMC and discusses the significance of the *Goldmark Report* in shaping the PUMC's unusual emphasis on public health and baccalaureate education. It also introduces the PUMC's most recognized alumnus, Vera Nieh, and analyses early controversies at the Beijing Health Station that foreshadowed conflicts to come. Chapter 2 (1932–40) focuses on the PUMC and Chinese nursing, examining the impact of the Japanese invasion and the Nationalist government's requirement of Chinese leadership at the helm of all organizations. It includes analyses of the shift in leadership at the Nurses Association of China and Vera Nieh's uneven path to the deanship of the PUMC School of Nursing. Chapter 3 (1936–40) focuses on Canadian missionary nursing at the WCM, considering how nursing's social identity shifted as nurses responded to war-related phenomena such as the mass migration to West China, relentless air raids, and diminishing resources. It also discusses how these factors – coupled with the destruction of the WCM Women's Hospital and consular calls for the evacuation of missionaries from China – contributed to the erosion of Canadian missionary nursing across China. Chapter 4 (1940–42) analyses the devastating impact of Pearl Harbor on PUMC and WCM nursing. The attack resulted in the Allies, including the United States and Canada, declaring war against Japan, triggering the immediate arrest and internment of

Westerners in Japanese-occupied territory and the dramatic takeover (and, ultimately, closure) of the PUMC.

Part 2 begins with Chapter 5 (1943–45), which examines the migration of PUMC nursing faculty to Sichuan and the political manoeuvring between groups keen to host the elite school. It describes the early days of the refugee PUMC while also tracking the denouement of Canadian missionary nurses and their traditional forms of nursing education. Chapter 6 (1943–46) examines escalating clashes between Dean Vera Nieh and virtually every male administrator in her reach, largely due to her insistence on standards and structures similar to those in Beijing. It analyses the resultant relentless (yet ultimately unsuccessful) schemes to force her resignation, and considers how gender, race, class, nationality, and other social constructs figured in the conflicts. Chapter 7 (1946–49) explores the return of Canadian missionary nurses to China and of PUMC nurses to Beijing, and the residual controversies and opportunities sparked by both. It also examines the WCUU's attempted shift from lower-grade to university-level nursing education in 1946, a change catalyzed by and modelled after the refugee PUMC but fraught with controversy once the PUMC departed. It explores the growing rift between missionaries and Chinese nursing students and staff, drawing on interviews of nursing alumnae to analyse shifting postwar allegiances and expectations. Chapter 8 (1949–51) examines the shift in understanding nursing as an expression of altruism to one of patriotism, exploring how the rising tide of Communism both supported and threatened nursing as a patriotic act. It traces the last days of modern nursing at the PUMC and the WCUU, describing how at the very moment that Chinese nurses were coming into their own – separating out Chinese from Western ideals while also selecting which Western practices and relationships furthered their ideals – the Communist government was finding ways to purge Western influences from China. It describes the Communist takeover of the PUMC and the WCUU in 1951 and their subsequent shutdown, and includes a postscript of what has happened in the intervening years. The Conclusion highlights salient themes and new insights, asserting that the departure of Western nurses and the parallel dissolution of modern nursing was as inevitable as it was painful. Western nurses always asserted that their aim was to eventually turn nursing over completely to their Chinese protégées. They did not envision that the unsettled years of Japanese occupation would give way to their abrupt departure, and the complete eradication of higher education for nurses in China – that is, eradication of the outcome that they had been most proud of.

Part 1

Before the Closure of the Peking Union
Medical College

CHAPTER ONE

China Calling (1914–33)

Missionaries, Western Nursing, and the Rockefellers

When the China Medical Board of the Rockefeller Foundation made
the decision to purchase the Union Medical College of Peking, rather than
to start a new college, they did so because "the creditable beginnings
made by the missionary societies" should not be discarded.

> — *John Z. Bowers, Western Medicine in a Chinese*
> *Palace, 1972*

Missionary doctors and nurses were generally a breed apart from the run-of-
the-mill evangelists. They expressed their faith through their fingertips, rather
than in street-corner preaching. They measured their success not so much in
souls saved as in bodies healed, diseases conquered, and hospitals built.

> — *Alvyn Austin,* Saving China, *1986*

In 1914, in an era when China was searching for an educational model
for its modernization efforts,[1] three events opened a path for Chinese
women to become key players in the dramatic and complex modern history of nursing in China. First, the Rockefeller Foundation (RF) established the China Medical Board (CMB), its primary commitment being
to establish and operate the Peking Union Medical College (PUMC) in
Beijing. Second, the West China Union University (WCUU) established a medical school, causing Yuan Shikai, the president of the new
Republic of China, to note that "science may be said to have permeated
the world when it has become an integral part of higher learning in as
remote as spot as [Chengdu, Sichuan]."[2] Third, in this year, the modern
Chinese nurse was named into being, when American missionary nurses
in the newly established Nurses Association of China (NAC) adopted the

term *hushi* (literally, "caring scholar") to describe the new professional role being taken up by their Chinese protégées.[3] When Chinese nursing faculty from the PUMC School of Nursing took up refuge at the WCUU between 1943 and 1946 after the Japanese army closed the PUMC in Beijing, the threads of these auspicious 1914 events were drawn together.

This chapter provides the context for the later story of Chinese, Canadian, and American nurses in Japanese-occupied China. To understand the significance of the refugee PUMC years in Chengdu (1943–46), it is helpful to get a sense of what was happening in Western medicine and nursing in China in the years leading up to the eight-year Sino-Japanese War (1937–45). Following a brief commentary on early missionary nursing, this chapter will focus on the early years of nursing at both the WCUU and the PUMC.

When Elizabeth McKetchnie, the first trained nurse in China, arrived in 1884, there was no equivalent in Chinese culture to the conceptualization of nursing popularized by Florence Nightingale – that is, as a vocation for unmarried, God-fearing women who were educated through a strict, hospital-based, residential apprenticeship program.[4] The missionary ideal of nursing as an honorable profession was so novel that the Chinese had no word in their language to express it.[5] However, at the NAC conference in Shanghai in 1914, Elsie Mawfung Chung, a Chinese graduate from Guy's Hospital, London, having consulted with sinologists, proposed the term *hushi* for "nurse," and *husheng* for "student nurse."[6] *Hu* means to care, protect, and look after, and *shi* stands for intellectual or scholar. *Hushi*, then, means "caring scholar."[7]

In the traditional healing system in China, caring for the sick was a family responsibility with well-established gender norms and a status hierarchy: only members of the family or household who were the same gender as, and had lower status than, the patient could provide care.[8] Early missionary nurses found a professional niche that was socially acceptable both in China and at home by working in women's hospitals, where the work was focused primarily on obstetrics and gynecology. Women's hospitals, in turn, established training schools for nurses, and nursing students provided much of the day-to-day care of patients.[9] The women's hospitals were typically funded by women's missionary societies, as were missionary nurses. When the Canadian Methodist (later United) Church Mission in Chengdu opened its newly built Women's Hospital and School of Nursing in 1915, it was completely administrated and funded by the Methodist Woman's Missionary Society (WMS).

For women who became missionary nurses, the decision to go to China was generally viewed as a sacred calling from God. It involved an awareness of the needs of people in parts of the world considered unreached by the Christian gospel, a concern for both the spiritual and physical well-being of strangers, and a willingness to give up the comforts of life at home to serve others. Such a calling was typically understood as a life-long vocation. For some – such as long-serving North China Mission (NCM) nurse Margaret MacIntosh – nursing was a means to an evangelical end; MacIntosh was criticized by later missionary nurses for the lack of progress of nursing in Henan during her thirty-eight-year tenure, due to her focus on evangelizing.[10] For others, missionary nursing was a practical expression of the gospel: missionary nursing was simply an extension of Christ's mandate to the early church to care for the sick and vulnerable. In this sense, the shift in focus at the NCM from evangelism to service in the 1920s was not a new ideal but a reflection of an ancient one. As Christoffer Grundmann notes, "the justification of medical [and, by extension, nursing] missions as an expression of Christian love in witness to God's love is part of a tradition much older than the mission strategy argument. Even historians of medicine recognize the church's work of caring for the sick as integral to the Christian faith of individuals and congregations from the very beginning."[11] In the case of Anglican nurse Susie Kelsey, her ongoing evangelistic focus did not diminish her commitment to modern scientific nursing or her interest in advancing nursing as a profession; healing bodies and saving souls were coherent expressions of her calling.

To Caroline Wellwood, a long-serving nurse in the West China Mission (WCM), concerns about women's education and their right to social and economic independence were inextricably tied to her understanding of her particular calling from God. Her passion was evangelism and nursing education – both of which served to provide women with a new understanding of the world they lived in. For Wellwood, modern nursing was a liberating movement for Chinese women: "Heretofore there seemed to be only one avenue open to women," she wrote in 1926, "that of gaining a husband who would be responsible for her support ... The numbers of women who seek an avenue for escape are many, and ... who have a dream that by gaining an education they might become self-supporting, and thus be freed from slavery of both body and soul."[12]

Caroline Wellwood's career in Chengdu spanned thirty-seven years. She played a key role in the development of the WMS nursing school, which graduated its first class (of three nurses) in 1918.[13] It was a complicated venture. Wellwood's vision to train young Chinese nurses started in 1907, when she visited a hospital in Hangzhou and found there that "a number of Chinese girls [were] being successfully trained as nurses."[14] There were two Canadian mission hospitals in Chengdu at that time – the Women's Hospital (at Hsin Hang Tsi), started by Dr. Retta Gifford Kilborn in 1895, and the Men's Hospital (at Si Shen Tsi), started by her husband, Dr. Omar Kilborn, a year earlier, in 1894.[15] The Women's Hospital was operated by the Woman's Missionary Society, the Men's Hospital by the Foreign Mission Board (FMB). Thus, although the two hospitals were geographically close and part of the same Canadian mission, they were staffed and administrated independently. The Men's Hospital had rudimentary training for male nurses. In 1909, Caroline Wellwood trained two young Chinese women to dispense medicine and change dressings at the Women's Hospital, hoping they would become nurses. Unfortunately, one died the following year of tuberculosis. The other, Wu Ueh Bin, eventually graduated from nursing, and worked at the Women's Hospital for over forty years.[16] When Caroline Wellwood died in 1947, she included a financial gift to Wu in her will.[17]

EARLY MISSIONARY NURSES AND THE NURSES
ASSOCIATION OF CHINA

In 1907, during her first year in China, American Methodist missionary nurse Cora Simpson wrote to the president of the China Medical Association, asking about the state of nurses' work in China. He answered that "as yet there was no organized nurses' work, but that he hoped the nurses would soon be organized."[18] Simpson's letter to the president was printed and "sent to every medical person in China."[19] Simpson reported that nurses across China agreed with the idea of uniting their work, but that distances and limited means made it difficult to get together for meetings. Despite the challenges, in 1908, a fledgling nurses association met for the first time and, a year later, the Nurses Association of China was established, with Mrs. Caroline Maddock Hart of Wuhu (the head nurse of Wuhu Hospital from 1905 to 1913)[20] as president.

In 1912, Cora Simpson and "many nurses" found themselves unexpectedly gathered together at the Kuling Mountain. They were in exile from the Chinese Revolution, a political upheaval that would result in the overthrow of four thousand years of imperial rule, and the establishment of the new Republic of China. The Chinese government, under the rule of the Manchu Qing Dynasty, was considered enfeebled and out of step with the rest of the world. The Empress Dowager Cixi Taihou, who had ruled China for forty-seven years, died in 1908, leaving two-year-old Aisin-Gioro Puyi to ascend the Qing throne. A revolution was predicted. Some missionaries, finding themselves under threat by local and spreading violence, evacuated to safer regions. Others expressed taking "comfort in rebel warnings that anyone caught meddling with foreigners, or their possessions, would be beheaded."[21] However, the British consul in Chongqing predicted that "an outbreak of anti-foreign feelings could only be a matter of time."[22] Canadian missionaries who returned to Chengdu in September 1911 after vacationing at the resorts on Mount Omei found the situation so "explosive" that they asked the commander of the Manchu forces for protection from danger.[23] In response, the general confined them to their own compounds for three full months before they were allowed to evacuate downriver.[24] Their evacuation was as part of a flotilla of forty ships carrying 149 foreigners along with their servants. The ships, flying Union Jacks, were fired upon several times, and five-year-old John Jolliffe, son of Canadian WCM missionaries Lena and Richard Jolliffe, was killed.[25] American missionaries in Fuzhou exited the city on 31 October 1911.[26] Women and children had been "hustled to the relative safety of the foreign settlement outside the city wall and close to the U.S. consulate while men stayed in the mission compound and were joined by six bluejackets from the *USS Bainbridge*."[27] Other missionaries, including Cora Simpson, were evacuated to Kuling Mountain.

The "many nurses" at Kuling took advantage of their new proximity by planning a coordinated approach to nursing education in China.[28] They held "very helpful and enthusiastic meetings,"[29] which resulted in the development of a recommended program of study and examination plan for nurses' training schools. These were sent to the Medical Association in Beijing. Afterwards, a joint committee of nurses and physicians finalized the program.

In 1913, Simpson reported that there were thirty members in the Fujian Branch of the new association of nurses. They anticipated starting a nursing journal as a means to communicate with each other across the country. In the meantime, they were provided space in the *China Medical Journal* to print and discuss reports. Classic American textbooks were translated and made available in Chinese – including, for example, Isabel Adams Hampton Robb's *Principles and Practice of Nursing* and Lavinia Dock's *Materia Medica*; staples in American and Canadian schools of nursing.

Cora Simpson would become known as one of the early nursing leaders in China. From 1907 to 1922, she worked at an early women's hospital in Fuzhou. Interested in nurses' training from her earliest days, she helped found the nursing school in Fuzhou in 1909. In 1913, Simpson reported in the *American Journal of Nursing* that "Chinese women are at liberty to study any profession they choose and in the new Republic have equal rights to men in matters of education." Nurses' training schools, she noted, were opening up all over China. "Many of them are not up to the standard we desire," she wrote, "but these are days of beginning in China, and we do not forget how very few years nursing has been known in America and England."[30] Instrumental in the early days of standardizing nursing education (and therefore practice) in China, Simpson would later take on the role as the executive secretary of the Nurses Association of China in 1922.

WEST CHINA MISSION

The United Church of Canada operated three missions in China – the North China Mission (NCM) in Henan, the West China Mission (WCM) in Sichuan, and the South China Mission (SCM) in Guangdong. The NCM and SCM were started by the Presbyterian Church in 1888 and 1902, respectively, whereas the WCM was started by the Methodist Church in 1892. They joined together under one umbrella in 1925, when Canadian Methodist, Presbyterian, and Congregationalist churches joined together to become the United Church of Canada. Despite this union, each of the missions retained characteristics of their founders. Although physicians were among the first missionaries at each site, and although each founded hospitals and nursing schools, the NCM emphasized evangelism, whereas the WCM emphasized education. The SCM was started primarily with the support of Chinese Christians in Canada, and its work remained limited. The SCM started a men's hospital and a women's hospital, both with nursing schools.[31] The NCM started three hospitals and nursing schools. The WCM started seven hospitals, including a men's and a women's hospital, all with nursing schools (see Table 1.1).[32] The NCM participated in the founding of the medical school at the Shandong Christian University in Jinan (in 1918), but for the most part was not involved in university education. The WCM stood out from the other Canadian missions in its commitment to the founding, in 1910, and operation of the West China Union University, which included a medical school.

In 1891, when Reverend Dr. Alexander Sutherland, general secretary of the Methodist General Board, determined that Canadian Methodists should start a mission in China, there were already a handful of Canadian Methodists in the country, serving with American Methodist missions.[33] Adeline Galliland (later Hart) was the first Canadian missionary in China, arriving in 1865. She was sponsored by the same church in Farmersville, Ontario, that, in 1875, sent out Dr. Leonora Howard. Dr. Howard was the second female missionary doctor to be sent out by any denomination. According to Alvyn Austin, it was Mrs. Adeline Hart, wife of the Reverend Virgil Hart, who was instrumental in founding the

TABLE 1.1 Canadian hospitals in China

Mission	Province	City	Hospital type	Date established	Nursing school established
North China Mission	Henan	Anyang	General	1897	1932
		Weihui	General	1922	1922
		Huaiqing	General	1920?	1932, combined with Anyang
West China Mission	Sichuan	Chengdu	Men's	1894	1913
			Women's	1895	1915
		Rongxian	General	1910	1920s
		Jiading	General	1928	n/a
		Ziliujing	General	1907	1920s
		Chongqing	General	1910	1920s
		Fuzhou	General	1915	1920s
South China Mission	Guangzhou	Guangdong	Men's	1924	1924?
			Women's	1912	1915

SOURCE: Cheung, *Missionary Medicine in China*, *11–15*; Austin, *Saving China*, 40; Grypma, *Healing Henan*, *85; 90; 125*; Mindon, *Bamboo Stone*, 26–39; Service, W. (1924): West China Mission Stations. UCCA 78.096C box 7: 1–2.

Canadian Methodist (later United) Church mission to West China. She and her husband had started the Central China mission of the American church at Wuhu in 1881, moving further inland until they reached Sichuan in 1886. They retired in 1888 due to his ill health, but came out of retirement to return to China in September 1891 as members of the first Canadian Methodist mission in China. They opened their first dispensary in 1892.

Between 1892 and 1913, the West China Mission established ten central stations and eighty-one outstations in Sichuan.[34] Each of the carefully selected central stations was a focus of political or economic activity. Chengdu, Chongqing, and Ziliujing were the largest stations, with the most developed medical service. In 1910, the Canadian Methodists became one of five participating denominations in the founding of the West China Union University in Sichuan.[35] The importance that the WCM attached to educational work explains its foundational role in the establishment of the WCUU as well as the fact that, of all the founding groups, it contributed the largest share to the WCUU's finances and personnel.[36]

In his study of the SCM and WCM before 1937, Yuet-wah Cheung concluded that the WCM was the more cosmopolitan of the two. While the SCM was "only a minor effort," in response to a request from some Chinese Christians in Canada for a mission in their homeland, the WCM was *the* mission in China opened by the Methodist Church in Canada.[37] Its most important feature was its "overriding emphasis on secular education as an integral part of its missionary endeavors."[38] Cheung argues that this was due to the strong social gospel influence on Canadian Methodists, which rested on the premise that "Christianity was a social religion, concerned ... with the equality of human relations on this earth. Put in more dramatic terms, it was a call for men to find the meaning of their lives in seeking to realize the kingdom of God in the very fabric of society ... The gospel mandate required response to concrete human needs."[39] Their emphasis on the role of social reconstruction, argues Cheung, is why the Canadian mission in West China was more involved in education and social reform than were the NCM and SCM, which were sponsored by Canadian Presbyterians. By the time the Methodists and (most) Presbyterians became the United Church of Canada in 1925, the distinction between them had already been set.

The ten WCM central mission stations in Sichuan occupied a strip of territory running from north-west to south-east in the centre of the province. Varied in width, it was 700 miles in length (see Table 1.2 for the central stations).[40] One of the primary medical stations was in Chongqing. That city, which was 1,500 miles from the sea, was considered the great commercial metropolis of Sichuan.[41] It was a significant receiving and distribution centre for all upriver traffic (to the coast) and a clearing-house for downriver merchandise (to Sichuan). Chongqing itself, according to Canadian missionaries, was not an attractive city in which to live or work. It was overcrowded, with narrow, winding, dirty streets, and unending steps – "a city of steps and swear-words," according to one missionary[42] – and was filled with smoke from "tens of thousands of soft coal fires."[43] It was a city of dire poverty and great wealth – the extremes seen everywhere in China. Chengdu, another main medical station, was,

TABLE 1.2 Stations of the West China Mission, ca. 1920s

Year established	Location	Distribution of beds in hospital or dispensary	Key early personnel	Nursing school opened
1892	Chengdu	150 (Main/Men's Hospital, 1894) 60 (Women's Hospital, 1895)	Dr. Kilborn and Dr. Retta (Gifford) Kilborn; Dr. C.B. Kelly; Dr. R.B. Ewan; Dr. C.W. Service	1913 1915
1894	Leshan	30	Dr. H.M. Hare	n/a
1905	Rongxian	60	Dr. W.E. Smith	1920s
1905	Renshou	25	Dr. J.R. Cox; Dr. F.F. Allan	n/a
1907	Ziliujing/ Zigong	150	Dr. Wilford; Dr. A.E. Best	1920s
1907	Pengxian	25	Dr. A.J. Barter; Dr. E.K. Simpson	n/a
1908	Luzhou	25	Dr. Ferguson	n/a
1910	Chongqing	60	Dr. R. Wolfendale	1920s
1911	Zhongzhou	20	Dr. W.H. Birks	n/a
1913	Fuzhou	25	?	1920s

SOURCE: Yuet-wah Cheung, *Missionary Medicine in China: A Study of Two Canadian Protestant Missions in China before 1937* (Lanham, MD: University Press of America, 1988); "The Central Stations of the West China Mission," *Vic in China*, 2015, Victoria University Library, http://library.vicu.utoronto.ca/exhibitions/vic_in_china/sections/missionaries_and_mission_stations/the_central_stations_of_the_west_china_mission.html.

in contrast, a walled city built on a vast plateau with half a million residents. The Canadian mission covered about one-quarter of the city itself and also included four *hsiens* (districts) in the city's suburbs.[44] The city was important commercially but, as the provincial capital of Sichuan, it was also a significant admistrative centre. In addition, Chengdu was the site of the WCUU, whose campus was located at the south gate of the city, contributing to its status as an educational centre for China.[45]

In 1914, the Medical College was opened at the WCUU. It required good-quality hospitals for the training of medical students, and these hospitals were staffed by missionary and student nurses. Two new hospitals with training schools for nurses were built by the WCM in Chengdu at about this time – the Men's/Main Hospital, in 1913, which trained Chinese men, and the Women's Hospital, in 1915, which trained Chinese women.[46] Over the years, the WCM became increasingly invested in medical service, operating as many as eleven dispensaries and small hospitals in Sichuan – six of which had nursing schools.

In 1938, the Men's Hospital and Women's Hospital in Chengdu were combined into a single entity called the United Hospitals of the Associated Universities in Chengdu. This was in order to service the growing needs of the WCUU medical school, which at that time was hosting two refugee medical schools. The two nursing schools associated with these hospitals were combined to become a single School of Nursing of the United Hospital. Although not a university school, the school of nursing was recognized as a WCUU "affiliated institution,"[47] and for many years the staff of the WCUU assisted in the teaching of nurses. The entrance requirements for the nursing school were graduation from a registered junior middle school, and the passing of an entrance exam. The nursing program was three and a half years, the first six months being a probationary period. The biggest change came with the new admissions policy. Although the Men's Hospital had run a nursing school for men since 1913, after 1938, the United Hospitals accepted only female students.

The Kilborn Family

One cannot properly write about medicine and nursing at the West China Mission without discussing the Kilborn family. Three generations of Kilborns served in mission hospitals in China and Hong Kong between 1891 and 1963, including missionary nurse Cora Kilborn, who served for twenty-six years in China. In 1891, Dr. Omar Leslie Kilborn and his wife, Jennie Fowler, joined Dr. Virgil and Adeline Hart as part of the nine-member pioneer group of missionaries who travelled from Canada to China.[48] Jennie Fowler died of cholera in 1892. Two years later, Omar Kilborn married Dr. Mary Alfretta (Retta) Gifford, one of the first missionaries appointed to West China by the Woman's Missionary Society, in 1892. Omar Kilborn helped to establish the Men's Hospital (1894), the

WCUU (1910), and the College of Medicine (1914) in Chengdu.[49] Retta Kilborn opened a WMS dispensary and Women's Hospital in 1895 in the same city. The two hospitals established by the Kilborns were, for many years, the principal teaching hospitals of the WCUU. Omar Kilborn died of pneumonia in 1920. Retta Gifford Kilborn continued to practise medicine and served as a faculty member at the WCUU until her retirement in 1933.[50]

The Drs. Kilborn had four children, three of whom were born in China: Leslie Gifford (1895), Constance Ellen (1898), and Roland Kenneth (1901). Their second daughter, Cora Alfretta (1899), was born when the family was on furlough in Canada.[51] Leslie Kilborn graduated in medicine from the University of Toronto in 1921. That same year, he headed for Chengdu with his wife, Dr. Janet McClure – daughter of pioneer NCM missionary Dr. William McClure and sister to NCM missionary Dr. Robert McClure. Their child Robert McClure Kilborn was born in 1923. In 1925, during a period of warlord-related political instability, Leslie Kilborn was shot while returning from holidays at Mount Omei, and the wound left him with a permanently disabled left shoulder.[52] The couple had three more children, Mary Eleanor (1925), Frances Margaret (1927), and Jean Alfretta (1930). Leslie Kilborn took administrative responsibility as director of the College of Medicine from approximately 1930 to 1950, during most of which time he also served as dean of medicine. When the WCUU hosted evacuated universities between 1937 and 1945, Leslie Kilborn was responsible for arranging accommodation and teaching facilities for contingents from Jinan (Qilu), Nanjing (National Central), and Beijing (PUMC; Yenching). After Janet Kilborn died while the family was on leave in Canada in 1945, Leslie Kilborn returned to China. Two years later, in 1947 in Hong Kong, he married Dr. Jean E. Millar, a Canadian missionary sent to West China in 1932 to take over the work of retiring Retta Kilborn at the WMC Women's Hospital. Leslie and Jean (Millar) Kilborn returned to Chengdu from furlough in Canada in October 1949, accompanied by Leslie's daughter Mary Eleanor, a nurse. Mary Eleanor began work at the WCUU University Hospital, but when Chengdu surrendered to the Communist army on 25 December 1949, there was so much disruption and disorganization that she returned to Canada in 1950. Leslie and Jean Kilborn left Chengdu in March 1952, and were among the last six Canadians to depart Sichuan.

It was within this family context that Cora Kilborn served as a missionary nurse in Chengdu. Having grown up in China, she graduated with a BA (honours) degree from Victoria College in Toronto in 1920 and then trained at the Toronto General Hospital School of Nursing.[53] Following that, she studied public health nursing at the University of Toronto, where she also completed a program in teaching and administration. In 1926, she became a United Church of Canada missionary, working in the Women's Hospital established by her mother in Chengdu. In 1940, while she was in Canada caring for her ailing mother (who died in 1942), the Women's Hospital was destroyed by fire. Once back in China, Cora Kilborn dedicated herself to the project underway to develop a new baccalaureate program for nurses at the WCUU, although only two graduated before the Communist takeover of the WCUU and closure of the nursing program. Cora Kilborn returned to Canada and transferred to home mission work before her marriage to Benjamin Cannell in 1952.

PEKING UNION MEDICAL COLLEGE

In 1914, the China Medical Board, which consisted of members of a number of mission hospitals and medical schools, requested funds from the Rockefeller Foundation to build and operate a new medical school and hospital in Beijing, which would be one of four medical centres in the country.[54] In 1915, the CMB purchased the Union Medical College in Peking from the London Missionary Society, assuming full support of the college on 1 July 1915.[55] Thereafter the Union Medical College in Peking would be known as the Peking Union Medical College (PUMC). Recognizing the magnitude of the project it had undertaken, the CMB sent a (second) China Medical Commission to the country in 1915. The first commission had suggested a vision of what might be. The second intended to give that vision form and substance. The aim was "to create as good a medical college as can be found anywhere in Europe or in America ... with an excellent staff of teachers, well-equipped laboratories and a good teaching hospital and dispensary ... [and] a training school for both male and female nurses."[56]

PUMC programs would have high standards for both students and faculty and would be taught in English – members of the commission were convinced that it was "impossible to train students properly in modern medicine through this tongue [Chinese]."[57] Admission requirements would be similar to those adopted by the majority of the better schools in the United States. Finding the existing Union Medical College students "quite unfitted by their lack for preliminary training and ignorance of English to participate in the new order of things," the commission worked out plans to transfer the 128 remaining students to other institutions to complete their medical education. At the same time, some of the faculty were assigned to other mission posts in China. Others were given the chance to return as PUMC faculty after study abroad. To the commission, it would be impossible to maintain "this higher order of medical school" on the low scale of missionary salaries: salaries, benefits, and pensions would need to be adjusted to attract elite faculty.[58]

Canadian architect Harry Hussey, principal of a Chicago-based firm, was the designer of the extravagant PUMC Hospital. Before designing the PUMC, he had designed two others: the Peking Central Hospital and the Church General Hospital at Wuchang.[59] According to historian Michelle Renshaw, both buildings were geared toward the work of medical missionaries, including dispensaries that consisted of examining rooms, bathrooms, surgeries, and offices for Chinese and missionary doctors. Dispensaries were usually the first point of contact between the Chinese patient and the medical missionary. Hussey's dispensary design was in line with the principle of "not frightening the natives": entrances, through matching gatehouses, as well as waiting rooms and offices would feel familiar and possibly even welcoming to potential patients. Presumably, by the time patients were admitted to hospital, they would be sufficiently familiar with the atmosphere to be undeterred by the foreign appearance of the hospital proper.[60]

Hussey also was attentive to the need to separate men from women to meet Chinese ideas of propriety. This could be done by building separate men's and women's hospitals. Keeping "young women in the Women's department and young men in the Men's department" would serve to "relieve the general tensity among the staff workers and especially the nurses" and "control nurses who are being trained."[61] Furthermore, "in order to insure even a fair degree of safety, provision must be made to by which the necessity, and even the possibility, of any considerable contact between men and women nurses in training should be eliminated."[62] As it turned out, there was an easy way to eliminate the concern of male and female nurses living in "tensity": the PUMC decided not admit any male nursing students after all.

As Hussey designed it, the PUMC hospital interior would be thoroughly modern, but the exterior thoroughly Chinese, using the same architectural style as Beijing's Forbidden City. He used large bricks from the ancient wall of the original palace, glazed imperial tiles that emulated the Forbidden City roofs, and added traditional embellishments such as huge ornaments on the ridges and eaves. By December 1919, the estimated costs of the PUMC hospital had risen six-fold from the original estimates, to $6.88 million. Hussey's contract was terminated, but the costs continued to rise. The final figure was $7.55 million. The RF board of trustees had two alternatives: close down or press on. They chose to press on.[63]

The premedical school was opened to men in 1917 and to women in 1919. The PUMC was the first co-educational medical school in China. The PUMC Hospital supported clinical training of both physicians and nurses. The Medical College admitted its first class – seven students – in 1919. The School of Nursing admitted its first class – three students – on 28 September 1920.[64]

PUMC SCHOOL OF NURSING

The first dean of nursing, Anna D. Wolf, was appointed PUMC superintendent of nurses in 1919. Part of her role was to organize the Nurses Training School (later the School of Nursing). During her years as a student at the Johns Hopkins School of Nursing, Wolf had begun to see the limitations of apprenticeship-style nurses' training, which convinced her of the need for higher education for nurses.[65] Her view was subsequently reinforced by Adelaide Nutting and others at Columbia Teachers College, where Wolf completed her master's degree in 1916. The new position at PUMC provided Wolf with an enticing opportunity to put to the test her vision of establishing baccalaureate education for nurses. With this in mind, Wolf took up the role as dean of nursing.

The first group of American nurses to go to Beijing with Anna Wolf in 1919 were appointed as "graduate nurses"[66] (see Appendix 2 for the names of the PUMC nursing faculty). While the new PUMC buildings were under construction, students studied Chinese and served at the old Hsin Kai Lu Hospital. Nursing students completed a pre-nursing year in the basic sciences. The American nurses were in charge of the new PUMC Hospital wards, where the students learned clinical practice.[67] By 1922, Anna Wolf had established two programs, one that led to a diploma, and another that led to a diploma from the PUMC plus a bachelor of science degree from Yenching University. The nursing program by itself would be three years and nine months. The combined program of study would take six years and eight months – four for liberal studies at the university, and the rest at the PUMC doing practical work. Through this combined program, the PUMC hoped to "attract women of ability, who will be able to fill the more important of the executive positions of institutions at the end of their education."[68] The exclusive nature of the PUMC was noticeable right away; as one observer commented, "It is not expected that there will be a great number of [qualified] applicants."[69] The PUMC School of Nursing "has been more fortunate than [even] most American schools in regard to its historical background and economic status."[70] Blessed with Rockefeller funding, PUMC students could enjoy an education "comparable to the best that Europe or America have to offer."[71]

Over the first decade, the PUMC class sizes – and therefore total number of graduates – were small (Figure 1.1). By 1931, the PUMC School of Nursing graduated thirty-nine nurses. Of those, seventeen were involved in institutional (hospital) and nursing education, nine in midwifery, eight in public health, one as a PUMC instructor in dietetics, and one in private duty; three others were not in active service – of these, one had died. Of the thirty-six alumnae who were in active service in 1931,

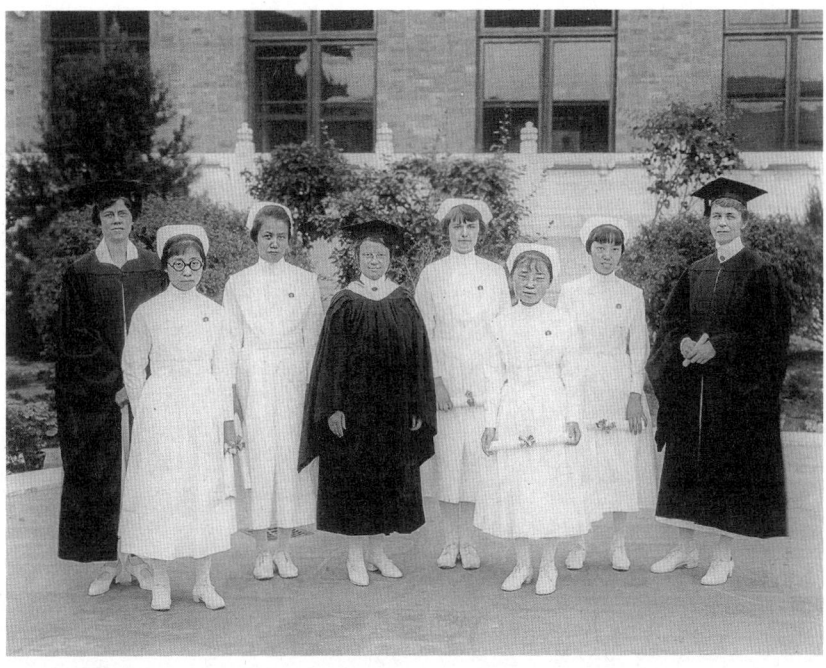

FIGURE 1.1 PUMC School of Nursing graduating class, 1926. The graduates are Bernice Chu, Civili Sinhanetra, Svea Lindberg, Evelyn Lin, and Ravenna Tien. Dean Ruth Ingram is in the centre of the photo. | Courtesy Rockefeller Archive Centre, RAC-CMB-FA065_ S1048_B31_F36.

more than a third (thirteen) were employed as PUMC faculty. Most of the others were employed in affiliate health programs in Beijing[72] (see Appendix 4).

By 1931, the PUMC had increased its affiliations with universities, adding the Gining in Nanjing, Soochow in Suzhou, and Lingnan in Guangdong, each of which could provide a pre-nursing year of study. One reason for the pre-nursing requirement was that English was the language used throughout the PUMC and it was considered exceedingly difficult to find women "with adequate language to benefit by the opportunities of the [PUMC] School."[73] Furthermore, since parents of prospective PUMC students were "prejudiced against nursing," much preferring their daughters to go into medicine, the PUMC School of Nursing, by requiring a pre-nursing year, was attempting to "emphasize the opportunities open to educated women in the nursing profession

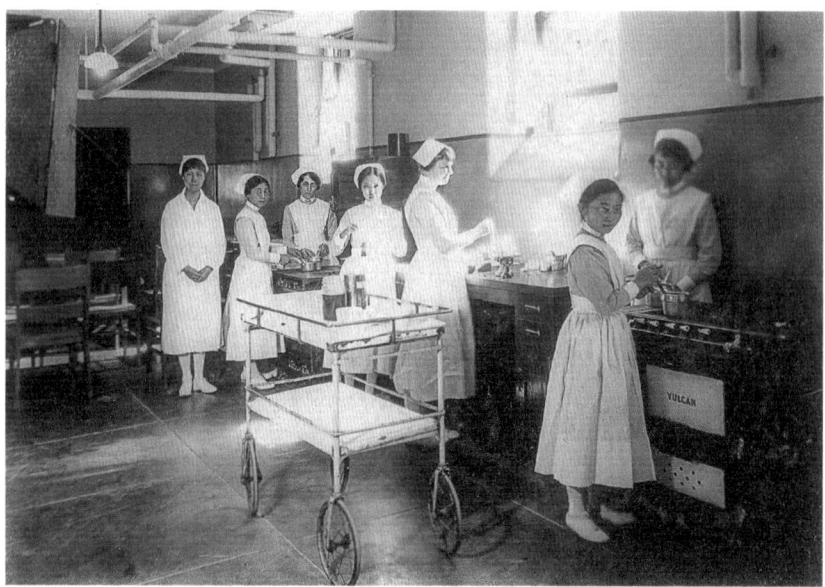

FIGURE 1.2 PUMC senior class practicum, 1926. Vera Nieh is fourth from left. | Courtesy Rockefeller Archive Centre, RAC- CMB_FA065_S1048_B30_F330_00.1.

also."[74] Promotional materials were geared to parents "who are the type most apt to send their daughters to college."[75] The content of the promotional materials gives a sense of how PUMC personnel understood nursing, what they saw as the value and distinctiveness of the PUMC program, and what they thought would be the priorities of parents from Chinese gentry. Three areas of emphasis stand out: how well the students would be cared for, how a PUMC nursing education would prepare their daughters for both a vocation *and* marriage, and that the public health emphasis of the curriculum would prepare students to be good citizens. These are examined in turn.

First, in terms of how nursing students would be treated, promotional materials reassured parents that their daughters would work no more than forty-six hours per week, that the dormitory was under the direction of a competent matron, and that the dining room served well-presented Chinese food.[76] "If your daughter comes to [PUMC]," the pamphlets assured them, "she will lead a well-balanced life which allows for eight hours of work, eight hours of sleep, and eight hours for recreation."[77] In other words, their daughters would be well taken care of. Photos of the new facilities and the PUMC Hospital confirm the high quality of the institution (see Figure 1.2).

Second, PUMC students would be taught skills that were transferable to their personal lives, making them not only eligible for steady work, but also attractive for marriage. There was no subtleness here: in marketing documents from 1931, one draft is entitled "The Nursing Profession as a Preparation for Marriage."[78] In it the author notes, "in this day and age when background and training are essential to any profession one feels that the greatest of all professions for women, that of marriage and the care of a home and family, has been somewhat neglected in so far as education and preparation are concerned."[79] In contrast, nursing "is one of the best preparations for homemaking that one can find today."[80] And this is why:

> The girl who gets her nurse's training at the Peiping [Peking] Union Medical College learns not only the essential household arts of caring for her home and children and preparing meals, she also learns self-reliance and is capable of efficiently directing and managing a household whether large or small. The student nurse has learned obedience to authority as well as the ability to take responsibility for herself. She has learned to care for and prevent illness. She is herself healthy and well and had learned the best methods of guarding against illness. She is an intelligent young woman with many and varied interests, able to take her play in any community and be an interesting and helpful companion to her husband.[81]

PUMC views on marriage fit well within the social norms of the day. In that era, marriage and nursing were mutually exclusive. Nursing students, while required to be single, were also of prime marriage and childbearing years. It was common for graduates to marry shortly after graduation. This may be part of the reason why hospitals during this era (the PUMC was a notable exception) were staffed mostly by students; once married, nurses had to quit the profession. Students and avowed single women formed a more predictable and reliable workforce. It was not until the Sino-Japanese War started in 1937 that these views in China began to shift. With the wartime nursing shortage, married nurses became full participants in the nursing profession.

The third area that stands out in the promotional material is the PUMC's emphasis on public health as a distinctive program. Learning how to care for the health of the nation prepared nurses to be good citizens. Appealing to the nationalist ideals of parents while also reassuring them about the motivations of an American university was crucial for the success of the PUMC. According to a 1931 report, the PUMC School of Nursing was set apart from the outset by its arms-length relationship with the affiliate hospital (that is, students did not staff the hospital, but rather were there as learners), its strong affiliations with universities, and its cutting-edge focus on public health. There was a "crying need" for prevention of disease in China, and, given the scientific medical knowledge available, it was "obvious" that "every program of administration and education must inevitably recognize this as its first objective."[82] The recruitment strategy included an appeal to nationalism and patriotism: "The young women of China today are preparing themselves to help in the work of making China a strong and healthy nation. They are educating themselves to take responsibilities and to be leaders. The nursing profession needs women of education and ability to help in this great work of rebuilding China."[83]

This part of the recruitment strategy struck a cord and linked back to the reason that the PUMC promoted public health as a priority: "The strength of a nation," one pamphlet posited, "depends on the health of its citizens. To make China a strong and powerful nation, Health Centers must be established where the sick may come to be cured and taught how to remain healthy and strong."[84] Of all that the PUMC could offer students, the preparation of nurses as patriotic citizens would prove most enduring.

THE PUMC AND THE *GOLDMARK REPORT*

In 1919, the Rockefeller Foundation sponsored a Committee for the Study of Nursing Education, headed by Dr. C.E.A. Winslow of Yale

University.[85] Its comprehensive examination of nursing and nursing education in the United States came on the heels of the devastating Spanish influenza pandemic of 1918–20, which killed fifty million worldwide. The "Spanish flu" had an enormous impact on nurses' collective psyche; it was nurses who were the first line of defence during the pandemic.[86] In Canada, as elsewhere, nurses and nurse leaders collaborated to bring the attention of the country to two glaring deficits in society, particularly in the aftermath of the Great War: the poor level of physical health of individuals, and the poor health of the community.[87] Numerous countries, including Canada, the United States, and China, developed departments of public health, recognizing that nurses could provide not only symptomatic relief from infectious diseases such as the Spanish flu but also preventative measures and education that would be beneficial to improving the overall health of the population of entire nations.[88] The study of nursing education, with Josephine Clara Goldmark as principal investigator, examined seventy schools of nursing over a four-year period. The resultant *Goldmark Report* (1923) would have a strong influence on the priorities and values that shaped the PUMC approach to nursing education. "The PUMC School of Nursing was started," one writer noted in 1931, "after that illuminating report."[89]

According to the Rockefeller Foundation, the recommendations of the *Goldmark Report* "proved crucial in subsequent RF funding decisions."[90] In the United States, the Yale School of Nursing became the first American school to receive Rockefeller Foundation funding to improve the education of public health nurses, while in Canada the "influential program" at the University of Toronto became a "model program" and important centre of training.[91] Both institutions would become sites for Rockefeller-funded postgraduate fellowships for PUMC nursing staff, including Vera Nieh. By following recommendations in the *Goldmark Report*, the PUMC set itself apart not only from missionary programs in China but, indeed, from the status quo of nursing around the world. However, while the *Goldmark Report* helped to create an elite school in China, it did not take root as a model for the world.

From the outset, the PUMC curriculum planned to prepare graduates for both public health and institutional (hospital-based) work. It also offered programs for postgraduate work. To the PUMC, strong nurses needed to know the cause of and cure for diseases, but also how to prevent them, and they had to understand the people they would teach about preventing disease. They learned this in the PUMC Hospital and outpatient department, as well as at the Beijing municipal Health Station. The PUMC School of Nursing controlled the provision of nursing service in all of these sites, either directly or "through the power of appointment of teaching personnel and the direction of the educational policies."[92] The *Goldmark Report* showed "the advantages which the nurse had over other types of workers" in terms of public health, as well as the "many weaknesses in her education as it then existed." The PUMC was "acutely aware of these deficiencies" and determined to avoid them at its new facilities. Of primary consideration was to ensure that the nursing program was "free from the economic pressure of a hospital upon student nurses for services." The PUMC wanted to avoid any appearance of providing cheap labour for the PUMC Hospital. That the School of Nursing could claim that the PUMC Hospital "has never depended for its care of patients upon student nurses for services" was an indicator that it was, indeed, a cutting-edge program.[93]

Educating Vera Nieh

One of the PUMC's earliest and most celebrated alumnae was born in the resort village of Beidaihe in Hebei Province in 1905.[94] Brought up in a well-to-do family, Vera Nieh (Nieh Yuchan) had three brothers and an elder sister.[95] Her father, Nieh Chi-shuan, was, as Vera Nieh described him, an "old intellectual person" with a traditional education who was "very broad-minded," "well-learned" and "far-sighted."[96] He had travelled extensively through China and believed strongly in education as important for the country's future. According to Nieh, "he gave me a very good education at home. He told me at that time that he thought China had four basic problems. First, poverty. Another is ignorance. The third is weakness – weak health is not very good; people are unhealthy – and fourth, selfishness. That's all. At least at that time the four points were thought as the main, basic problem of China."[97] These four problems, which eighty-year-old Vera Nieh would associate directly with her father's teachings, were also the four main problems of rural reconstruction identified by the Mass Education Movement of the 1920s and 1930s: ignorance, poverty, (physical) weakness, and selfishness.[98]

With her father's support, Nieh decided to become a physician. She took the entrance examination at the PUMC but, while there, met "two important friends" who eventually persuaded her to change from the study of medicine to the study of nursing. One was a high school graduate who was in her third year of nursing at the PUMC; the other was Nieh's high school friend whose mother was an operating room head nurse. "They told me about the importance of nursing," Nieh later recalled, "just as important as doctors."[99] They impressed on Nieh that nursing was a very good profession for women, and she was aware of the excellence of the PUMC's university-level nursing education program, the only one in China. Her friends convinced her to reconsider her goals – and thus began Nieh's impressive career. Her transfer to the PUMC School of Nursing in 1923 would open doors to remarkable educational and professional opportunities (see Table 1.3), challenge her gendered, national, and class identities, and test the limits of her self-determination.

At her 1923 entrance interview, the twenty-one-year-old Vera Nieh impressed the interviewer as being a "very bright, alert young woman [with] excellent knowledge of English."[100] Nieh had attended Keen Memorial High School – also called the Anglo-Chinese Girls' School – that was part of the Methodist Episcopal Mission.[101] On her PUMC application, she identified her "belief" as "Christianity."[102] She was not among those who earned a bachelor's degree at PUMC; the degree program had started only in 1922, and it is possible Nieh was not interested in doing a pre-nursing year of university.

Over the four years of her schooling at PUMC, Vera Nieh would continue to impress her instructors as someone who was smart, thorough, reliable, and well mannered. She was variously described as "considerate and sympathetic" to patients, "very genteel" to officials, "most courteous" to colleagues, and "dignified and thoughtful" to domestic staff.[103] She had musical talent as a singer, as well as a "talent in mimicking," which made her "the most popular figure in parties" and left her audience

TABLE 1.3 Vera Nieh's education and work experience

	Organization	Place	Dates	Title
Education	PUMC	Beijing	1923–27	Diploma in nursing
	University of Toronto	Canada	1929–30	n/a
	Columbia University	New York	1930–31	Bachelor of science Degree
	University of Michigan	Ann Arbor	1936–37	Master of science
	Various US universities		1947	4-month visiting fellowship
Positions	PUMC Hospital	Beijing	1927–28	Staff nurse
	Beijing Health Station	Beijing	1928–29	Staff nurse
	PUMC School of Nursing	Beijing	1931–33	Instructor, public health nursing
	Beijing Health Station	Beijing	1932–33	Chief, visiting service
	PUMC School of Nursing	Beijing	1933–34	Instructor, nursing
	(No work)	China, USA	1934–36	n/a
	PUMC School of Nursing	Beijing	1938–39	Instructor and assistant supervisor of nursing
	PUMC School of Nursing	Beijing	1939–40	Assistant dean of nursing
	PUMC School of Nursing	Beijing	1940–52	Dean of nursing
	Nurses Association of China	China	1947–49?	President

in tears of laughter.[104] According to a biographical piece written after the war, Nieh took up the profession of nursing at the inspiration of her father, "who believed that only through practical education could China become strong."[105] In this way, Vera Nieh's family values aligned well with the values espoused by the PUMC.

As a student, Vera Nieh was considered bright, even brilliant.[106] She also demonstrated that she had a mind of her own. She did not disguise her lack of interest in some subjects or required activities. One instructor reported that Nieh had taken advantage of her inexperience as a "young head nurse & went off the ward during her case study hour more than once."[107] If Nieh thought something else was more important, she would neglect her primary duties. For example, in 1927 her instructors "felt her heart was in her [Nurses Association of China] examination rather than in her work here."[108] Considered "one of the most promising nurses

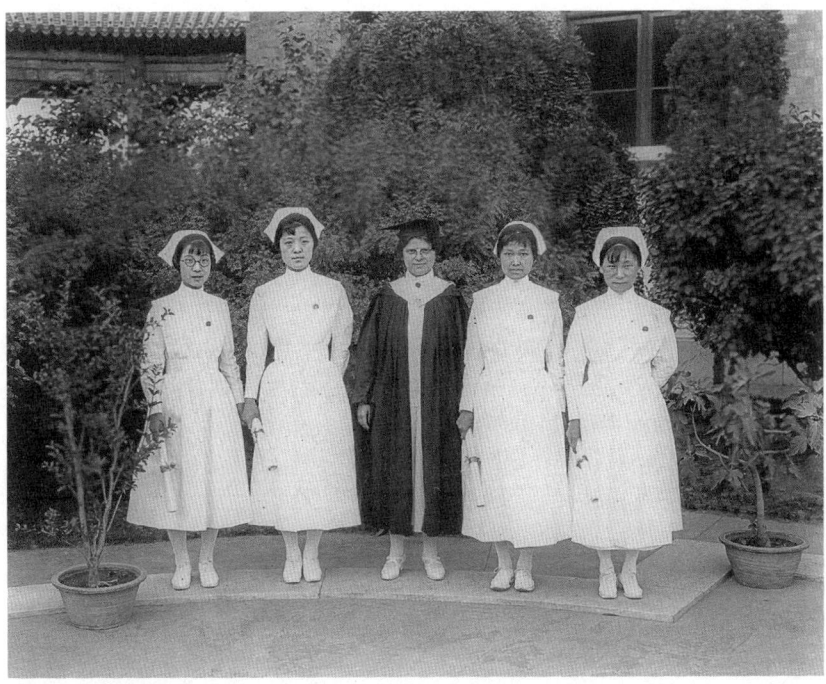

FIGURE 1.3 PUMC graduates, 1927. The graduates are Chao Hwei-ming, Vera Nieh (2nd from left), Cheo Chia-ih, and Liu Su-chun. Dean Ruth Ingram is in the centre. |
Courtesy Rockefeller Archive Centre, RAC-CMB-FA065_S1048_B31_F37_002.

produced by the Class of 1927,"[109] Vera Nieh passed her NAC exams with honours and was immediately appointed as a PUMC staff nurse, on 1 July 1927 (Figure 1.3).

In addition to praise for Nieh's intellect and character were concerns about her physical and mental health. A cycle of illness, psychological distress, withdrawal, and return would become a recurring theme. An early sign of this occurred in September 1927, when she became ill from "Hong Kong foot" – a type of ringworm – with a secondary infection.[110] By March 1928, she was "so thin, nervous, tired and pepless" on a week-end visit to Tianjin that her friends wrote Ruth Ingram, the PUMC dean of nursing, that they "were all quite worried about the change in her."[111] Ingram, too, was concerned. "I do not know whether this is due to over-work," she responded, "or to certain other factors that have nothing to do with her work."[112] Nieh had a thorough physical exam, and Ingram was keeping a close watch on her. "I talked with her sister Marion about her last Saturday," Ingram noted, "and I think her sister realizes that we are doing all we can to overcome this depression and bring her back to her usual state of health and spirits."[113] But it was not quite clear to anyone exactly what was the matter. Ruth Ingram arranged a vacation for Nieh. Following the vacation, Nieh resigned from her staff position at the PUMC Hospital on 14 June 1928. She requested, and was granted, a transfer to the PUMC's Health Centre to work as a public health nurse.[114]

While she awaited the transfer to public health, Vera Nieh's work performance in the hospital was inconsistent, evidence of her distracted state. On the one hand, she was considered reliable, resourceful, ambitious, interested, able to accept criticism, and a helpful coworker. She also possessed "dignity in administration."[115] On the other hand, she lacked interest in helping young nurses and had "fits of abstraction" during which she seemed to lose interest in her work.[116] In these instances, she exhibited "poor judgment."[117] Mary Purcell, the superintendent of nurses at PUMC, put it this way: "I have always felt that Miss Nieh was [affected?] by something outside of her work and that probably if placed in a different environment would do much better in many ways. Here she seems to be in a daze all the time."[118] A change in work settings, Purcell thought, might prove more satisfactory.

PREPARING FOR CONTROVERSY

The Beijing Health Station was created in 1925 by Dr. John B. Grant, a member of the Rockefeller Foundation's International Health Board and an associate professor of public health at the PUMC.[119] It was created as a "social laboratory" for training public health professionals and medical students. Vera Nieh had been in her new position as a public health nurse for only a couple of years when the China Medical Board recommended that she apply for an RF fellowship to study abroad. Since a senior position at the health station had recently become vacant, the idea was to "prepare Miss Nieh for a responsible [read: leadership] position in public health nursing."[120] In exchange for the fellowship, Nieh agreed to return for a minimum of two years of service at the Health Station – and preferably longer.[121] The fellowship gave Nieh important insight into what it meant to be connected to an elite organization like the PUMC and, more specifically, what opportunities being associated with the RF could open up for a bright, ambitious nurse like her. She returned from the fellowship to an administrative position, only to find herself immediately embroiled in a conflict with John B. Grant. By all accounts, Grant was difficult to work with. Nieh, together with two PUMC graduates, would resign in protest – a demonstration of solidarity that would come to characterize Nieh's approach to conflict during the refugee PUMC years in West China.

Before turning to the conflict with Grant, it is helpful to first get a sense of what requirements and expectations were associated with RF fellowships for Chinese nurses. The CMB worked diligently to avoid investing in someone who would not live up to her end of the bargain – whether by absconding to the United States or, just as disappointingly, getting married and thereby cutting short her nursing career. To reduce these risks, Anne McCabe, the chief of the Visiting Service Division at the Beijing Health Station (and Vera Nieh's boss), and Roger Greene, the resident director of the CMB in Beijing, worked to mitigate the culture shock arising from time spent in the United States.[122] McCabe noted, for example, that Vera Nieh should study at the University of Toronto rather than at the Columbia Teacher's College in New York, primarily because the RF's East Harlem Project in New York, where Vera Nieh would do her clinical learning, was too well-financed by private capital and therefore not a suitable model for China. "It is an exceptional student," McCabe wrote Greene, "who does not have great difficulty in adjusting to environmental conditions on returning, and unless they possess common sense, and the power of discrimination, they are liable to go thru a period of discouragement and unhappiness, before they are able to find a balance."[123] The idea was to find a relatively impoverished setting in the United States for Vera Nieh's clinical experience.

There were also concerns about social distractions in New York. McCabe recommended against Vera Nieh living in the International House on Riverside Drive in New York; it might give her a "wrong conception of values."[124] The concern that Nieh would be unduly tempted by a luxurious lifestyle in New York was echoed by the PUMC dean of nursing. "Miss Ingram feels very strongly," wrote Margery Eggleston, CMB secretary, to Roger Greene, "and I am certainly inclined to agree with her that the social life in New York and the special interest that so many Americans take in these attractive young foreigners make work at the Teacher's College advisable only for the more mature of our students."[125]

Finally, there was the concern about marriage. Of all the students eligible to go abroad, Vera Nieh was the only one who "gives evidence of remaining in the ranks" – that is, not marrying.[126] Indeed, John B. Grant himself wrote a memo confirming that Nieh "states that she considers a two year period of service [following her fellowship] as minimum and that she 'hopes she will never marry.'"[127] The preference was to support those without "matrimonial risk."[128] The pressure placed on single women is exemplified by another PUMC alumnus, Bernice Chu, who was granted an RF fellowship to study public health nursing at the Bedford Women's College in London, England.[129] Like Vera Nieh, Bernice Chu had agreed to give the PUMC two years of service on her return.[130] To do so, she had deferred her marriage. Although CMB administrators assured themselves that Chu's marriage was "an initiative [that] came entirely from her family and her fiancé," they were nonetheless aware of the limitations it placed on Chu's future in nursing: "As she is engaged to be married," Margery Eggleston noted, "she cannot be counted upon to remain in the service" beyond the required two years.[131]

One of the most significant benefits of the Rockefeller fellowships was that they exposed young Chinese women to other cultures while also providing opportunity to develop relationships with some of the most capable nursing leaders in the world. Because the RF was involved in fifty-three nursing schools around the world, Chinese nurses became part of an international nursing elite poised to raise the standards and prestige of nursing across the globe.[132] Success did not come easily to Vera Nieh. She struggled on a number of levels – with various courses, living in residence with unfamiliar women, speaking and studying primarily in English, and eating primarily foreign food. She was also exposed to new dangers and, in 1931, was "the victim of a 'hold-up'."[133]

"How sorry I am to hear this," Anne McCabe wrote Vera Nieh. "I hope you are not suffering in any way as a result of your sad experience."[134] Vera responded: "It was quite an unusual experience happened to me the other night. However, I presume that one has to be ready to meet all kinds of experiences in one's life-time, pleasant and unpleasant. I am very grateful for not being injured in any way."[135]

However unintentionally, the Rockefeller fellowships abroad helped to prepare Chinese nurses for the conflicts that lay ahead, most obviously during the Japanese Occupation, but even before. The fellowships in-stilled identity-shaping values such as commitment to profession over marriage, dedication to the welfare of one's home country, an inter-national mindset, and independent thinking. They also helped emerging nursing leaders to see themselves as equal partners with, not subservient to, others in authoritative positions. As it was, PUMC nursing graduates gravitated toward influential positions. For example, after the NAC con-ference in Shanghai in 1930, PUMC alumna Hilda Wang was elected vice-president of the NAC, Elizabeth Kong was elected Chinese editor of the NAC nursing journal, Bernice Chu was elected chair of the Com-mittee of Public Health, and Ravenna Tien became a member of the Curriculum Committee. "The next three to five years in China," Anne McCabe predicted, "are going to be the nucleus of great changes in Medical and Nursing Education" – and PUMC graduates would be at the fore.[136] Indeed, a core of China's future nursing leaders cut their teeth at the Health Station in Beijing in 1931, including Bernice Chu, Hilda Wang, Chou Meiyu, and Hsu Ai-chu. Vera Nieh would soon join their ranks.

CONFLICT AT THE HEALTH STATION

John B. Grant, a central figure in the development of public health in modern China, spent the 1920s and 30s establishing a Department of Public Health at PUMC. This department would train public health professionals, create health stations to study local health conditions and deliver health services, and assist the central government in establishing state medicine.[137] Both a PUMC professor and a member of the RF

International Health Division, Grant criticized the separation of curative and preventative medicine. Determined to integrate these two aspects of medicine, Grant designed a "community-based" model of public health education where students could directly engage in studying public health problems in the real world.[138] He helped establish the Public Health Experimental Station of the Metropolitan Police Department of Beijing – a collaborative endeavour of the PUMC, the Central Epidemic Prevention Bureau, and the Beijing Metropolitan Police – otherwise known as the Beijing Health Station.[139]

On 14 November 1931, Vera Nieh came on staff at the Health Station – initially as a PUMC nursing instructor, but then later replacing Anne McCabe, who was on furlough, as the head of the public health nursing program. The Health Station had seven divisions, each with its own chief: Sanitation, Vital Statistics, Nursing, Medical Services, Communicable Diseases, Public Health Visiting, and Administration. After Anne McCabe left and Vera Nieh was put in charge of the public health nursing program, a number of misunderstandings developed, partly because of the frequent absences of Dr. John B. Grant and Dr. Li Ting-an.[140, 141] Vera Nieh became the chief of the Public Health Visiting Division and was responsible for health visits to schools, factories, homes, and maternity cases. She was not, however, in charge of public health nursing. This fell to the chief of the Medical Services Division, Dr. Sohtsu G. King, who also had authority over school health, maternity health, and infant health.[142] Vera Nieh was furious that a physician was given authority over these nurses and that she herself now had "little or no real authority."[143] To Nieh, such abdication of authority was a step backward in the progress of nursing, and inconsistent with PUMC nursing ideals.

Grant did not support progressive nursing ideals. For example, he disagreed with the idea that nurses would regard themselves as a profession separate from that of medicine. While this approach might work in the United States, he surmised, it was "not tenable in China." If nurses persisted in such an approach, he argued, it would be a "detriment to the interests of the community and of public health."[144] Nor did Grant support university-level education for nurses.[145] His solution to the concerns raised by Vera Nieh was not to reinstate the Division of Nursing but rather to transfer public health nursing to the PUMC Department of Public Health – that is, the department of which Grant himself was the head.[146] Vera Nieh, of course, disagreed.

The power struggle would have to be resolved; there was much at stake. It is difficult to overstate the extreme value of and need for public health care in China during this period. In 1931, the rural population in China was reportedly poor, ignorant, superstitious, and haunted with frequent sickness and disease.[147] Ninety percent of the population was illiterate, and most lived in "mud huts, blackened with soot and smoke, swamped with flies, mosquitoes, bedbugs, fleas and rats."[148] Health knowledge was low, and available medical facilities "nil."[149] There were few or no trained physicians available in the various counties. The annual death rate in China was estimated at 7 per 1,000.[150] The main causes of "controllable excess mortality" were smallpox, gastro-intestinal diseases (dysentery, typhoid, cholera), tuberculosis, and tetanus neonatorum – a severe form of infectious tetanus occurring during the first few days of life caused by factors such as lack of maternal immunization and unhygienic practice in dressing the umbilical stump or in circumcising male infants.[151] In rural China, maternal deliveries were "conducted on beds made of mud bricks by untrained persons with unwashed hands and long dirty fingernails. The cord is cut with unboiled scissors and the bleeding is controlled by applying mud or ash. Finally, the cord is wrapped in dirty cotton and rags."[152]

One of the earliest responses to the public health crisis was the Mass Education Movement (MEM). Organized by Dr. Y.C. (Jimmy) Yen, the original aim of the MEM was to bring literacy to the Chinese masses. By the 1930s, however, the MEM had moved past "merely" teaching illiterate persons to read, to educating them "for modern citizenship."[153] The MEM turned to the villages of China to organize Rural Reconstruction Projects – most famously in Dingxian county. There, MEM public health workers aimed to improve the mortality rate by teaching the rural population to attend to simple health measures such as clean water, personal hygiene, and proper disposal of human excreta. It also encouraged immunization against diseases such as smallpox. Seared into the consciousness of the public health workers were four main "problems" to resolve:

ignorance, poverty, weakness, and selfishness – the same list that Vera Nieh later attributed to her father. The PUMC Department of Public Health was particularly responsible for the third problem – physical weakness. The idea was to build up "a strong virile people through the promotion of health education and the practical application of curative and preventative medicine."[154]

An address delivered to the PUMC graduating class in 1929 by Hu Tun-wu, a second-year nursing student at the college, exemplifies the influence of the public health movement. Reiterating the purpose of the PUMC – to train leaders, and to do this primarily through preventative medicine – Hu noted that, at this critical stage in China's history, PUMC nurses had an obligation to attend to the health of Chinese people as a whole. Recalling her student experience at the Health Station, Hu noted,

> I'll never forget seeing one day a file of blind soldiers, six of them, one after another, each holding by the coat of the man in front. [People] laughed at them and let them pass unhelped, but I can never forget it. [I wanted] to know the cause of their blindness, so I asked the eye specialists [who said] it came from living on carbohydrates alone. Is it not a tragic [picture] of what ignorance there is of diet?[155]

Hu Tun-wu also described seeing mothers come into the Health Station every day, bringing their babies "in deep coma" either from meningitis, measles, or scarlet fever.[156] "Why did you not bring your child to the hospital earlier?" she would ask. The mothers would eventually admit that "they have [gone] to the temples for a prescription from the gods, and some ... drugs said to be good for the disease."[157] They would come to the Health Station only after traditional methods, including visiting the traditional Chinese doctor, had failed.

Hu Tun-wu's address is a zealous call to the gospel of soap and water.[158] "No matter what our special work may be," she exclaimed, "our duty, or responsibility, is the [t]eaching of health and the prevention of disease, in one word, the socialization of modern medicine." By carrying out such ideals, Hu contended, PUMC nurses would be able to "save lives and souls."[159] Shortly after graduation, Hu Tun-wu became a faculty member at the Health Station.

In 1933, the conflict between Vera Nieh and John B. Grant had grown to involve other nurses and physicians. It came to a head on 21 February 1933, when Nieh submitted her resignation "in order to improve the situation for the nursing school at the health station."[160] Roger Greene recommended that she take an early vacation or extended leave of absence instead, hoping he might be able to arrange for a reinstatement of the Nursing Division under the head of the Health Station, Dr. I.C. Fang. If it seemed that "no sincere effort has been made to recognize our problems and to assist in solving them," Greene assured Nieh, "we will be unwilling to continue our cooperation at the health station, even though there is a promise of a division of nursing which is, of course, necessary."[161] On that promise, Vera Nieh remained. However, on 6 June 1933, she submitted a second letter of resignation. "After a long and careful consideration," she wrote, "I still feel that for the benefit of the [nursing] service and my health, I have decided to resign."[162] PUMC alumnae Hu Tun-wu and Hsu Ai-Chu submitted their resignations as well.

Although Greene had committed to re-establishing a Nursing Division, Vera Nieh felt that there was too much friction for her to continue. Hu Tun-wu was reluctant to take over responsibilities from Nieh "and to face the double allegiance involved under which she was partly responsible to Miss Hodgman and partly to Dr. I.C. Fang," and she accepted a position from the National Health Administration in Nanjing.[163] Hsu Ai-Chu, in turn, received a "very flattering invitation" from Dr. F.C. Yen to go to Shanghai with the view of eventually becoming the dean of the School of Nursing associated with the National Medical College of Shanghai.[164] Gertrude Hodgman, who was on furlough in the United States, was furious at the news that three of her faculty were resigning. She held John B. Grant responsible.[165] She recommended the immediate withdrawal of nursing students from the Health Station, and their transfer to the PUMC Outpatient Department.[166]

Roger Greene, reflecting on the ongoing conflict, started to realize that the administrative structure at the Health Station was not the only problem. How things were organized at the PUMC also complicated matters. When public health nursing was first introduced at the PUMC in 1925, it was organized under the PUMC Department of Health rather than the School of Nursing. This was because Ruth Ingram, the dean of nursing at the time, had no experience in public health nursing "and was unwilling, therefore, to assume responsibility for its development."[167] John B. Grant, Greene noted, had maintained that this would be a temporary arrangement, as he hoped that Ingram or someone else in charge of the School of Nursing would eventually have sufficient knowledge of public health to take over responsibility for the public health programs at the Health Station. "We had this in mind when we selected Miss Hodgman to succeed Miss Ingram," Greene noted, "and Miss Hodgman's appointment was with the distinct understanding that she should have charge of public health nursing, and particularly of teaching in that field."[168]

Anne McCabe remained supervisor of public health during Gertrude Hodgman's first year as dean. "Having always been responsible to Dr. Grant," Greene wrote, McCabe "did not take naturally to the new organization under which ... she was supposed to be under Miss Hodgman."[169] This resulted in a great deal of friction, with things being done at the Health Station without consultation with Gertrude Hodgman. Furthermore, the young physicians "seemed to fret at having any outside influence like that of the Dean of the School of Nursing to consider in making their plans."[170]

Despite the resignations of Vera Nieh, Hu Tun-wu, and Hsu Ai-Chu, Roger Greene was unwilling to abandon or reduce public health nursing at the Health Station. Instead, he suggested that such nursing be separated from any direct relationship to the dean of the School of Nursing, and that Hodgman's contribution instead be made through her membership on the Committee on Health Stations. John B. Grant, I.C. Fang, and the acting dean of nursing, Miss Parsons, agreed to try out the plan. "I myself believe," Greene wrote, "that it might result in a better relationship between Dr. Grant and Miss Hodgman."[171]

Gertrude Hodgman remained frustrated. In a letter written to the associate director of the RF International Health Division, Mary Beard, Hodgman vented her anger. "Never have I felt so futile and discouraged about anything as I do about this situation," she confided. "We are playing checkers, instead of building a house with blocks. The nurses," she mused, "have no kings and few men."[172] If Vera Nieh, Hu Tun-wu, and Hsu Ai-Chu were leaving, it would be impossible to continue teaching nursing students at the Health Station (as part of their education at the PUMC). Hoping that they might change their minds, Hodgman stalled. "Perhaps," she concluded in her letter to Beard, "we can zigzag across one of the corners for a while."[173] It was not to be. Vera Nieh resigned on 10 July 1933, and Hu Tun-wu on 1 September 1933. Hsu Ai-Chu, "the last foreign-trained public health nurse," had resigned to take effect on 1 October 1933, but Hodgman had managed to convince her to stay until 1 December.[174] The friction between Gertrude Hodgman and John B. Grant would continue, and eventually result in her being edged out of her position as dean of nursing.

* * *

To be a nurse in early twentieth-century China meant being instilled with a sense of belonging to something greater than oneself. For Canadian missionaries and other Christian nurses, nursing provided a tangible opportunity to emulate Christ and serve God by serving others. This was most readily done through work in one of the myriad modern hospitals scattered throughout urban regions or in dispensaries in rural areas. In missions like the United Church of Canada West China Mission, staff nurses worked closely with physicians within complex medical systems modelled after Western approaches to diagnosing and treating illness and injuries. Missionary nurses lived in community with other missionaries, with their homes and places of work in close proximity, often on the same mission-owned property. As in Canada and the United States, hospital-based nursing in China necessarily entailed teaching nursing students. Since student labour was typically required for staffing hospitals, part of the role of missionary and other graduate nurses was to instruct students. In this way, nursing education was central to modern nursing; to be a nurse in a modern hospital involved both education and practice.

For PUMC and other Chinese nurses during this period, nursing provided an opportunity to develop – and to themselves become – strong

Chinese citizens. Determined from the outset to be a cutting-edge institution geared toward developing Chinese nursing leaders, the PUMC drew on its strong links to persons of influence to advance a progressive view of nursing that aligned well with some of the most innovative thinking of the day. While PUMC nurses identified strongly with PUMC ideals, they decidedly resisted being part of the medical community, sensing that collaboration with medicine inevitably meant losing power. Influenced by American values of independence, PUMC nurses viewed nursing as a completely separate discipline from medicine, and they strived to maintain nursing control over nursing practice and education.

Through reading institutional archives of both the WCM and PUMC, one cannot necessarily tell the extent to which China's sorrows spilled into the work of nurses like Vera Nieh and Gertrude Hodgman. Yet, the unsettled socio-political landscape is precisely what defines the need (and opportunities) for nursing care. Between 1914 and 1935, China was convulsing from unrelenting socio-political upheaval. Significant events included the pneumonic plague in Manchuria (1911), which opened up confidence in Western medicine and science; the transition from a dynastic kingdom to a new republic (1912), which opened opportunity for relationships between Westerners and government; and the Warlord Era (1916–27), which followed the death of Yuan Shikai, the first official president of the new republic. Events also included the May Fourth Movement (1919), which exemplified and exacerbated anti-imperialist sentiment, and the Nationalist Northern Expedition (1927), with Chiang Kai-shek's march to Nanjing. While rife with violence (and triggering the great missionary exodus of 1927), the Northern Expedition ushered in a decade of stabilization as the new Nationalist government centralized health and education into state-run departments. But Japan's invasion of Manchuria in 1931 foreshadowed the most devastating socio-political upheaval yet – Japan's occupation of northern China in 1937 and the resultant eight-year Sino-Japanese War.

Throughout these events, ordinary Chinese citizens struggled against poverty, illness, flood, and famine. Nurses in China, in the best tradition of the profession, saw it as their responsibility to attend to those most profoundly affected by these conditions, whether by providing (together with physicians) curative treatments, or by trying to prevent or mitigate the illness or injury that sprang from difficult living conditions. And institutions like the West China Mission and the Peking Union Medical College provided educational avenues that allowed aspiring nurses to do just that.

CHAPTER TWO

Unsettling Nursing (1932–40)

Japanese Invasion and the Shift to Chinese Leadership

Nursing is still in the newborn stage of development, and they have a sympathetic central Ministry of Health at [Nanjing]. I wish that more of the upper class women would consider nursing, but this they will not do, until we raise the educational requirements and standards, and it ranks as a profession.

> — *Anne McCabe, PUMC chief, Visiting Nurses, 1929*

Within a reasonable period of time the institution [PUMC] should be taken over, maintained and operated by the Chinese, its Board, faculty and personnel having gradually become predominantly Chinese.

> — *John D. Rockefeller, upon his retirement from the PUMC Board, 1940*

The decade leading up to Japan's full-scale invasion of China was a period of tentative peace, the threat of war always looming on the horizon. As the new Nationalist government focused on stabilizing, centralizing, and standardizing social services from its headquarters in Nanjing, reports and rumours of the movement of Japanese troops instilled fury and fear. Missionaries and PUMC leaders alike kept attuned to local and international newspapers and radio broadcasts, trying to find patterns and predictions in the unfolding events. For example, in March 1933, Roger Greene, the acting director of the Peking Union Medical College (PUMC), noted in a letter to Rockefeller Foundation (RF) vice-president Selskar M. Gunn that "I am waiting with some anxiety to learn what the effect of the stiffer resistance put up by the Chinese troops as Hsifengkou ["The Great Wall"] on Japanese military opinion is going to be."[1] Recognizing the significance of the local hostilities, he concluded (correctly as it turned out) that "there seems to be danger that this might lead to much more active and wide-spread military effort on the part of the Japanese, inspired partly by a desire for revenge."[2] By 1936, there was no ignoring the signs. In a letter dated 7 February 1936, Gertrude Hodgman, the dean of nursing at the PUMC, wrote to Mary Beard at the RF, "the political situation seems to be one of apprehension as to what will happen next. There is a considerable exodus of the well-to-do Chinese from the city [Beijing]. Our hospital receipts for six months are down about $35,000 chiefly as a result of this, I presume. When the embassies move to [Nanjing], as they doubtless will, in the relatively near future, we will be high and dry up here."[3] While the focus of this letter was on the economic impact of losing wealthy, private patients who helped cover the cost of running the PUMC Hospital, it also reflected the general unease in 1936. Something was coming.

This chapter examines how nurses responded to wartime challenges from the outset of the Japanese Occupation and through the end of 1940. It traces the reflections, experiences, and decisions of ordinary nurses who sought to teach the next generation how to prevent, relieve, and help find meaning in suffering, even while suffering themselves. It also explores the Nationalist-mandated shift to Chinese leadership in nursing, considering ways in which social and political events acted variously to accelerate and impede the transition.

VERA NIEH AND THE SHANGHAI INCIDENT

A sense of impending disaster was a familiar feeling in China. Ongoing skirmishes between Nationalist and Communist factions, together with natural calamities (floods, drought, famine) kept China off balance – a situation the Japanese army was eager to exploit. The first significant push by the Japanese was the Mukden Incident, which Japan used as a pretext for its invasion of Manchuria, on 18 September 1931. Within days, Japanese forces took other cities, effectively securing control of Liaoning and Kirin provinces and, with them, China's entire northern border with Korea. The threat continued, with Japan bombing Shanghai on 28 January 1932, a military action that became known as the Shanghai

Incident. The response of Chinese PUMC faculty, staff, and students to the Shanghai Incident reveals how a new generation of local leaders was already emerging. The incident, and the PUMC's response to it, imbued Chinese nurses such as Vera Nieh with the confidence to step into leadership roles independent from American benefactors, and also, if necessary, in opposition to them.

By 27 January 1932, the Japanese military had concentrated a number of ships, airplanes, and troops on the shoreline of Shanghai, and, on 28 January, Japanese aircraft bombed the city. On 14 February 1932, Chiang Kai-shek sent the Fifth Army to Shanghai. Around the same time, "in view of the national crisis," a group at the PUMC organized a Medical Corps for field service.[4] One hundred and thirty personnel signed up, including six surgeons, two physicians, eleven other medical officers, thirteen nurses, and fifty-two interns and medical students, among others. Indeed, "the entire student body has joined the Corps in daily training under C.T. Loo," the students each paying for their own brown uniforms and full kit.[5] Vera Nieh, who had started teaching as an assistant instructor in public health nursing at the PUMC on 1 January 1932, sat on the Finance Commission of the corps.[6] On 26 February 1932, a group of fourteen members of the commission put out an announcement "for all Chinese staff members, professional and non-professional" to appeal "to every Chinese member of the college" to "make a [financial] contribution" to the corps "as a patriotic duty."[7] There was an immediate need for $15,000 to cover medical and surgical supplies, and the PUMC Medical Corps recommended that all (Chinese) staff and faculty contribute a percentage of their salary for three months to cover this cost. The College Pay Office was authorized to deduct a specific amount from salaries, ranging from 3 to 10 percent, depending on the size of the salary. The idea was that all Chinese would participate, although the announcement note that, "if anyone finds real difficulty in contributing ... [they should] send a written statement to the Secretary." If the commission did not hear anything within one week, "it is understood that you agree to participate in this financial plan."[8]

The desire among Chinese nursing and medical faculty and students to assist in the resistance against Japanese aggression in 1932 is striking –

particularly since this was five years before what is typically referred to as the start of the Sino-Japanese War, in 1937. It presaged what was to come in terms of the Japanese threat, and the readiness of the PUMC alumnae, including Vera Nieh, to support the Chinese cause. In addition to helping out with the Medical Corps, PUMC nurses were finding other ways to provide patriotic support. In a letter to Gertrude Hodgman dated 24 February 1932, British missionary nurse Gladys Stephenson noted that she had received a letter and radiogram from a Dr. J.H. Lui (in addition to one from Hodgman) asking for male and female nurses to go to Shanghai. Although they would not be paid, they would be fed.[9] Gladys Stephenson had been a Methodist missionary in China since 1915. She was also actively involved in the Nurses Association of China (NAC), serving as its president in 1924.[10] At the time of the Shanghai Incident, Stephenson was working at the Union Hospital in Hankou. While she does not spell out in her letter to Hodgman what the situation was that required nurses, it was presumably to provide humanitarian relief in Shanghai. "Other nurses are asking to go," Stephenson noted, and "I hope to wire you the number of graduate men who can go after this first group have got off."[11] She also noted that "our repairs are proceeding merrily & our wards are busy" – possibly a reference to violence in Hankou as well. In March 1932, Hodgman and Stephenson corresponded regularly about the PUMC nurses. On 2 March 1932, Hodgman informed Stephenson that the PUMC had enough nurses for its "unit" and that "if we need additional nurses we will telegraph you."[12] What Hodgman seems to be referring to is a "unit" of PUMC medical and nursing staff and alumnae who were assisting in Shanghai. "I doubt the PUMC will be willing to finance anymore," she noted. "Therefore, any further calls for nurses will probably come directly from Shanghai."[13]

Regardless of whether the PUMC would finance it, there was a strong desire on the part of its nurses to assist the bombed city. In a letter to Hodgman dated 7 March 1932, Stephenson notes that nurses reached Shanghai a few days previous, and, while "I made it clear to them that I did not know whether they would be needed in the PUMC unit, they all offered to go in response to Dr. Liu's wire for no salary, so I do not [think] there should be any difficulty if they were not needed in your unit."[14]

Stephenson, in the meantime, was busy in the Union Hospital. "We are getting repaired gradually," she noted, "all wards are available now and we have a class of thirty new students."[15] She loved her work. "It is glorious work," she wrote, "and I am so happy to have the privilege of doing it."[16]

The organization of PUMC faculty and staff into the Medical Corps and the collaboration between the PUMC and American missionaries at Hankou are striking, primarily because they suggest that Chinese nurses' decisions whether to work independently from Westerners (in the Medical Corps) or collaboratively (through the Hanzhou mission) were pragmatic rather than ideological ones. In the case of the Medical Corps, rising anti-imperialism and related nationalism made it necessary for Americans to tread carefully, while also not joining directly into movements that could further agitate the Japanese. In the case of the missionaries, it was part of their mandate to care for the ill. Working with PUMC nurses, then, was politically acceptable to Gladys Stephenson. In other words, Chinese nurses, including Vera Nieh, found ways to leverage their relationships with wary Westerners toward patriotic aims.

Nurses Association of China: From Missionaries to PUMC Alumnae

In November 1936, the Nurses Association of China was in full swing. Having just completed a "very successful" national conference in Nanjing, there was already excitement about the International Council of Nurses conference in London the following year, and in Chengdu, Sichuan, in 1938. Nursing education, administration, and public health were among the "great themes" of the conference, which signified a national desire for a shift toward university-level nurses' education, as it was at the university level that nurse educators, administrators, and public health nurses received their education. The aim of the NAC was to register all schools of nursing with the Ministry of Education, and all graduate nurses with the National Health Administration. In other words, the Nationalist government was becoming increasingly interested in the education and practice of nurses. Indeed, the 1936 conference included "many addresses by Government Officials."[17] The NAC leaders fully supported the move to government oversight, noting to its members that "our Government has now given [nursing] a place in the Nation, and nurses should speedily avail themselves of this opportunity to become registered nurses."[18] Toward this end, the NAC was planning a new administrative-hostel building, which would be completed that year.

From its inception in 1909, the main thrust of the NAC had been to raise the standard of nurses' training in China by the adoption of a "uniform course of study and examination."[19] In the absence of governmental authority on nursing education, the NAC took responsibility for setting the standard for all nursing schools in the country, formulating a model curriculum, and holding certification examinations.[20] By 1920, forty-eight Chinese graduate nurses had joined the NAC, fifty-two training schools had been registered, and 150 Chinese nurses had successfully passed the NAC examinations and received the NAC diploma.[21] That same year, the NAC commenced its own quarterly journal, the *Nursing Journal of China*, which carried each article in English and Chinese. Two years later, it formed the Committee on Nursing Education and became the first Asian country to be admitted to the International Council of Nurses. By 1926, 112 schools of nursing were registered under the NAC, with 2,000 students enrolled. Most schools were associated with American mission organizations; five were Canadian.[22] By the late 1930s, 6,000 nurses were registered with the NAC.[23]

In 1928, the NAC appointed its first Chinese president, Wu Zheying (Lillian Wu). In some respects, the shift from Western to Chinese leadership can be seen most readily through the transition of the NAC from a primarily missionary organization before 1920 to an increasingly nationalized organization. The early NAC was first a missionary organization, imbued with Christian ideals. The first foreign-trained Chinese nurse, Elsie Mawfung Chung, then the matron of the Government Hospital in Tianjin, highlighted this in her 1914 address to the NAC in Shanghai. Drawing on her own Christian faith as a call to solidarity and racial equity, she appealed to an audience of primarily (if not completely) missionary nurses to do the same, stating,

I beg each member – you who are giving your services so gen-
erously – to do it with the spirit of true helpfulness, to treat the
Chinese as human beings, to raise the standard of nursing, to
raise the people to enjoy that standard; forget race differences, for
are we not all Christian, brothers and sisters in Christ, whether
they be Negroes, Chinese, Americans or English? If God makes
no distinction, who are we that we should make one?[24]

This understanding of nursing as an act of Christian faith, as a vocation
(or "calling") that could, and should, be informed by Christian disci-
plines such as prayer, scripture reading, worship, and service, was common in the West during this period. Bible reading, prayer, and hymn
singing, for example, were conventional in Western nursing schools, and
were common well past the mid-twentieth century. It is no surprise, then,
that, in China, where modern nursing was initially introduced and established by Christian missionaries, Christian values, beliefs, and practices
would commonly have been woven into nursing education and leadership. The NAC, for its part, expressed its "theology" as late as 1926 in
seven words: "For God so loved that He gave."[25] It espoused a Western,
Christian understanding of nursing, encouraging schools of nursing to
"instill the highest ideals of nursing ethics throughout the profession"
and to "encourage Chinese nurses to regard their work as a true act of
service to God and to their countrymen."[26]

During the Nanjing Decade (1928–37) the Nationalist government
established the Ministry of Education, and the NAC came under government oversight and control. Part of the Nationalist requirement was that
Chinese, rather than foreigners, head organizations like the NAC. Given
the PUMC focus on leadership development, it is not surprising that so
many PUMC alumnae were among the Chinese presidents of the NAC
(see Table 2.1). Over time, an increasing number of Chinese sat on the
NAC board and committees; by 1936, the majority of NAC members
were Chinese. By that time, the NAC had two boards: a board of supervisors (with one American and four Chinese nurses) and a board of directors (with two American and nine Chinese nurses). Two of the American
nurses on these boards were the well-known Gladys Stephenson and

TABLE 2.1 NAC milestones and involvement of PUMC alumnae, 1908–2013

Year	Event	PUMC class
1908	First meeting of what became the NAC: Guling, Fuzhou	
1909	Second meeting of NAC, Fukien Branch: Guling, Fuzhou First president: Mrs. Caroline Maddock Hart[29]	
1912	NAC meeting organized Gulling, Lushan, Jiangxi President: Nina Gage	
1914	NAC commences recognition and registration of nursing schools	
1920	First quarterly issue of the *Nursing Journal of China*	
1922	NAC joins International Council of Nurses (ICN)	
1928	First Chinese president: Wu Zheying (Lillian Wu)	n/a
1930	NAC moves from Beijing to Nanjing	
1936–42	President: Lin Sz-sing (Evelyn Lin)	1926
1942–46	President: Hsu Ai-Chu	1930
1946–48	President: Nieh Yuchan (Vera Nieh)	1926
1949	China removed from ICN membership	
2013	China readmitted into full ICN membership (now called Chinese Nursing Association)	

Cora Simpson.[27] PUMC dean of nursing Gertrude Hodgman was invited to sit on a committee to revise the NAC constitution. The nature of the small and tight-knit nursing community in China is reflected in a letter that notes that the other members of the committee were all well known to Hodgman.[28] Perhaps most significantly, a number of PUMC graduates sat on the two NAC boards, including Evelyn Lin (PUMC 1926), Hilda Wang (PUMC 1932), Bernice Chu Chen (PUMC 1926), and Hsu Ai-Chu (PUMC 1930). Each of these PUMC alumnae, along with Vera Nieh, had or would receive Rockefeller fellowships to study abroad. And each of them would end up in Free China after 1942.

In 1934, the Ministry of Education organized the Central Board of Nursing Education; Vera Nieh was its first secretary.[30] The board took over the NAC's function of setting the curriculum and compiling textbooks and syllabi for nursing schools, and students who graduated from nursing schools had to pass board examinations. Between 1934 and 1936, over 5,000 nurses were granted diplomas, and over 160 schools were in the process of registering with the Ministry of Education.[31] This new interest by the Nationalist government was encouraging, but not without its difficulties. As Cora Simpson wrote to Gertrude Hodgman on 17 November 1936, the government now had a standard for regulations for all associations or organizations registered with it. The constitutions of all associations had to be approved by the government – something Simpson agreed with, despite the extra work it presented for the NAC: "You can readily see the need for this," she wrote, "when we consider the secret organizations that might spring up and cause no end of trouble for the Government at this time in the National History."[32]

The shift to Chinese leadership was apparent across China, including at the Canadian North China Mission (NCM) nursing schools. In September 1936, missionary nurse Cora Kilborn reported that the School of Nursing in Chengdu (Renji) had hired its first Chinese principal.[33] "It is true," the report noted, "that this step was necessary and inevitable as they are registering with the Government, but we are glad to be moving with the times and more glad and proud that we have someone capable of filling this position."[34] The West China Mission (WCM) also hired its first Chinese head nurse, Dju Shu Chwan, a graduate of Renji who had done postgraduate work in Hankou and Beijing. To the missionaries, Dju Shu Chwan was a good choice because she was older, mature, and, above all, "a splendid Christian."[35] To missionary nurse Jeanette Ratcliffe, this change signified a significant marker in Chinese nursing history: "All this meant far more than raising standards of education for our nurses, it meant that nursing had won a battle for recognition throughout China, that schools had been standardized, and that the allegiance of educated and high-minded Chinese womanhood had been enlisted."[36]

In 1937, the number of registered nurses in China dropped: only 575 nurses were registered with the government, although thousands had graduated from accredited nursing schools.[37] This was likely a result of the unsettled conditions in China. In June 1937, the new NAC headquarters opened in Nanjing, ten years after Nanjing became the capital of China.[38] It was a three-story building, opened debt-free; paid for by nurses. Japan's invasion of China happened shortly after the NAC headquarters opened. The Chinese government moved to Chongqing, and all other official agencies followed it. However, the NAC felt their work was urgently needed in the occupied regions. Many of the hospitals were overwhelmed with sick and wounded, and it was important that schools of nursing continue to educate and train nurses.[39] Although the Ministry of Education had taken over the NAC registration exams, it now asked the NAC to resume charge of this work for all of the occupied regions of China. Part of the NAC went to Free China. Its secretary, PUMC alumna Ravenna Tien (in Nanjing), and an augmented board of directors (in Shanghai) took responsibility for occupied regions. Gladys Stephenson was the last missionary nurse serving on the board of that time; the others were all Chinese nurses. After Stephenson was interned by the Japanese, the NAC board consisted completely of Chinese nurses. At that time, sixty hospitals and schools of nursing were still functioning in occupied cities and towns that had been captured by Japan, from Beijing to Guangdong.

Remaining behind in Nanjing, Ravenna Tien had to verify repeatedly that the building was Chinese property; the Japanese constantly tried to prove it was American property so that they could seize it. Although postal communications were destroyed, Tien managed to keep in touch with nurses, sending letters, examination forms, and diplomas secretly on the persons of "loyal friends."[40] Cut off as they were from the rest of the NAC in Chongqing, Tien and the board in Shanghai were obliged to take full responsibility for the schools in the occupied regions. Tien travelled every few months to Shanghai to meet with the board. According to Stephenson, each board "meeting began with earnest prayer for guidance and for protection for the nurses about whom they were anxious."[41] In these challenging times, they embraced "their association motto, 'With God nothing is impossible.'"[42]

THE INDOMITABLE GERTRUDE HODGMAN: LEADERSHIP CRISIS AT THE PUMC

Gertrude Hodgman became PUMC dean of nursing in 1930. A graduate of Vassar and Johns Hopkins Hospital School of Nursing (BA) and the Teachers College of Columbia University (MA), she taught at Yale University before joining the PUMC.[43] Unlike Ruth Ingram (PUMC dean of nursing from 1918 to 1929), Hodgman had a strong background in public health nursing education.[44] The Yale University School of Nursing had been founded through a gift from the Rockefeller Foundation after the 1923 *Goldmark Report* highlighted the importance of this area of nursing. Yale was the first American school to receive RF funding to improve the education of public health nurses.[45] (Not incidentally, the co-author of the report, Dr. C.E.A. Winslow, was a professor of public health at Yale.)[46] A condition of the gift was that the graduates should be prepared to enter the field of public health nursing.[47] That Gertrude Hodgman was known in her own right as a leader in public health nursing is evident in a 1929 article she authored in the *American Journal of Nursing* detailing the public health nursing program at Yale.[48] Her disagreements with Dr. John B. Grant in the early 1930s, then, over the administrative structure of the PUMC Beijing Health Station were rooted in a particular understanding of the best way to teach and learn public health nursing. Yet her tenacious stance on this and other issues, however well founded, earned her a reputation as someone difficult to get along with. By 1937, colleagues were quietly agitating for her resignation.

The rift between Hodgman and Grant that had started in 1933 had, by 1936, widened rather than being resolved. Their mutual distrust is exemplified by an exchange of letters between Hodgman and her RF colleagues in New York, Selskar Gunn and Mary Beard. In a letter to Gunn, Hodgman expressed her disagreement with Grant's decision to appoint a nurse, Miss Hu (likely Hu Tun-wu), to replace Vera Nieh on the Rockefeller-funded Commission for Medical Education. Surmising that Grant favoured the appointment because Hu was a good scholar and would have been able to translate Chinese texts, Hodgman asserted that "the needs and opportunities which this possibility offers to the development of nursing work should require a much more comprehensive program than the mere writing and translation of text material." Furthermore, Hodgman commented, Hu's "emotional instability and certain other qualities which have been apparent to those who know her, make me feel that ultimately she will not be acceptable to those who represent the best nursing work in China." Hu's appointment would, therefore, "cause much unnecessary friction where cooperation is essential" and would be "a serious embarrassment to both the PUMC alumnae and School of Nursing."[49]

In a second letter enclosed with the first, Hodgman tells Gunn that she "would much prefer that the enclosed letter which I have written to you may not be shown to Dr. Grant."[50] In the second letter, she states that she had already expressed her view to Grant, and, in her experience, she did not believe that Grant would give any consideration to her opinions. She was writing to Gunn, therefore, to "register with you my protest against this appointment which I understand will be made on funds from the Foundation."[51] Hodgman also complained to Mary Beard. In a letter dated 7 February 1936, Hodgman confided her opinion that Hu was "not loyal to anyone – but to her own ambitions and her not entirely healthy self."[52] Hu had started a new nursing organization of public health nurses, which, to Hodgman, "seems to be very much a political move on her part."[53] It seems likely that Gertrude Hodgman's view of Hu Tun-wu stemmed from her experiences at the Health Station in 1933, when Hu, together with Vera Nieh and Hsu Ai-Chu, had resigned. Hu had then moved to Nanjing to accept a position in Health administration there.

The point is that neither Gertrude Hodgman nor, as will be seen, others associated with wartime nursing in China were shy about giving frank (and sometimes deleterious) opinions regarding the capability of others. Nor were they exempt from being on the receiving end of such sentiments. Indeed, Gertrude Hodgman, Vera Nieh, and Cora Kilborn each experienced pressure to resign at different times, usually because of a pooled resentment against them from within their own organizations. For Cora Kilborn, it came from her Chinese nursing colleagues and students within the WCM, and resulted in her departure from China. For Vera Nieh, it came from Chinese Medical Board and West China Union University administrators, both Chinese and Western. In the early part of her career, Nieh had resigned from stressful positions of her own accord before the conflict escalated too far. However, by the time she was dean of nursing at the PUMC, she pushed back against the criticism levied against her, strategically garnering support within her varied networks. One of her strongest critics during the PUMC refugee years would eventually exonerate her, expressing warm admiration for her by war's end. In this sense, Nieh fought (and won) her own war of resistance.

For Gertrude Hodgman, pressure to resign came from PUMC and RF administrators. Having experienced four years of frustration, she agreed to step down at the end of her term, in October 1937. However, as it turned out, war interrupted her departure plans. First, the Marco Polo Bridge Incident[54] on 7 July 1937 that marked the start of the Sino-Japanese War indefinitely delayed an American replacement. Hodgman wavered, wondering aloud whether departing immediately would prove too disruptive for the PUMC. Without an American replacement, it was not immediately clear who should – or could – replace her. As it turned out, despite her agreement to resign in 1937, Gertrude Hodgman stayed in her position until 1940, when she was finally replaced by Vera Nieh.

Although ongoing conflict between Gertrude Hodgman and John B. Grant had been evident for years, it was not until 1937 that Henry Houghton, acting director of the PUMC, stepped in. Writing to Dr. Wilber A. Sawyer of the International Health Division (IHD) of the Rockefeller Foundation (on 18 March 1937, Houghton noted that, regarding proposed changes aimed at keeping nursing aligned with government views of nursing needs in China, "the head of our School [i.e., Hodgman] does not view with favor what is being considered. It has been so difficult to secure her cooperation, indeed, that I am not sure she will want to stay beyond the expiry of her present term of service (autumn of 1937) or alternatively that the officers of the College will want to renew her appointment."[55] In apparent anticipation of Hodgman's resignation, Houghton recommended that the RF send IHD assistant director (and nursing consultant) Elizabeth Tennant to China for two years. During that time, Tennant would "act as an adviser in nursing education, and ... start off one of our own promising Chinese graduates at the head of the School."[56] By 3 May 1937, considerable discussions back and forth between New York and China had ensued, with all involved agreeing with the idea of Tennant taking over for Hodgman. At the same time, Sawyer and Tennant were themselves "anxious that these suggestions should not influence the decision with regard to the continuation or termination of Miss Hodgman's service to PUMC. If is it independently decided that she will not renew her contract, then we should be inclined to assign Miss Tennant to PUMC, if requested by you."[57] Dr. Grant was also pleased with the possibility of Elizabeth Tennant coming to the PUMC – and undoubtedly of Gertrude Hodgman departing.[58]

In the meantime, war intervened. The Marco Polo Bridge Incident escalated into a battle between Chinese and Japanese troops. A decision about Tennant was delayed until the end of September 1937. In a letter to W.A. Sawyer on 29 September 1937, Henry Houghton apologized for the delay, noting that the "sudden changes taking place here" have made it "difficult to plan very far ahead, particularly with respect to the outcoming of foreign personnel."[59] However, since Houghton was now in a position to make a decision, he sent a return telegram "earnestly" requesting that Tennant come for two years, commencing 1 February 1938.[60] He was not concerned that the fighting in northern China would affect the PUMC: "there appears to be not the slightest likelihood of any military disturbances taking place within [Beijing].[61] In Houghton's view, Beijing was "safe and quiet, and the conditions of life are essentially normal, apart from the presence of a good many soldiers. These are well-disciplined and well behaved, however, and their pervasiveness is at most slightly annoying."[62] On the political front, therefore, Houghton saw no reason not to go ahead with plans for Tennant. However, the social front was a different matter.

Gertrude Hodgman was starting to feel reluctant about departing the PUMC in October 1937 as planned. She felt that "her going at this time would suggest a personal retreat" and furthermore "might be bad for the morale of the school."[63] Houghton agreed. He suggested she extend her service to the PUMC until 1 March 1938, with the understanding that Tennant ("or whoever is to come as adviser") would be sought for beginning a service about the first of February, allowing time for an overlap. By then, Houghton predicted, the PUMC ought to have "two or three excellent choices of Chinese graduates to head up the School."[64]

It was not to be. By the time Henry Houghton's message reached New York, the RF had already decided not to send Elizabeth Tennant after all, due to the uncertain wartime conditions.[65] Furthermore, even if Beijing was considered safe, "the political separation of the area in which the [PUMC] is situated from the greater part of China, would prevent the carrying out of essential parts of [Tennant's agreed-upon plans] related to visiting other programs" in other regions of China. Given the wartime conditions, "it would seem that Miss Tennant would not be able to maintain the necessary contacts, through travel or otherwise, for advising Dr. Grant on the development of public health nursing in his field or adjusting the education of nurses at [the PUMC] to the actual field conditions in China."[66] The plan fell through.

The PUMC School of Nursing was now in a difficult position, and John B. Grant was worried. One solution would have been to ask PUMC alumna Chou Meiyu to take over the deanship. Initially she agreed. She was certainly well qualified. Chou Meiyu had left the PUMC in 1931 to work with the Mass Education Movement (MEM) in Dingxian, and then went abroad on a Rockefeller fellowship to study at the Massachusetts Institute for Technology, where she earned a master's degree in 1935. Gertrude Hodgman supported recommending Chou, as did the senior members of the School of Nursing faculty.[67] Returning to Dingxian, Chou became an honorary instructor in the PUMC School of Nursing on 1 July 1937, just days before the Marco Polo Bridge Incident.[68] Then the Japanese invasion started in earnest, with conquest of regions in northern and eastern China. Nurses fled from occupied regions, hospitals and nursing schools were closed, and the demand for emergency care of wartime wounded increased.[69] In September 1937, Chou Meiyu and her nurses fled Dingxian as Japanese soldiers advanced. She relocated to Changsha with the rest of the MEM group. She decided to join Dr. Lim Khosheng (Robert Lim) at the newly formed Emergency Medical Service Training School at Guiyang.[70] Likely because of the unsettled conditions, her starting date as the first Chinese dean of nursing at the PUMC was deferred from 15 March to 1 October 1938. Yet, at a conference in Hong Kong in September 1938, just days before she was to about to start into the new position, Chou informed Gertrude Hodgman that she "refused to accept the position."[71] Chou had "been given very important duties under the Red Cross in Changsha and felt she could not leave under the present conditions.[72] In her stead, Gertrude Hodgman recommended Vera Nieh.[73]

PATH TO THE PUMC DEANSHIP

While Gertrude Hodgman was working through the complications of her role at the PUMC, Vera Nieh was working through career complexities of her own. Having resigned from the Beijing Health Station in 1933, she moved from job to job, unsatisfied with any. In 1935, she was offered a post in Nanjing, "probably the headship of the visiting nurses at the Nanking Health Station."[74] According to Nieh's recollection, the Ministry of Public Health wanted her to join in its work, specifically assisting the ministry on a new committee on nursing education. Her role involved inspecting "all the nursing schools in China. To see whether or not they are up to the standard. And then, if they are up to the standard, then they can be registered in the government."[75] Schools that did not meet the standard were considered "unqualified" schools.[76] By 1936, Nieh was considering a position at the Canton Hospital, which was the first Western hospital in China, started by Dr. Peter Parker in 1835. The hospital was planning to hold a short summer school for school nurses (nurses who work in grade schools) and hygiene teachers that July involving "practically all the important mission schools in Canton"[77] A nurse was needed to oversee the work and to help the hospital determine how many nurses the summer school could accommodate and what extension of the work would be possible by the following July. "At any rate," her employer, Dr. Oldt, noted, "there will be enough doing to make plenty of work for Miss Nieh."[78]

Vera Nieh was not ready to make a decision about Canton Hospital. She was, it seems, experiencing another bout of depression. "I fear Miss Nieh is not going to be able to make a decision about her future work just at this time," wrote Gertrude Hodgman in response to Dr. Oldt. "She is very much discouraged and says that it is with herself that she is discouraged."[79] Vera Nieh was in a state of uncertainty, and was even, rather unrealistically, considering a trip to Honolulu. "Much as I wish to hurry her in her decision," Hodgman continued, "I feel that this is impossible." To Hodgman, Nieh was "in a sense something of a problem to herself and to us at the present time." That said, Hodgman also impressed on Dr. Oldt that "I would not have you think for one minute that I consider her nervously or mentally ill. Actually, she has very good control and judgement and I think her only difficulty is that she has been put in a difficult place and sees too clearly the difficulties of it."[80]

Whether Vera Nieh was mentally ill or just restless, by the fall of 1936, she was at Qilu University in Jinan, taking premedical courses (anatomy) with an eye toward studying medicine again. "What I find here," she wrote to Gertrude Hodgman," is exactly what you told me." In other words, everything was "in a bad shape," presumably a comment comparing the facilities at Qilu to those at the PUMC.[81] However, she liked the university campus and the fresh air. Furthermore, a number of staff at Qilu used to be at the PUMC and were kind to her. She was hoping to transfer to a better medical school, preferably in the United States, when the opportunity arose, and she had submitted various applications for admission and scholarships.

Four days after penning that letter to Hodgman, Nieh suddenly changed course again. On 16 October 1936, she wrote to Hodgman that she was heading to Tianjin that evening to get her passport, with the idea of sailing from Shanghai to an undefined destination on 3 November 1936.[82] Her brother would accompany her. She had decided to travel to the United States "at her own expense for further study."[83] Nieh had "made this decision somewhat suddenly in order to take advantage of the opportunity of traveling to the United States with her brother who is going at this time and she has therefore had no time for exchange of correspondence with any institution in the United States about her admission for advanced studies."[84] She would be entering the United States as a "non-quota immigrant."[85]

Once in the United States, Nieh started applying to different universities, while Hodgman provided reference letters. One, to the University of Cincinnati, gives some insight into Nieh's situation at the time, as understood by Hodgman:

[Vera Nieh] has not been entirely happy or satisfied in nursing work as she is impatient of the difficulties in this pioneer field [of public health] and somewhat intolerant of other people's ideas. It is possible that she will be more satisfied and therefore ultimately more successful in the field of medicine than nursing. Her difficulties in nursing have been more on her own side than in any criticisms which other have made of her or her work.[86]

As it happened, Nieh was accepted into the University of Michigan at Ann Arbor, where she spent a year and a half completing a master's of science in public health. According to Nieh herself, her ultimate desire was to obtain a PhD. In an interview in the 1980s, Nieh suggested that she would have stayed in the United States longer to pursue a doctorate, but the Japanese invasion of China changed her plans. "I am rather patriotic," she recalled, and she felt she could not "stay any longer outside [of China] to study when my country is invaded by Japan. I couldn't study anymore and I thought it was my duty to come back as a nurse. [I] came back to join the war [effort] and do something. That is where my thoughts [went]. After I finished [her courses at the University of Michigan], that is 1938, I came home."[87]

Originally planning to go into "the interior" (i.e., Free China) to work, Nieh first stopped in Beijing to say goodbye to her mother. According to Nieh's recollection, "When I arrived [in Beijing] the news [that I was there] reached Dr. Houghton ... Director of PUMC at that time. He wanted to see me and of course I went to see him."[88] Dr. Houghton tried to discourage her from going to the interior, saying that so many people had gone there and some of them could not find work. He was afraid that she might not find work either. "What our plan is," he asserted, "is that you stay here, and we would like you to take the position of Gertrude E. Hodgman."[89] At first Nieh rebuffed Houghton, noting that, as a patriotic Chinese, her desire was to join the war effort. Houghton appealed to her patriotism, however, with the question, "To train more highly educated nurses, isn't that an important job for your country?"[90] Nurses, he argued, were precisely the kind of personnel that China needed. Nieh took some time to think it over, to consult with family and friends. Her mother was happy to see her stay in Beijing. Her friends saw this as an important opportunity – that it was important for a Chinese nurse to take over the headship and for the PUMC to train more nurses. "So, I agreed."[91] This appointment had "the cordial approval of the [PUMC] officers and staff, and is particularly satisfying to the Nurse Alumnae, who will give her their undivided support and good will."[92] Henry Houghton had "no fears of the outcome of this appointment; Miss Nieh is a highly intelligent woman, our own graduate (in 1926), a Northerner of excellent family and connections."[93]

The plan was for Nieh to take a role as assistant dean so that she could learn the role, eventually taking over the full deanship. Gertrude Hodgman and others would mentor her. While the appointment to dean was neither official nor guaranteed, it was tacitly understood that this would be the next step. "She is one of the abler early graduates of the School of Nursing," one report noted, "qualified to assume a much more responsible position than proposed, if such a position were open for her at the present time."[94] Another noted that, "I think it very important that we should make some effort to secure Miss Nieh's services now with the possibility of having her permanently on our staff later in some important position for which she is qualified."[95] In the meantime, Hodgman prepared Nieh to succeed her. "In her office," Nieh recalled, "I learned how to conduct a school, under her leadership, under her guid[ance]."[96] It was, all together, a two-year apprenticeship. By the time Hodgman departed China in 1940, Nieh was ready.

Vera Nieh was appointed dean of the PUMC School of Nursing on 15 September 1940.[97] Gertrude Hodgman, as part of her earlier appointment as dean of nursing, had agreed that she would "train one of the senior Chinese members of the faculty of the School of Nursing to succeed her at the conclusion of the appointment."[98] This is exactly what she did, thereby bringing the PUMC to a milestone in developing nursing and women's leadership: "It is a matter of gratification that the School of Nursing has now reached a time when one of its own graduates can assume the important responsibility of its administration as Dean. Miss Nieh is the choice of the faculty of the School and of her fellow-alumnae who have unanimously expressed their support of her."[99] The PUMC board of trustees passed the historic motion to appoint the PUMC's first Chinese dean on 27 March 1940.

* * *

Japan's invasion(s) of China unsettled nursing practices and plans while also providing opportunities for a new cadre of Chinese nurses to prepare to step into the looming leadership gap. Japan's first foray into China, in 1931, gave Chinese PUMC faculty a glimpse of their collective political strength as they responded quickly, decisively, and patriotically to the Shanghai Incident. Nurses and physicians found ways to serve the cause of their country through organization of their time and energy in ways independent of their American counterparts. Although there were years of reprieve before Japan would invade again, the looming threat solidified the desire to strengthen and prepare Chinese citizens to take up leadership roles in nursing and medicine. This included a shift from Western to Chinese leadership in the NAC, the Beijing Health Station, and the nursing deanship at the PUMC. Having been prepared for leadership positions as part of their education at the PUMC School of Nursing, PUMC alumnae were ready to take up the call. Leadership, however, did not come without a toll. The conflict between Gertrude Hodgman and Dr. John B. Grant eventually resulted in her departure. Vera Nieh, having resigned from the Health Station due to her own conflict with Dr. John B. Grant, became untethered for a while, floating from place to place, turning down opportunities to work and taking up opportunities to study – eventually rediscovering herself through master's education in the United States. Her uncertainty was replaced by a sense of purpose when her PUMC colleagues Henry Houghton and Gertrude Hodgman called her to take up a leadership role at the PUMC. Although the years ahead would also be filled with conflict, she was never as despondent as she was before the breakout of war in 1937.

Patriotism is a strong theme running through this chapter. From the PUMC staff's impassioned response to the Shanghai Incident, to Ravenna Tien's determination to keep the NAC buildings from Japanese hands, to Chou Meiyu's determination to work with emergency services rather than take up a prestigious position as PUMCs first Chinese dean, to Vera Nieh's decision to cut short her PhD dreams to return to China – each of these decisions was underpinned by a fervent desire to see China made whole. The PUMC's experimental approach to education, which set leadership development and public health as its core mission, was paying dividends.

CHAPTER THREE

Shifting Missions (1936–40)

The Erosion of Missionary Nursing in West China

Gradually the Province [of Sichuan] became united [under the Nationalists] and the Communists seemed to fade away; we ceased at any rate to hear about them.

— *Dr. W.E. Smith*, A Canadian Doctor in West China, *1939*

Here after three and a half years of war, transportation difficulties, soaring prices, our hospital supplies are almost down to rock bottom which makes effective medical work, particularly in the nursing department, very difficult.

— *Adelaide Harrison, Woman's Missionary Society secretary, Chengdu, 1941*

The early years of the War of Resistance in West China were extremely challenging, albeit in a different way from in the Japanese-occupied regions. Whereas those living in the occupied regions suffered from the violence of the Japanese military on the ground, those living in so-called Free China suffered from the violence of the Japanese military in the air. Conditions in occupied regions triggered the mass migration of millions of Chinese to Free China. Refugees lost their homes and possessions and faced months of horrific travel conditions, often on foot, to reach the relative freedom of provinces like Sichuan and Yunnan. West China, however, was by no means a haven. Living in West China meant unrelenting air raids, overcrowded living conditions, and lack of food, proper clothing, running water, and heat. West China had no choice but to accept, accommodate and adapt to the influx of refugee "downriver" folk. In this chapter, I take a closer look at the changing social and political context in West China, and how this influenced missionary work in general and missionary nursing in particular. After considering ways in which nursing's social identity shifted during this period, I examine how war-related phenomena such as mass migration, relentless air raids, and diminishing resources contributed to the erosion of missionary nursing in West China well before Canada and the United States declared war on Japan at the end of 1941. This, in turn, set the stage for the entrance, in 1943, of the Peking Union Medical College (PUMC) School of Nursing into the narrative arc of Canadian missionary nursing.

SHIFTING IDENTITIES: RELIGION, RACE, AND GENDER

Religion, race, and gender were important social constructs in nursing in the early twentieth century. Nursing in pre–Second World War Canada was almost exclusively a profession for young, unmarried, Caucasian women. While it was not essential to identify as Christian in order to be accepted into nurses' training, nursing as a professional practice reflected the dominant religious culture of Canada, with Christian (Protestant and Catholic) ideals infusing how nursing was understood, taught, and practised. The assumption was that students, too, were Christian. Thus, the idea of integrating faith and nursing was not unique to Canadian missionary nurses – it was a familiar approach to nursing. Nor was the notion of Christian duty reserved for the mission field; it was a central aspect of nursing education and practice as a whole. Early nursing leaders in the United States and Canada envisioned the development of nursing into a standardized, moral profession for intelligent women; missionary nurses enacted that vision. From a professional nursing perspective, the "gospel of intelligent caring" was not at odds with the gospel of Christ; it was a natural extension of it.[1] And that belief extended to the PUMC as well.

Although the West China Mission (WCM) was *expressly* Christian, the PUMC echoed Christian values in subtle ways. It had a chapel. Chinese staff were familiar with hymns.[2] Admission forms asked applicants to identify their "belief." Staff publicly expressed "thanks to God" when feeling a sense of being protected through dangerous times.[3] After all, the Rockefeller Foundation (RF) also had Christian roots: the devout Baptist faith of John D. Rockefeller Jr. had fuelled his philanthropic energies, which included the support of a handful of mission colleges through the 1920s.[4] It was China, however, that most captured the collective RF imagination and led to the establishment of the China Medical Board (CMB) under the auspices of the foundation. The idea was not to replicate or replace missionary medicine in China, but rather to augment, expand, and improve it. In 1914, the RF decided that any program undertaken in China should be in medicine (and, by extension, nursing) and that such work should be based in existing agencies, whether missionary or governmental.[5] The CMB would aim to improve Western medicine in China, missionary and otherwise, by emphasizing the scientific aspects of healing bodies, and decidedly *not* the religious aspects of saving souls.[6] By 1933, the RF had spent over $37 million in China, more than in any other foreign country. And most of this was spent on the PUMC.[7]

The religious norms that helped shape nursing identity at the WCM and, to a lesser degree, the PUMC, had started to shift by the 1930s. Critics, both inside and outside of missionary circles, started to question the missionary emphasis on conversion – and particularly the view of missionary medicine as a wedge meant to open Chinese homes and hearts to the Christian gospel.[8] Second-generation missionaries at the Canadian North China Mission in Henan were inclined less toward saving souls and more toward a social gospel – a larger vision of using Christian principles to combat injustice, suffering, and poverty. As China-born Canadian medical missionary Dr. Robert McClure neatly described it, emphasis on temporal rather than spiritual concerns was more satisfying: medical missionaries *knew* when they were functioning well; evangelists "merely hoped."[9] In a similar way, a 1932 report entitled *Re-Thinking Missions: A Laymen's Inquiry after One Hundred Years,* noted a "gradual shift in attitude ... on the part of many missionary doctors away from the use of the hospital for public and direct evangelism."[10] A commission chaired by William Ernest Hocking and comprising men and women representing seven Protestant denominations based this report on a comprehensive review of missions in India, Burma, China, and

Japan.[11] Notably, one of the members of the commission was Henry S. Houghton, acting director of the PUMC. It offered four principles as a basis of religious activities in mission hospitals:

1 Service rendered in love, responding to conscious need, given without inducement, offering disinterested relief of suffering, fulfills with nobility the obligations of a Christian physician to those whom he serves.
2 The spoken word may have its appropriate place in the hospital. It is not possible always to dissociate bodily from spiritual requirements; the wise physician, responsive to the unspoken needs of his patients, is often able through intimate conversation to enlarge and enrich the professional service he has given, and to convey hope and assurance to troubled minds.
3 But the use of medical or other professional service as a direct means of making converts, or public services in wards and dispensaries from which the patients cannot escape, is subtly coercive, and improper.
4 Clear-minded experimentation in the religious phases of hospital work is urgently needed. Much evangelistic work is casual and perfunctory; some of it is stupid and unworthy.[12]

According to Hocking, "we believe that the time has come to set the educational and other philanthropic aspects of mission work free from organized responsibility to the work of conscious and direct evangelism ... Ministry to the secular needs of men in the spirit of Christ *is* evangelism.[13]

In the view of the Commission, the focus on evangelism could actually be a liability to medical mission work. Indeed, by 1930, the professional work of the modern mission medical centres was considered "too often inferior to the nearby government and other non-missionary hospitals."[14] This was unacceptable. As Canadian missions opened hospitals with training schools for nurses, the centrality of medical work to mission policy became more apparent. According to Canadian missionary Margaret Brown, "the change in purpose came so gradually as to be almost imperceptible. Medical work was no longer to be a mere means to an evangelistic end. It was in itself to be a living expression of the

Christian Gospel and, therefore, had to maintain the highest standards. It was the age of the Social Gospel, and Medical work could be the strong arm of this Gospel."[15] In terms of religion as a social construct, then, any differences between PUMC and WCM nurses began to level out well before the refugee PUMC came to West China.

Like religion, race was also a consequential social construct in nursing in China. In Canada during this period, segregation of patients and nurses based on race was a common occurrence. When Canadian missionary nurse Margaret Gay took nurses' training in 1926, the Vancouver General Hospital had a "foreign ward" occupied by Chinese, Hindu, Mexican, and Japanese patients.[16] Indeed, as Helen Vandenberg has noted, several Asian wards were established in British Columbia hospitals at the turn of the twentieth century in response to racism and related harsh economic, political, and immigration restrictions.[17] Schools of nursing effectively barred women of Asian, Indigenous, and African descent. As Kathryn McPherson described it:

> Whether Black women in Nova Scotia, Japanese Canadians in British Columbia, or Native women anywhere, women of colour rarely were accepted in training programs on the grounds that White patients could not be entrusted to the care of non-White nurses. When Chinese- and Japanese-Canadian women were admitted to the Vancouver General Hospital [nursing program] in the 1930s, their entry was predicated on the assumption that they were needed to work in "their own" communities, which were poorly serviced by the formal health-care system.[18]

For Canadian missionary nurses in China, then, the idea of working with persons from other races and ethnicities, though an obvious part of their vocation, was not something they had much experience in as students in Canada.

Their work included the responsibility to adapt to local conditions, and learning to read and write Chinese was an important foundation for their work. They had been teaching and mentoring Chinese women for over two decades by the time the Nationalist government called for a shift to Chinese leadership. In terms of racial identity, both Chinese and Western nurses in China were influenced by the values, beliefs, and practices of the other, criticizing and admiring each other in equal measure. While the Western influence on Chinese values is evident throughout this book, it is worth noting that racial attitudes in Canada also shifted somewhat during this period – something that was likely attributable, at least in a small way, to the flow of Canadian missionary nurses between Canada and China. For example, one of the first schools in western Canada to open its doors to Asian students – the Lamont Hospital in Alberta – was a United (previously Methodist) Church of Canada mission hospital. In 1925, a question was put to the Lamont nursing students as to whether to admit Asian women to the School of Nursing. In a secret ballot, the students unanimously voted in favour. Over the years, Lamont Hospital – run by the same organization (and individuals) that supported Canadian missionary nurses in China – would graduate twenty-two students of Chinese, Japanese, and Korean descent.[19]

The bicultural nature of nursing in China complicated ethnic or racial assumptions. PUMC graduates such as Vera Nieh, Hsu Ai-Chu, Chou Meiyu, Evelyn Lin, and Bernice Chu Chen spent their formative years in higher educational institutions in large cities in the United States, Canada, and England, and were fluent in English and well versed in certain aspects of Western culture, such as food, clothing, and Protestant religious observances. Missionary nurses, a number of whom spent decades in China, were also bilingual and bicultural. Most interesting are the Canadian "mishkid" nurses – born in China to missionary parents and returning to China as missionaries themselves after going to nursing school in Canada. "Through a process of osmosis," Marion Menzies Hummel described it, "we grew up feeling comfortable in both Western and Chinese ways."[20] WCM nurses Cora Kilborn and her sister Mary, along with Dorothy Boyd, were mishkid nurses. They returned to China with a unique insight into Chinese ways.

Also of interest are nurses born in China who, after being reared in Canada, returned to China as nurses. One of these was Agnes Chan, the first Chinese nurse to graduate from a Canadian school of nursing.[21] Chan was born in China to a poor family in the late 1880s. After being sold to two different families in China, she was sold to a woman in Victoria, British Columbia. In that city, she ran away to the Women's Rescue Home for Chinese girls, established by the Methodist Church in 1887. After graduating from the mission school in 1920, she applied to – and was rejected by – several nursing schools in western Canada. She eventually graduated from Women's College Hospital in Toronto, in 1923.[22] She took a postgraduate program in Detroit before returning to China to work in a large Methodist mission hospital and school in southern China. While little is known about her work in China, she did serve on the Educational Committee of the Nurses Association of China, and, in 1945, the Women's College Hospital Alumnae Association (Toronto) heard of her "harrowing experiences in China" and sent her an award of one hundred dollars.[23] Another Chinese-Canadian nurse who returned to China as a nurse was Margaret Lee. As will be seen, Lee joined the Canadian WCM in 1940 and became a bridge between the Canadian mission and the refugee PUMC nurses.

Along with religion and race, gender was a significant social construct in nursing in China that shifted at the WCM during this period. In the early days of nursing in China, Canadian missionary nurses provided nursing care to males in the presence of male physicians. Later, they adapted by separating male and female patients into separate wards and even separate hospitals. The WCM in Chengdu had separate training programs for men and women (at the Men's and Women's Hospitals, respectively). In 1934, the WCM tested the idea of co-educational training by accepting a class half of women and half of men. Canadian nurse Muriel McIntosh noted that "hospitals with both men and women patients trained both men and women as nurses, but never before had women been trained to care for men."[24] It marked a new era. Parents had "considerable misgivings" when their daughters entered the co-ed training school. One unanticipated problem occurred when a graduate male nurse at the Men's Hospital fell "head over heels in love" with one of the new female instructors. However, overall the new scheme satisfied the Canadian missionary nurses, even though it lasted only two years: by 1936, the entire class entering nurses' training at the Men's Hospital happened to be female. In 1948, Canadian missionary Kenneth Beaton exclaimed, "there are practically no men left in graduating classes anywhere in West China to the great advantage of patients and the delight of the doctors."[25]

In contrast, the Canadian North China Mission (NCM) in Henan integrated male and female students into its nursing programs from the beginning and held fast to that approach. For example, when the Men's Hospital at the NCM was being restored after the Nationalist 30th Army occupied it during Chiang Kai-shek's Northern Expedition, staffing was problematic; there was a nursing shortage, with no male nurses to work with the male patients.[26] Noting that "the community is hardly ready for girl nurses in the men's ward," the mission instead hired three boys with no experience.[27] In the meantime, as already noted the PUMC, while initially planning to accept both male and female students, in the end admitted only female students.[28]

MASS MIGRATION AND WEST CHINA REFUGEES

Scarcely a month after the first shots were fired near Beijing in July 1937, educational institutions in East China had to make decisions regarding their immediate future.[29] Japanese warplanes seemed to be intentionally targeting educational and cultural institutions. To faculty and staff of those institutions, remote Sichuan suddenly seemed an attractive province.[30] Institutions started sending requests to the West China Union University (WCUU) for refuge.

On 23 October 1937, the United Church of Canada's Woman's Missionary Society (WMS) in West China received word that forty students and eight teachers from Qilu medical school had left Shandong a couple of weeks earlier, enroute to Chengdu, "where they will carry on in connection with the Medical College of our West China Union University."[31] The National Central University Medical College and Dental College were also on their way from Nanjing. "This will more than double the number of students at our University," the WMS secretary wrote. "A big problem and a wonderful opportunity."[32]

National Central University in Nanjing had been one of the early targets of Japanese air raids. After being severely bombed on 19 August 1937, faculty and staff migrated to West China, with plans to join the WCUU's

College of Medicine and Dentistry in Chengdu.[33] They arrived in October 1937 with staff, students, and equipment. The following month, staff and students from the Qilu College of Medicine at Shandong Christian University arrived. They, however, had no supplies. Bringing personal baggage over the Lunghai Railway was a difficult task, and packing equipment and books was "out of the question."[34] The Qilu students, therefore, shared the equipment, books, and supplies of the WCUU. Whereas Qilu staff and students became students and staff of the WCUU, the National Central University ran a parallel operation.

In 1938, John B. Grant, the head of the Public Health Division at the PUMC, noted that the effect of the war on medical education had been "almost incomprehensible. Only 5 of the 33 medical, pharmacy and dental colleges existing before the war continue unaffected." The remainder had either been "suspended, destroyed, or forced to remove, in instances thousands of miles ... This is almost a complete national disruption."[35]

By June 1939, forty-seven institutions had moved to Free China, an additional twenty-one moving to Shanghai. The WCUU became home to five universities: Qilu Medical College, Yenching (Yanjing) University, Ginling Women's College ("a pioneer in women's higher education in China"), National Central University ("one of the strongest medical universities in China"), and Nanjing University.[36] Prior to 1937, the WCUU was not well known beyond the borders of Sichuan province, as it was isolated from the rest of China. By 1939, as a result of hosting evacuated universities, it was widely known.[37] "The record of the spirit of West China Union University in opening its gates to admit the weary refugees from war areas will be outstanding in the history of Christian war service," noted one missionary.[38] The student body at the WCUU had increased from 350 to 570.

Over the course of the war, millions of individual Chinese fled to western provinces (Yunnan, Sichuan, Guizhou, Gansu), as did whole universities, factories, government offices, and consulates.[39] Leslie Kilborn, dean of medicine at the WCUU, set the estimated total number of migrants to Free China at between 20 and 60 million.[40] This mass migration by boat, bus, cart, and foot over more than a thousand miles of dangerous territory was, as C.H. Corbett described it, "one of the most astonishing phenomena in the struggle against Japan."[41] Canadian missionary nurse Clara Preston described the trek of Yenching students this way:

> They escaped from Peking – they jolted in a bus – they trudged along the road – they climbed the hills – they stopped to earn a little money, they rode in rickshas [sic] when possible or even went by wheelbarrow or boat – they hid when the planes came over – sometimes tired, ill, and penniless – then as wraiths, clothes in shreds, they arrived on the refugee campus in high spirits, determined to take up the studies that will prepare them to become the leaders New China so desperately wants.[42]

When Yenching students first arrived in West China, they were able to continue their studies at the newly opened "Emergency University" in Chengdu. Clara Preston, who had relocated to Chengdu from Japanese-occupied Henan in 1940, visited the students there. The WCUU was doing everything to support the students who had trekked so far for their education; when Preston visited, they were making two hundred desks. Yenching retained its high standards. As Preston wrote, "there is something unexplainable about the Yenching spirit ... It would have done any University credit in pre-war times. It was an inspiration to hear young professors say 'we must not let the refugee situation be our excuse for poor work, lowering of standards, or in any way interfere with our doing a good job of teaching and expecting a good grade of work from students.'"[43] The same would later be said of the PUMC.

When new students arrived at the WCUU, the first order of business was accommodations. At the WCUU, the Nanjing students were housed in a building that had been intended to become the laundry of the proposed University Hospital, while staff were housed "in a building that is ultimately to be used as the residence and teaching building of a new school of Agriculture."[44] Canadian missionary Marnie Copland and her family were among a group of North China missionaries who evacuated to West China. She noted that some of the evacuated universities and schools lodged in temples and empty buildings or put up temporary quarters.[45] As she saw it, "whatever our nationality, all of us down-river people were refugees in a strange land."[46] Copland was a mishkid; she had been born in China to missionary parents, and was conversant in Chinese. "The Szechwanese could tell we were down-river as soon as we opened our mouths. A Peking or Honan accent is as different from a Szechwanese as a Newfoundland is from a prairie accent."[47] Just as many refugees considered the "backwoods" of Sichuan as "quaint and somewhat shocking,"[48] the local people found the "downriver" people to be peculiar in both language and customs.

The Coplands' refugee experience in Sichuan was different from that of the university students and professors. The family was assigned an empty house. Originally, when they arrived in 1939, they had "the normal roster" of three servants (a gardener, cook, and amah); two years later, inflation required a reduction to one. "In Canada," Marnie Copland wrote, "one servant doesn't sound like any great hardship; three sounds a bit ostentatious."[49] However, she defended the necessity this way: their house in Leshan was ninety-eight steps above sea level. All of their water had to be carried up those steps from a well along the street, two buckets at a time, swinging from a carrying pole across the gardener's shoulders. The gardener also carried their youngest child, who was not able to climb so many steps. All of their laundry was done by hand. In a hot, damp climate, with two small children and many houseguests, there was daily washing and ironing. When Marnie Copland studied, taught, or went out, someone had to mind the children. "Chinese families didn't need babysitters," she noted, "they had relatives. We hadn't relatives, so we had an 'amah.'"[50] A cook was necessary, "unless I was willing to spend all my time in buying and preparing food," which she was not. There was no refrigeration. Everything in the market was in its natural state. Grain was sold whole, vegetables had not been washed of soil, chickens and fish were alive, pork carcasses lay on the market tables to be chopped into the required pieces, wheat had to be ground into flour, peanuts roasted and ground into butter. "Even such a simple thing as keeping up the supply of drinking water – the boiling, filtering and cooling," she wrote, "took time and energy."[51]

Leshan, the Canadian mission outstation where the Coplands lived, was home to the refugee Wuhan University, which had moved from

Hangzhou early in the war. The Coplands mixed easily with the evacuated professors, sharing meals and friendship. Marnie Copland helped Helen Sun, a young student from Henan, who was attending Wuhan University, to improve her English while the student helped Copland improve her Chinese – written and spoken.[52] From Sun, Copland learned of some of the difficulties refugee Chinese students endured as they followed their universities across China to the western provinces. As Copland recalled, "finding accommodation, settling down to study in a strange province with no family or relatives to support them, took determination and fortitude. But it paid off."[53] Helen Sun had her graduation dinner with her classmates on the Coplands' porch and lawns.

According to Alvyn Austin, all the missions in West China benefited from the influx of coastal refugees – and money.[54] The United Church of Canada mission, the largest in Sichuan, expanded considerably. The Canadian mission hospital in Chongqing, the largest in what was now the capital of Free China, had outgrown its "dank premises" within the city during the 1930s, and now moved to a new building across the river, "using the old hospital as a 'feeder' clinic."[55] The hospital acquired two nursing schools from the occupied areas and opened a new fifty-bed tuberculosis wing. Dr. A. Stewart Allen was the only foreign doctor on staff – and, for a while in 1938, the only foreign doctor in all of Chongqing.

Hosting refugee medical colleges (as well as individual refugee medical students) intensified the WCUU's need for a new hospital for medical teaching. For thirty years, the WCUU had mostly used the various Canadian mission hospitals for its clinical training. Now the WCUU considered the lack of a hospital of its own to be a serious issue. The construction of a new University Hospital had been in the works since 1935; by 1939, it was finally underway.[56] A University Hospital would allow the WCUU and its associated refugee medical schools to accept larger classes of medical and dental (and, later, nursing) students. In addition to the staff and students from five universities, the WCUU also received individual refugee students from about a dozen other medical colleges in the war zones. The WCUU therefore lifted its previous limit of sixteen medical students (and twelve dental) and was now taking in about four times that number. In September 1938, prior to the completion of the new

University Hospital, the Chengdu hospital board affected a "complete union" in clinical work between the three medical colleges (Qilu, Nanjing, and the WCUU) through the creation of a "United Hospital(s)" under the Chengdu hospital board – that is, a coming together of the various mission hospitals under one administrative structure. All of the medical and dental institutions in Chengdu were now under a director, general superintendent, and treasurer appointed by the Chengdu hospitals board. The three colleges worked under a unified curriculum (the National Central University followed its own curriculum). Similarly, the former two Canadian mission schools of nursing (Renji, in the Women's Hospital at Hsin Hang Tsi, and the Men's Hospital training school at Si Shen Tsi) were united under one principal.[57] These structural changes would affect the refugee PUMC School of Nursing when it arrived in 1943; whereas, in Beijing, the PUMC School of Nursing had acted fairly independently under a dean of nursing who was also the superintendent of the hospital, in Chengdu, the principal of the School of Nursing reported to a medical director and general hospital superintendent.

There had been practically no increase in missionary personnel at the WCUU and what were now called the Union Hospitals. Instead, the number of staff was augmented by the addition of Chinese teachers. Had this not happened, "the war would have found medical education in China in a much more precarious position."[58] In 1939, the WCUU suggested that "the fact that two Christian medical colleges and a national Government institution have been able to effect such complete cooperation and union is perhaps one of the most significant recent developments in Christian-mission work in China."[59] The WCUU was grateful for the recognition of and support for its work in West China. However, missionaries were also "all conscious that in this rapidly expanding work we may lose sight of our Christian aim."[60] The sudden expansion was throwing a great administrative burden on the missionary staff, which in the past year had been reduced in numbers by death, ill health, and withdrawal. This was particularly true with respect to Canadian missionary nurses, whose numbers had decreased from a high of sixteen to just ten in 1939. One of these was Cora Kilborn, who, in May 1938, returned to Canada to attend to her elderly mother, pioneer missionary physician

Retta Gifford Kilborn.[61] Cora Kilborn was away for four years, returning after her mother died, in 1942.[62] By the time the war ended (and the refugee PUMC left Chongqing), there were just two Canadian missionary nurses in West China, including Cora Kilborn.

BOMBING WEST CHINA

In November 1938, the Nationalist government moved from Nanjing to Chongqing. The diplomatic and military missions, as well as the news media, naturally followed. The city was officially designated as China's wartime capital on 6 September 1940. Two cities with the largest Canadian medical missionary presence, then – Chongqing and Chengdu – were significant political centres as well: Chengdu was the capital of Sichuan; Chongqing had become the capital of China. Situated on a narrow peninsula at the confluence of the Jialing and Yangtze Rivers, Chongqing had direct river access to China's east coast. It also had an airstrip and road access – both of which were improved during the war for movement of personnel and supplies. As the Canadian missionaries described it, Sichuan was cut off from the rest of China for many hundreds of years by its geographical position and lack of communications. The Yangtze River was its main link with the outside world. The early missionaries made the trip from Shanghai to Chongqing by river steamer and then houseboat. According to Marnie Copland, "bandits and warlords added to the natural hazards of the trip. The baby of one Canadian family we know was shot by a bandit as he lay sleeping in his basket."[63] Since, until the late 1930s, all outsiders came to Sichuan by river, the Sichuanese called missionaries "downriver people."[64]

During the first three years of what the Canadian missionaries called "Japan's undeclared war of aggression on China," there were scores of air raids on cities and towns in Sichuan, particularly Chongqing.[65] "These are cruel days," wrote Margaret Outerbridge. "The Japanese air force is scientifically reducing each city they attack to utter ruin. We all wonder how soon we'll get ours."[66] The mission stations at Chengdu, Leshan, and Luzhou also suffered greatly.[67] At least one-third of Luzhou and Leshan was in ruins and ashes by 1940. Hundreds of civilians were killed, hundreds more wounded, and thousands made homeless. The Canadian mission hospital and residences at Luzhou were burned, the church and other residences destroyed. At Leshan, downtown property that housed the church and an outpatient clinic was destroyed by fire. In Chengdu, extensive damage was done to a number of WCUU buildings and houses.[68] It was Chongqing, however, that was worst hit.

Chongqing became known as the most heavily bombed region of China. According to records kept by the Chongqing Air Defence headquarters, in the forty-three months from 30 January 1938 to 1 September 1941, there were 193 enemy air raids targeting the city.[69] An aggregate of 5,553 enemy planes took part in dropping 11,181 demolition bombs (designed to demolish buildings and structures) and 1,800 incendiary bombs (meant to start fires).[70] The first major bombing in Chongqing was two years into the War of Resistance against Japan, on 3–4 May 1939. In the first raids, the loss of civilian life (and practically all deaths were among civilians) was, in the words of Canadian missionary Gerald Bell, "appalling."[71] Although, in Bell's opinion, the government policy of evacuating from the cities all civilians who could possibly leave, as well as the setting up of more effective measures to clear the people out when alarms sounded, eventually greatly reduced the number of casualties, the first bombings were horrific.[72] Canadian missionary Dr. W.E. Smith recorded the first bombing of Chongqing on 3 May 1939 this way:

> Twenty-minutes after the air-raid warning, we heard the unmistakable drone of the heavy bombers and following that the swish of falling bombs and the thud of explosions ... The next day, May 4th, at six o'clock in the evening, in roared twenty-seven Japanese planes, their usual squadron, flying low and right over our heads. Just as soon as they reached the city, they commenced to unload their murderous freight, and cut a swath through a densely populated part of the city about one hundred yards from us ... The horror of the whole thing was fierce and indescribable in language – all brought upon innocent people. The casualties were very high for the two raids, probably five thousand, all civilians of course.[73]

To Smith, "the hope of the Japanese military party is, of course, to break the morale of the people in the rear and make them willing to sign a peace at any price."[74] Breaking the morale seemed likely. In a news release from an entity self-described as the China Information Committee on 5 May 1939, the authors wrote, "In a fit of wanton fury, the Japanese air force on May 4th transformed the midtown section of the inner city of [Chongqing] into a mad inferno of flames in which thousands were immolated ... [They] left a trail of incendiary and demolition bombs that marked the most merciless air raid in the history of the war."[75]

Doctors and nurses were immediately involved. At the Canadian mission hospital, Dr. Stuart Allen

> did yeoman service far into the night as he endeavoured with the unceasing stream of wounded people that poured past him. The sisters of the Mission of Franciscan Sisters in the consular district also threw open their doors to hosts of the suffering. Daybreak found a tired-eyed Mission community that had battled against almost overwhelming odds and was still undaunted in its determination to bind up and heal the wounds inflicted by a savage barbarism.[76]

The Chongqing Municipal Hospital was also hit. A bomb landed close to the wall of the main building, and the 220 patients had to be moved out of the building, even before the planes had completed their attack. The nurses and doctors of the hospital remained on duty to receive the "long stream of wounded that poured in for treatment."[77]

Bombing continued through the summer. Various missionary reports – be they diaries, memoirs, or circular letters home – all had a similar theme: the Japanese were barbarian; the American and Canadian governments were complicit through their ongoing trade with Japan; the Chinese were resolute in their resistance. Writing in her diary from Mount Omei on 11 June 1939, Margaret Outerbridge recalled conversations with other missionaries. "The Endicott's," she wrote, "have been through a rather bad time." James Endicott, who had served in the last war, "says the Japanese bombings are the most horrible thing he has ever experienced. [Chongqing] is literally going underground, digging huge caves for shelter. Jim believes that [Chengdu] is next on the list of major targets."[78] He was right. Later that same day, Chengdu was attacked. It was a beautiful, clear sunny day. "We [felt] so secure," recalled missionary Mrs. Gerald S. Bell. "The Japanese were far away; the city lay low in the plain, many-treed and inconspicuous."[79] The air raid siren started. The people in the streets were getting "jumpy." "Poor things," Bell thought. "Every time the 'Get-ready' is signaled little bundles such as one can carry are collected, children run home and the wise ones close shop and house and make for the open country, over the city walls, through the city gates."[80] The streets were crammed with "terrified people," jostling pushing, cursing. Then, "out of the north they came, on spread wings, twenty-six of them in wedge-shaped formation."[81] The thuds of the falling bombs came next.

The following day, Bell set out to survey the bombed WCUU campus. Damage included the destruction of the Baptist Middle School dormitory, which had been a refuge for "down-river university folk."[82] Refugees from Nanjing were again out of a home, as was the president of Nanjing University. Miss Whang, a pharmacy student, and Harold Hsu, a Christian pastor, were both killed. Hsu had been at the New South gate when the planes came and apparently went into a wayside tea shop for shelter before a bomb completely destroyed the place.[83]

For Bell, one of the most shameful aspects of the bombings was that Canada and the United States played a role in supporting the Japanese by supplying material that could be used in creating the bombs: "Japanese bombs filled with – can you bear it? – Canadian metals perhaps?"[84] She could not hide her disgust with Western governments:

> From self-interest, if from nothing else, the people in Canada and the United States ought to wake up to the fact that Japan is no gentle, exotic oriental maid, but an implacable military power bristling with an outspoken hatred for Britain and all that is British, and scarcely hiding her contempt in the suavity of her bowing and protestations of "a mistake I assure you" over the many breaches of international good will.[85]

Altogether, the WCUU campus had been hit by five bombs in the initial raid. "One bomb landed amid a group of students at the river's edge," noted missionary Margaret Outerbridge, "killing and wounding I don't know how many. Another blew out all the windows and doors at the unfinished medical complex, the machine shop, the Canadian School and nearby residences (Mrs. Liljestrand was wounded by the flying glass)." One girl was killed when a dwelling constructed of woven bamboo mats was "blown to bits." Two other girls were in "poor condition" in hospital with shrapnel wounds to the head."[86]

As the bombing continued over the next few months, conditions became "simply indescribable."[87] Winifred Harris, secretary of the Woman's Missionary Society in Chengdu wrote, "We hear that two thousand babies have already been unearthed and buried. Rescue work is still going on; but things here are in a terrible condition. It appears that the bombs were meant for Chengdu but that they were turned back by pursuit planes and so they delivered this inferno to [Leshan]."[88] On 19 August 1939, Margaret Outerbridge heard the "low roar of airplanes" and the "sound of heavy machine guns."[89] Close to three dozen Japanese bombers were circling in the distance, firing at a Douglas passenger plane due to land in Chongqing from Hong Kong. The Douglas was "like some hunted bird," dipping, banking, and dodging. The Douglas escaped. However, when Margaret and her husband Ralph, a missionary doctor, went to an outlook that commanded a view of Leshan, "our hearts sank ... A dark mist hung over the city, and what seemed a definite column of black smoke was rising."[90]

In response to the bombing of Leshan, Ralph Outerbridge organized an emergency medical team. He set out in the evening down the mountain with another Canadian doctor, two other missionaries, and two wagons full of supplies. They started to walk, through the dark, expecting to walk all night. Margaret worried, knowing that Leshan "at the moment was infested with malaria, cholera, encephalitis, meningitis, infantile paralysis, amoebic dysentery and, of course, typhus."[91] From the distance of Mount Omei, the city of Leshan was a red glow from the incendiary bombs.

As Ralph later recalled to Margaret, the group walked all Saturday night. Nearing Leshan in the morning, ten hours later, they encountered crowds still hurrying to safety with their belongings. Inside the town, people were digging through the smoldering ruins. Well over one-third of the city had been completely levelled; charred bodies everywhere. "Suddenly," Margaret wrote, "someone started the cry (false as it turned out) that the Japanese planes were returning. Everyone began to run, the less agile literally trampled to death by the crowd, driven by sheer animal terror."[92] Ralph and the others were horrified.

They found the mission hospital. The injured, "many of whom had been dragged from under collapsed houses," lay on shutters, boards, or doors they had been carried in on. Most astonishingly, "all of the medical personnel who were supposed to be on duty were asleep in their respective quarters, apparently quite unable to cope and unwilling to try."[93] While the doctors responded to the admonishments of the Canadian team, the nurses refused. The missionaries operated all day and late into the night (the two non-medical missionaries giving anaesthetic). At midnight, James Endicott arrived with a Red Cross team from Chongqing, comprising two surgeons, an operating room nurse, and a dresser. The next day their "coolies" were not available to help them return up the mountain; the military had seconded them to help bring more than two thousand charred corpses to a mass grave beyond the city gates.[94]

So it continued into the fall, with missionaries reporting the bombing of Luzhou on 11 September 1939. With the Canadian mission hospital destroyed, the downtown hospital was used "to treat the worst cases," and some of the Canadian medical workers assisted there. To missionary Gordon Jones, "so far as the Canadian Mission is concerned and perhaps from every point of view this appears to have been the worst disaster yet."[95] James Endicott agreed. The bombings left about 2,000 families homeless, "and already the mission compound is crowded with refugees."[96] About 400 had been killed and 400 wounded. In addition to the mission hospital, two of Luzhou's three other hospitals were burned.[97]

The unrelenting bombing would leave an indelible mark on the Canadian WCM, placing missionaries in danger while testing their resolve regarding the extent to which they could meet the medical needs of others. The air raids were part of Japan's attempt to occupy all of China. Canadian missionaries viewed the Chinese response to the bombings as a testament to their tenacity and resolve. To Canadian missionary Dr. W.E. Smith, "resistance is stiffened rather than weakened, and back areas that really knew little of the horrors of war and the cruelty of the Eastern Ocean military invasion are beginning to know what it means, and so are becoming the more determined to resist it."[98]

NURSING IN WEST CHINA

The years 1936 to 1940 were extremely difficult in Free China. Although Sichuan was not under Japanese occupation, it was the target of ongoing air raids, which, together with a severe lack of resources (food, running water, electricity, heat) made for grim living and working conditions. During these years, there was a steady turnover of Canadian missionary nurses at the West China Mission (Table 3.1). By 1940, four had departed, one was on leave, and five had arrived. Of those who stayed, all were long serving, having been in China for between eleven and thirty-four years, for an average of twenty years. Of the five newcomers, three (Dorothy Boyd, Margaret Gay, Clara Preston) were seconded from the Canadian North China Mission after the mission hospitals in Japanese-occupied Henan were forced to close in 1939. Another 1939 newcomer was the Canadian mission's first Canadian missionary nurse of Chinese origin, Margaret Lee. By 1945, only three remained – all from the long-serving group; the next year, there were only two: Cora Kilborn and the newly arrived Julien Bessie. War had taken its toll.

The crisis in WCM nursing started almost as soon as war broke out in China's north, in 1937. By early 1938, refugees and their horrific stories streamed into West China. "If one tenth of what we hear of the suffering of the people and the cruelties of the other side are true," WMS secretary Adelaide Harrison wrote, "even that would be dreadful beyond words."[99] Refugees from downriver were coming by the thousands.[100] A private press column dated 18 February 1938 compiled observations by foreigners about the refugee crisis in Japanese-occupied areas. One noted:

TABLE 3.1 Nurses at the WCM, 1936–41

Name	Year Arrival	Departure	Notes	1936	1937	1938	1939	1940	1941
Caroline Wellwood	1906	1944		×	×	×	×	×	×
Susan Haddock	1913	1941		×	×	×	×	×	
Irene Harris	1921	1945	On furlough 1940	×	×	×	×		
Geraldine Hartwell	1914	?	In Chengdu in 1940	?	?	?	?	×	?
Alma Tallman	1924	1945	On furlough 1941	×	×	×	×	×	
Cora Kilborn	1927	1950	On leave 1938–44	×	×				
Mary Crawley	1929	1942	On furlough late 1941	×	×	×	×	×	×
Marguerite McLeod	1930	1939		×	×	×	×		
Hilda Dunkin	1932	1938		×	×	×			
Janet McIntosh	1931	1937		×	×				
Lillian Hilton	1933	1936		×					
Dorothy Boyd	1939	1941	Seconded from NCM				×	×	
Dorothy Fox	1939	1943					×	×	×
Margaret Lee	1939	1944						×	×
Margaret Gay	1940	1941	Seconded from NCM					×	
Clara Preston	1940	1943	Seconded from NCM					×	×
Total number of nurses at WCM				10	9	7	8	10	5

SOURCES: "West China Nurses" UMSAC, Beaton fonds; "Missionaries of the Woman's Missionary Society, West China Mission." UCCA, WMS, 83.058C, series 5, box 60; Grypma, *Healing Henan.*

Terror still stalking [in Nanjing]. No single word is adequate to describe actual conditions. The Japanese army not only refuse to feed the 250,000 refugees, but also forbid relief to come from the outside. The bark of trees, grass etc. serve as edibles. There are neither cats nor dogs left in the safety zone. Conservative estimates place the number of civilians killed at 10,000. Cases of rape are estimated at at least 8,000. But the probability is a number of 20,000. On one compound alone 17 Japanese soldiers raped one woman successively in broad daylight. Japanese officers are guilty of the same excesses. 40% of all the buildings have been burned down. Every house in the city was thoroughly looted. From the Metropolitan and Fuchang Hotels everything, including fixtures, were taken. The flags of all nationalities, American, British, French, Italian, German, were torn down.[101]

In contrast, Japanese papers from Nanjing proclaimed:

The municipality of [Nanjing] is quiet as the streets of the dead. The sun's merciful rays shine forth with partiality for the refugee district in the northeast of the city. The crowds who fled for their lives from what was then the midst of death, have met the gentle soothing of the Japanese army. Before the Japanese troops entered the city, these people suffered from the oppression of the anti-Japanese armies of the Chinese. Indeed, not a grain of rice or millet could reach their hands. The sick could not get medical aid. The hungry could not get food. The sufferings of the good citizens were terrible. Fortunately the [Japanese] Imperial Army entered the city, put their bayonets into their sheaths, and stretched forth merciful hands.[102]

Canadian missionaries in Chengdu heard about the atrocities – Japanese propaganda notwithstanding – and looked for ways to help the refugees coming into West China. Missionary nurse Caroline Wellwood took charge to help convert the mission school property in Chongqing into a Christian hostel to help accommodate the "thousands and thousands of refugees that are coming or have already come from down river, and who arrive in [Chongqing], many without friends to receive them, or not knowing where to go from there."[103] In the meantime, NCM nurses Dorothy Boyd, Clara Preston, and Margaret Gay were in northern China, working under increasingly difficult and dangerous conditions. Dorothy Boyd was a mishkid born to Canadian missionary parents in Henan; she was one of six NCM mishkids who, after taking nurses' training in Canada, returned to China as missionary nurses. They were all in China during the war and included Dorothy's sister Mary (Boyd) Stanley as well as Elizabeth (Thomson) Gale, Jean (Menzies) Stockley and her sister Georgina (Menzies) Lewis, and Florence (MacKenzie) Liddell.[104] Dorothy was the only one who had not married; each of the others met and married missionaries and were therefore no longer under the auspices of the United Church of Canada WMS. When Dorothy came to China in 1938 to work at the NCM, the conditions there were considered too dangerous, and she was assigned various short-term projects in and around Tianjin and Beijing. When her parents evacuated from Henan to West China, she joined them.

In April 1940, Dorothy Boyd was appointed to the Chongqing hospital. "I think she will like it there," noted Winifred Harris, "for her work will be with foreign patients for the most part. [Irene] Harris's furlough is due and while we are hoping that [Clara] Preston will be able to relieve Miss Harris there is a great need also for a second nurse there."[105] However, the move to West China was difficult. As Winifred Harris wrote in April 1940, Dorothy Boyd "has not been well since she reached [Chengdu]. The journey from [Beijing] was a hard one and I think she was somewhat run down in health. She is now getting over the effects of a bad carbuncle on her face. It is so hard for these people to leave their homes and work, and re-establish themselves amongst new people and surroundings. Even the dialect is different."[106]

The difficulty of the journey from China's occupied regions to Free China cannot be overstated. The associated risks are exemplified in recollections of Canadian missionary Dr. Ernest G. Struthers who, in November 1940, departed Qilu to join his medical students and staff at the WCUU.[107] Struthers, unable to obtain a bus ticket for Chongqing, learned he could get a ticket from the post office granting permission to ride atop a truck filled with mailbags. The truck ended up in an accident, with Struthers injured. He described it this way:

> After fifty kilometers the driver, who had driven some distance the previous day and gambled all night in [Chengdu], lost control of the truck and threw several of us into a field a yard or so below the road. I found myself covered in mailbags and saw the truck overturn and fall on us. I expected to be killed immediately, and thought,

"What an inglorious way to die!" But the bags broke the fall, and the truck settled down on the bags. Finally I could not breathe at all, but the truck stopped settling. Cries from a woman near me brought four or five of those not injured to our rescue. They lifted the truck by hand, and pulled us out, in my case pulling on the fractured arm, the only time I felt pain. I collected my baggage and had my cot bed put up in a sheltered part of the field. Fortunately I had on a winter coat and had some bedding with me.[108]

Stranded with the other injured, Struthers tried to figure out how to get medical help:

I gave five dollars to a man to send a telegram to [Chengdu] for the Mission ambulance, but the telegram was never sent. About noon [Nanjing] engineers, on their way to [Chengdu] with a truck loaded with lumber, saw my plight, put the cot on top of the lumber and kept blankets over me until we reached [Chengdu] and had Dr. Wilford send for a stretcher. I was back in my own bed in Dr. Wilford's home by night and thanks to careful nursing by Chinese nurses both day and night for a while, and to the skill of the orthopedic surgeon, Dr. Chen, and good care by Drs. Wilford and Lenox, I recovered after two months in bed.[109]

While it is clear that Dorothy Boyd originally had every intention of completing her contract in China, she abruptly changed her mind. On 6 May 1941, she submitted a resignation letter to the WMS, and she headed back to Canada with her parents on 6 June 1941, having served only two years of her three-year term – none of it in Henan, the province of her birth.[110] The two other NCM nurses, Margaret Gay and Clara Preston, arrived in West China in 1940. They had both been in Henan through the difficult months of Japanese invasion, anti-foreign demonstrations, and the eventual evacuation of missionaries, in the summer of 1939. Preston had been in China for seventeen years when, in 1939, a local anti-British movement in Anyang, Henan – apparently instigated by the Japanese – resulted in her and a handful of other remaining Canadian missionaries barricading themselves within the walls of the Anyang Mission Hospital compound for three weeks. It was not until two grenades were thrown over the compound wall that they decided to evacuate, on 16 September 1939. Preston travelled to Beijing, where she did a month of observation at the PUMC before eventually going to West China to work as the superintendent of the WCM hospital in Chongqing, in April 1940.

Clara Preston started in West China with high hopes. She had travelled from Tianjin to Shanghai to Hong Kong, from where she took her first plane ride, to Chongqing. The Canadian mission hospital, built eight years earlier, was a four-storey building with electric lights but no running water, and no heating in the winter due to the high cost of coal. The hospital typically had 180 to 220 patients, and was headed by Dr. Stewart Allen. The hospital included care for "a ward full" of typhoid and dysentery patients, and had an obstetrics and pediatric ward. The chief work, however, was surgery.[111] The West China Mission hospital was designated the Fifth Red Cross Emergency Hospital in Chongqing. As such, it received cases from bombing in the area – as many as seventy-two at a time.

Like other nursing schools in West China during this period, the school at the Canadian mission hospital at Chongqing comprised mostly young women from other parts of China, "which complicated their training."[112] Some had started in other schools and, having travelled to Free China, were separated from their families without any means of support. The courses at Chongqing covered the same material that nurses in Canada would study at the time, as well as "English and Chinese literature."[113] The classes were difficult to schedule during the "bombing years"; Preston recalled one graduation "where we had to rush it through before the planes visited us."[114] Upon graduation, the nurses were conscripted by the Chinese government to work for one year in either public health, the military, or the Red Cross. The government allowed the Chongqing hospital to keep 15 percent of its graduates.

There were eleven doctors, twenty-four graduate nurses, and about eighty nurses in training at Chongqing. Preston liked her accommodations, which she shared with Dorothy Boyd, across the river from the part of Chongqing that was crowded with refugees. However, as Preston soon found out, the air raids were relentless – and started on the day she arrived. "Often a scouter plane would be seen in the morning," she later recalled, "and a warning would go up ... Then we would hear the first alarm, and everyone was hurrying to get the most essential things done, treatments completed, medicine secured, or food sent to the wards before the raid started." When the bombers came, it was, she wrote, "as if heaven was ripped open and hell let loose."[115]

When the alarm was sounded, hospital staff cancelled or hurriedly performed operations, evacuated patients from the wards, brought laundry in off the line, and scrambled to nearby dugouts. Patients from the third and fourth floors of the hospital were carried to the main floor, from where servants would take them on stretchers down the front ramp to the ground in front of the hospital Tuberculosis patients were left on the verandah, having signaled their preference to stay in their beds.[116] James Endicott later called Clara Preston "the unsung heroine of the war" because of her "constant heroism during raid after raid of Jap bombers, when she would sit by the side of patients, too ill to be moved to the shelters, to assure them that all was well."[117] Preston would leave China just under three years later; the wartime conditions were just too difficult. By the end of the war, in 1945, the Canadian mission hospital had an entirely Chinese staff supervised by a single Canadian working as superintendent and chief physician, Dr. Stewart Allen.[118]

Like Clara Preston, Margaret Gay had gone through a trying evacuation experience after the Japanese takeover of Henan. When the anti-British movement broke out in Weihui, Henan, in 1939, missionaries were given one day to leave.[119] She later wrote, "I had ten minutes in which to leave the place where for ten years I had worked amongst nurses and patients. Opening a drawer I gathered up a handful of vials of narcotics, and put them in my pocket. Then I went up to the storeroom on the third floor, where there were thousands of dollars worth of new goods [and gathered] as many new hot water bottles as I could [carry]."[120] After a month at Huaiqing, another Canadian mission site nearby, she was forced to evacuate again, this time given refuge by the Catholic mission in Xinxiang. After working with refugees in Tianjin for a number of months, she was asked to go to Sichuan to help out with the West China

Mission there. She arrived six months after Clara Preston, in October 1940, after a difficult journey.[121] Unlike Preston, however, who experienced air raids on her first day in Chongqing, Gay experienced them enroute. In total, it took Gay four months to reach Sichuan; she was delayed for weeks in Kunming, normally a one-hour flight from Chongqing.

When an air raid siren sounded in Kunming on the day after her arrival, Gay and another missionary hurried toward an open field with grave mounds and hid among the graves.[122] To their surprise, Chinese soldiers were also hiding there. As Gay later recalled, the women were placed under the guard of two bayoneted soldiers, who "made us lie down in a muddy gully, not allowing us to raise our heads" when the planes flew over.[123] They returned home to find that bombs had demolished their neighbourhood. Another missionary met them at the street corner and, together, by the light of his flashlight, the threesome "stepped along over piles of rubble, passing dead bodies here and there" before arriving at the missionary's house. There, they found "walls were smashed in, windows all broken, plaster and glass lying everywhere." Many of the surrounding buildings had been destroyed. After a restless night's sleep "in any corner that seemed safe," the cook's little boy awakened them at six o'clock in the morning. The first air raid alarm of the day had sounded: "the Japs," recalled Gay, "were coming again."[124]

By the time Margaret Gay got to Chongqing, she was mentally exhausted. She had a brief reunion with Clara Preston and Dorothy Boyd, and then headed off on the four-day journey (by bus, truck, and coal cart) to the Canadian mission at Rongxian, where she was to take charge of the WCM hospital. Although Margaret Gay later recounted that "we had a very happy time" in Sichuan and that her period at Rongxian was "one of the happiest times I had ever spent in China," she did have difficulty adjusting to the rigours of wartime work.[125] Correspondence between the WMS secretary in West China and the United Church of Canada home office in Toronto gives a sense of the difficulties. Gay went to Rongxian "on her arrival in Sichuan to work in the hospital there ... Our hospitals are very poorly equipped etc. in comparison with the ones in [Henan], and it was not easy for her to use makeshifts. It got on her nerves so it was thought best for her to come to [Chengdu] for a rest and change. Recently she has been helping in secretarial work at the Si Shen Tsi [General] Hospital and will likely continue with that until she leaves."[126] The WMS was aware of, albeit surprised at, the struggles the North China missionary nurses were having. On 18 February 1941, Adelaide Harrison wrote to Norman Knight, a NCM missionary working in Tianjin, that

> Misses Preston and Gay are finding conditions in our hospitals vastly different from [Henan] where they had ample supplies of all kinds to work with. Here after three and a half years of war, transportation difficulties, soaring prices, our hospital supplies are almost down to rock bottom which makes effective medical work, particularly in the nursing department, very difficult. Also we do not have modern conveniences like running water and central heating, as you have, and yet in spite of all these drawbacks they are doing a fine piece of work, and I don't know how our medical work would get along without them.[127]

Even for the seasoned North China missionaries, wartime West China proved too much. By 1941, Dorothy Boyd, and Margaret Gay had departed China. Clara Preston departed in January 1943. Like Dorothy Boyd, Margaret Gay made the decision quite suddenly, deciding to return to Canada "at once" to help care for her sisters.[128] According to the Foreign Mission executive secretary, Ruth Taylor, one of Gay's sisters "is finding it impossible to carry on at home without [Gay] because of the continued illness of her other sister."[129] Gay left Rongxian by sedan chair, travelling four days over the mountains to Chengdu, and then rode by mail truck driver for two more days to Chongqing, before flying to Hong Kong.[130] Whereas the trip to Chongqing had taken four months, the return trip from Chongqing to Hong Kong took only four days. She sailed for Canada on 14 May 1941 and was granted a leave of absence from missionary work. The leave was later extended indefinitely, and lasted until her retirement in August 1951.[131] Leaving aside the issue of the soundness of their reasons for departing, the North China missionaries' short tenure in West China left a poor impression on the West China missionaries.

In April 1941, Dr. Jean Millar was called to go to Rongxian to help out
with "an emergency situation" there. She was given a month's leave of
absence from Chengdu to sort things out there. "I might say confiden-
tially," wrote Adelaide Harrison, "that this emergency was partly due to
Miss Gay's inability to adjust herself to the work and Chinese workers
here in [Sichuan]."[132]

One of the other new nurses, Margaret Lee, determined to stay; she
was in West China for four years, much to the relief of the West China
Mission. In 1939, the WCM had received word that the Woman's Mis-
sionary Society might be, for the first time, securing a Canadian-born
Chinese nurse.[133] After a year of deaconess training in Toronto, Margaret
Lee was making travel plans from Montreal to Vancouver, to catch a
steamship to China in July 1940.[134] In a letter to deaconess students,
Margaret Lee described herself this way:

> I was born in Montreal and grew up in that city the same way that
> other Canadian girls do, going to Church and school and playing
> during my leisure time. Inspired by my parents and friends of
> China, I decided I would serve China, the home of my ancestors.
> With the type of qualifications I had, how would I be able to give of
> my best? I thought this over carefully when different vocations
> were presented to me. After much thought and prayer, I decided to
> answer the call and need for nurses in that great land.[135]

Margaret Lee's father was born in China and had immigrated to Montreal, where he met his wife, described as "the first Chinese girl born in
Canada East of the Rockies."[136] The Lees were among "that fine group
of Chinese Christians" who urged the Presbyterian Church of Canada to
open a mission in South China, in Guangzhou.[137] Margaret Lee took her
nurses' training at Women's College Hospital in Toronto – the same
school that had accepted Agnes Chan in the 1920s.[138]

The much-anticipated arrival of Margaret Lee came at the end of
October 1940. She, too, was faced with an air raid immediately upon
her arrival in Chongqing. "Thanks to the Japs," she noted, they had an
"exciting welcome."[139] With the air raid under way when they landed,

"passengers scattered into the fields," while Lee and her colleague hid in a clump of bamboo for an hour, then climbed into a bus to bring them back to the main airport. From there she boarded another plane, this one to Chengdu. She finally arrived in Chengdu on 26 October, one month to the day after departing Montreal.

To many, Chengdu was considered a bit of a backwater compared with other parts of China. "Chengdu is a somewhat backward city with regard to certain facilities," Margaret Lee wrote.[140] While much had changed in other parts of China in the previous fifteen years, rickshaws were still used in Chengdu, even though automobiles, buses, and airplanes were in common use. Despite the city's limitations, changes had happened so quickly that the local people "are still somewhat in a daze." While radios, telegrams, and telephones were common, spinning and weaving were still done by hand. "I must admit that I miss the lights and rush of a Canadian city," Margaret Lee wrote, "but I enjoy the quiet of this part of the world."[141]

Months later, Margaret Lee had not yet started work in the hospital. Her first order of business was to learn the Sichuan dialect, which she was studying five hours a day, five days a week.[142] "Of course I already know one dialect of the Chinese," she wrote – this was likely Cantonese, as most Chinese immigrants to Canada came from Fujian – "but it isn't of any use in West China."[143] Eventually, however, she served not only the WCCU but also ultimately worked on staff with the refugee PUMC, fulfilling her wish that, "under the leadership of Jesus, I shall be able to do my small bit toward alleviating the suffering and need in China."[144]

THE DESTRUCTION OF THE WOMEN'S HOSPITAL

On 30 March 1940, the WMS Women's Hospital training school for nurses in Chengdu had held a capping ceremony for nineteen probationers – that is, those who had successfully completed their probationary period. Of the ceremony, Geraldine Hartwell wrote:

> In China, everything is done to promote the dignity of the nursing profession. The Nurses Association of China initiated this

ceremony some years ago ... At our capping ceremony, the members of the Board, the stewards of the church, the teaching staff and the staff of the hospital were invited to the chapel. Several guests spoke, I put the caps on the probationers. Miss Dju Tein addressed the girls. Then each girl was given a candle, and I, representing Florence Nightingale, started the light with my lamp and all lighted their candles from one another. This typified spreading the light of good health to everyone.[145]

Within five weeks, the WMS hospital and training school for nurses would be dealt a devastating blow.

On 2 May 1940, just one month after Dorothy Boyd's and Clara Preston's arrival in Chongqing, and a few months before Margaret Lee's and Margaret Gay's arrivals (in July and October 1940, respectively), the WMS Women's Hospital building burned to the ground. The missionary community suspected (but never proved) that the fire was deliberately set. "Even yet it is very difficult for us to realize such a thing has happened," wrote WMS secretary Winifred Harris to the mission headquarters in Toronto.[146] From what Harris understood, at 2:30 a.m. hospital personnel who lived on the premises were wakened by the smell of smoke, which seemed to be coming from the basement. By the time they could investigate, the part of the hospital underneath Caroline Wellwood's office was "almost like a roaring furnace."[147] Staff immediately went to work evacuating patients from the second and third floors before the fire cut off the stairway. "Yeoman service was given by the nurses and servants and not one life was lost, a thing for which we lifted up our hearts in grateful thanks," wrote Harris.[148] When nurses and staff were asked how they knew how to get the patients all out of the big, four storey building so quickly, the nurses replied that it was because they had to evacuate patients so often when the air alarms came. Only two were injured. One of the older nurses, Wu Ueh Bin, fell and broke her arm when helping a patient down the stairs. The other, an operating room attendant, was hurt when trying to escape through a window. He had been trying to run down the stairs with instruments he had saved from the operating room. However, he "saw his way cut off and ran back and jumped from the window, injuring himself in the face and head."[149] The fire brigade managed to keep the fire from spreading to other buildings, but the nurses' residence was completely destroyed.

Mary Crawley, who had been a missionary nurse at the WCM since 1929, was stationed at the WMS Women's Hospital in Chengdu.[150] She was praised for her quick thinking on the night of the fire when, "by her courage and cool-headedness she salvaged quantities of valuable drugs."[151] An undated newspaper clipping from Toronto deemed her a "heroic nurse," quoting from a letter Crawley wrote to her mother in Toronto:

> With the building aflame, Miss Crowley [sic] went to the drug room to try to rescue valuable medicines. "Both my flashlights," she wrote, "failed to work and I had only one candle which I gave to Dr. Jean Millar. She emptied the poison cupboard which contained our very expensive medicines, while I handed out through the window the ether and the chloroform and filled drawers with precious tablets and ampules. Though working in the dark I knew just where things were and filled baskets with my scales balance and weights and whatever I could think of that was precious. When the drawers and baskets ran out I took a sheet and filled with bottles of tablets. With an effort we got it out the window." Dr. E.R. Cunningham of Winnipeg at that point called her to come out herself. Reaching for more medicines, Miss Crowley [sic] relates, she called for him to wait a minute. A moment later she felt herself being forcibly carried out the window and placed on the ground. A moment later the whole building caved in.[152]

As with most of the nurses working at the hospital, Crawley's belongings were destroyed.

The origin of the fire was a mystery. It had started in an unused bathroom, in which there was reportedly nothing that could start a fire (e.g., a fireplace or electrical wires).[153] However, about eighty straw mattresses were stored there for use during air raids. "Whether someone went in there with a lighted cigarette," Winifred Harris wrote, "or whether it was done purposefully we will never know."[154] The general feeling was that the fire was arson, commited by "Chinese agents working for Japan."[155] Laura Hambley, a Canadian missionary, noted, "Poor Miss Wellwood feels so badly. It was she who equipped the hospital and much credit was due her that it was the best furnished and the best equipped in West China likely. And oh! the fine stock of drugs gone, just now when they cannot be gotten into the province. It must have been spies for the enemy who did it."[156]

The loss was a "tremendous one" for many reasons, including that the hospital was, simply, a beautiful building, and "it makes one heartsick to see it in ruins."[157] The hospital had first been established as a small clinic by Dr. Retta Gifford Kilborn in 1895, and became associated with a nurses' training school after the new building was erected in 1915. In 1939, a total of 2,800 patients were cared for in the hospital, and 25,000 in the outpatient department. In 1940, the staff included on Canadian and eight Chinese physicians, and two Canadian and twenty-one Chinese nurses.[158] The Canadian members of staff were Dr. Jean Millar and nurses Caroline Wellwood and Mary Crawley. Alma Tallman was also on staff but was in Canada on furlough.[159]

Within two weeks of the fire, the obstetrical work of the Women's Hospital was relocated to the junior middle school property at Feng Chan Gai, while the medical and children's departments were housed on the third and fourth floor of the General Hospital (previously the Men's Hospital) at Si Shen Tsi.[160] The General Hospital had previously been for men only. After the fire, it had sixty-five beds for women and children.[161] The relatively quick relocation of the departments of the Women's Hospital meant that there was very little interruption in their work.[162]

Mary Crawley reportedly "threw herself with optimism and enthusiasm into the difficult task of renovating the building of the General Hospital and starting a hospital with practically no supplies and very little funds."[163] At the same time, she had a constant struggle with ill health.[164] "Professionally Mary is a good nurse," noted Adelaide Harrison of the WCM, "but just did not fit into the work here."[165] Crawley tendered her resignation in October 1941, before returning to Canada for furlough.[166] She started for home just as Canada became embroiled in hostilities with Japan, in December 1941, but made it back to Canada safely. By the end of 1941, the WCM had lost four missionary nurses: Dorothy Boyd, Margaret Gay, Alma Tallman, and Mary Crawley.

* * *

The war years had a devastating impact on missionaries and others living in West China. Although considered safe relative to the Japanese-occupied regions, Free China was, in fact, an excruciatingly difficult place to live. Continual air raids took a particular toll. The fear of impending bombing wore on everyone's nerves, the effect of a direct hit being horrific beyond measure. Free China experienced new pressures as millions of Chinese refugees streamed in. Treating mass causalities, working from damaged buildings, responding to fire and air raid alarms, and seeing homes and hospitals destroyed weighed heavily on WCM nurses, both Canadian and Chinese. Each of these pressures, combined with a growing patriotism among Chinese nurses, unsettled the norms in Canadian missionary nursing at the WCM. Still dependent on Christian mores and finding meaning and comfort in their belief in a compassionate and just God, missionary nurses nonetheless started to disengage from their missionary work. Some married, and many evacuated China for various reasons, often illness (their own and family members'). Missionary nurses were part of a large group of missionaries in West China, and particularly on the WCUU campus. As missionaries adapted to the worsening conditions, missionary nurses drew and gave strength to members of the missionary community in Sichuan.

Gender, racial, and religious norms shifted during this period. Nicole Elizabeth Barnes has noted that the transition to Chinese staff at mission facilities throughout the country had a gendered component: "Whereas foreign male doctors consistently complained about their male Chinese colleagues' incompetence and unsuitability for leadership positions, foreign women generally celebrated their Chinese nursing colleagues' assumption of leadership roles and lauded their professional competence."[167] This rings true in West China. Irene Harris wrote from Chongqing that, between returning from furlough between 1941 and 1943, "I have filled a more or less nonentity position, the Chinese nurses having risen to the place where they can be heads of departments, Superintendents of Nurses, Principal, Dean of School of Nursing, etc., etc., and ... I have simply filled in, acting in an advisory capacity, standing behind them, making suggestions but letting them carry through."[168] Her 1943 report also included a description of the latest graduates of the Canadian mission hospital nursing school in Chongqing that confirmed her positive view of her Chinese colleagues' abilities: twenty-eight graduate nurses served on hospital staff, three in charge of the nursing school. Three worked full time in the mission's outpatient clinic in downtown Chongqing. One directed the health centre for a local cement factory with 300 employees. Another launched an entrepreneurial public health organization that employed student nurses to conduct immunizations in nearby firms and in schools with a combined 1,200 students.[169] The capability of Chinese nurses, combined with the toll of wartime conditions, meant that the WCM, like the PUMC, was ripe for Chinese leadership.

CHAPTER FOUR

Waiting to Exhale (1940–42)

Uncertainty, Internment, and the Japanese Takeover of the PUMC

Yesterday, December 7, 1941 – a date which will live in infamy – the United States of America was suddenly and deliberately attacked by naval and air forces of the Empire of Japan.

— *Franklin D. Roosevelt, radio address, 8 December 1941*

The selfish and the coward and the brave all stood out clear against the turmoil of those hectic days.

— *Dr. Stephen Chang, 1943*

In the months leading up to Japan's attack on Pearl Harbor in December 1941, Westerners in China veered between a sense of escalating danger and a stalwart commitment to strategic plans laid before the war. To Woman's Missionary Society (WMS) secretary Winifred Harris, "the enemy is now right up in the gorges and it looks as if the intention is to enter [Sichuan]. What the future holds for us and our work time alone will tell."[1] In the space between uncertainty and commitment stood individuals who were more adaptable to change than the bureaucratic structures they worked within. If the West China Union University (WCUU) and the Peking Union Medical College (PUMC) were to continue their mission of educating physicians and nurses, those on the ground had to figure out how to ensure that these institutions had adequate human and physical resources to meet the high standards of scientifically based, clinically oriented education. Under normal circumstances, energy and attention would be paid to improving curricula, administrative structures, and facilities. Under wartime conditions, energy also had to be put toward ensuring that patients, staff, and students were as safe as possible –

protected from everything from air raids to contaminated surgical instruments. No running water itself was an enormous problem – how does one clean wounds, sterilize instruments, and wash hands and linens without running water? Survival – of both individuals and programs – required adaptation and resiliency. Both the WCUU and the PUMC found themselves constantly adapting to local conditions during the first three years of China's War of Resistance against Japan. However, once the United States and Canada declared war against Japan, the situation in China became even more dire. Within hours, the Japanese army took over the PUMC, and all foreign staff (mostly American) were named enemy aliens and were subsequently interned. In this chapter, I examine how members of the West China Mission (WCM) and the PUMC persisted with their core aim of nursing education and practice in the period immediately before and following a defining wartime moment: the Japanese attack on Pearl Harbor on 7 December 1941.

WEST CHINA WAITING

In the year 1941, there was a sense of anxious waiting in West China. For some Canadian missionary nurses, wartime conditions in Sichuan were proving too much to endure, leading to early resignations. For the Chinese students studying at the WCUU – including refugee students from other universities – the waiting was getting difficult. In a letter written on 18 May 1941, William G. Sewell, a British professor of chemistry at the WCUU, observed that students "have a comparative security here on the campus and are immune from many of the war's dangers. They are denied by Government and pressure from their teachers, many of the opportunities youth the world over [are] now experiencing, and there is a danger of frustration for the individual who seeks a more positive outlet for his patriotism."[2] Missionaries were waiting, too. On the one hand, they were awaiting the next air raid. On the other, they were awaiting the end of the war. There was a sense of helplessness on a certain level – China's War of Resistance against Japan was not (yet) their fight, and their original mission had not changed: to provide medical and nursing care to the Chinese as both an expression of their Christian faith and an opportunity to bring others into that faith. A question underlying many interactions on the WCUU campus – which was the heart of the missionary community in Chengdu – regarded the degree to which wartime was helping or hindering them in fulfilling their mission. Providing tangible support to the Chinese through the provision of medical care was rewarding, as was the preparation of Chinese students to take over this type of work themselves. For those who managed to stay focused on the bigger picture, wartime was just a more complicated context within which to do the same work they had done since the WCUU opened almost thirty years prior. Problem solving had always been integral to missionary work. Wartime just made problem solving more complex.

Bombing continued unrelentingly through the summer of 1940. During this time, the Canadian mission hospital at Ziliujing was severely bombed, and little was left of it.[3] Constant bombing had reportedly left Chongqing in ruins.[4] The strain of the war was wearing on everyone. There was an epidemic of dysentery among the missionaries. One missionary child, Donald Campbell, was very ill, his condition considered grave. A young American doing research had recently died at the Canadian Si Shen Tsi Hospital, likely from typhus.[5] "We are trying to carry on as best we can," wrote Winifred Harris of the WMS, but "the problem of food is an acute one just now. The price of rice is prohibitive ... I am afraid there is trouble ahead unless something can be done."[6] A letter from long-serving Canadian missionary Dr. Ernest B. Struthers paints a picture of transportation conditions in Sichuan. Having just recovered from an earlier road accident, he had been sent to Ziliujing for a month in the summer of 1940 to relieve Dr. Sheridan. He wrote:

> No truck was available until the 8th of July. That morning after a very heavy rain we started off. There were seven of us perched on top of boxes with which the truck was loaded. As we rushed out of the city we were swished by the waterladen branches of the trees and had to duck to escape decapitation by the telegraph wires. About two hours out of the city the roads were dry and the sun so hot before evening [that] my hands were swollen with sunburn. The next morning I sat on my baggage, as did thirty others, in an

open public truck. The public bus, for which I did not succeed in getting a ticket, was packed so full that, in the midsummer heat, I was surprised some of the passengers did not suffocate. The road was good and we reached our destination in about 3 hours.[7]

Struthers reached Ziliujing in time for an air raid warning. All seventy patients in the mission hospital had been placed in an air raid shelter.[8] Five days previous, four bombs had been dropped in the mission compound, doing considerable damage to the houses and one end of the hospital; however, this part of the hospital had not been in use since it was damaged in an air raid the previous year. There were approximately four air raid warnings each week, and each time patients who could not walk would have to be carried out to a dugout close to the hospital. Five days after Struthers left, seven bombs were dropped in and around the compound. The roof was blown off and several wards became unusable. The hospital, Struthers noted, had a good nursing school under an "efficient" head nurse, Miss Chu.[9] It also had a number of graduate nurses who had trained in Chengdu. One of these nurses was a graduate of the Qilu Hospital training school in Jinan, Shandong – something especially gratifying to Struthers, as he had spent many years teaching medicine at Qilu. In fact Struthers' wife was still in Jinan, waiting to join him in West China. Waiting, and being at the ready, was the order of the day.

EQUIPPING THE WCUU UNIVERSITY HOSPITAL, 1941

During the "fourth terrible year of war in China" (1941), the WCUU had started to build the long-awaited new University Hospital in Chengdu.[10] The WMS Women's Hospital fire in 1940 was an unexpected impetus to keep the project moving. In February 1941, the staff of the Women's Hospital were trying to determine what would be best – to rebuild after the war, to unite with the Foreign Mission Board (FMB) at the General Hospital, or to become an integral part of the new WCUU University Hospital.[11] By this time, the WMS hospital had been carrying on its work for almost ten months on the top storey of the General Hospital at Si Shen Tsi, and in the junior middle school building at Fang

Chen Gai.[12] By the end of 1941, the WMS passed a resolution that its Women's Hospital in Chengdu would not be rebuilt.[13] The plan was to sell the hospital property but not the foreign residence.[14] The WMS staff would then continue their work as part of the new WCUU University Hospital. (See Figure 4.1: Plot Plan for the University Hospital and Medical Center, August 1941.)

Deciding to build a new hospital at the height of a war was an ambitious undertaking, with layers of complexity and, at times, conflicting agendas. The new hospital would be able to care for 300 inpatients and 400 outpatients every day.[15] Rev. James Endicott was the chair of the board of governors of the WCUU, which was concerned with raising funds to furnish the hospital. As part of the fundraising campaign, the board set up a fund to which donors in Canada could contribute from $50 (for a bed) to $7,000 (for a "heating plant and steam boiler") for the new hospital.[16] The initiative was called the Dr. Robert E. Brown Fund, after the anticipated director of the new hospital. A brochure published to assist with the fundraising efforts contains a peculiar preface – one that certainly reflected the views of Endicott, a politically active missionary, if not most of the thirty-three-member board. It mirrors the unease that some missionaries felt at being observers of Japanese aggression in China rather than active participants in the war to resist Japan – or, even worse, as (inadvertent) colluders with Japan. The brochure, as part of its appeal for funds for the new hospital, tapped into a sense that Canada owed it to China to commit funds to the hospital: "We earnestly commend to you this opportunity to atone in some degree to the Chinese people for the wrongs our [Canadian] countrymen have done in supplying the Japanese with the materials of war. It is not inappropriate that we should do our share in binding up the wounds of China."[17]

James Endicott was no stranger to stirring up controversy. A United Church missionary (and professor of English and ethics at the WCUU) who initially supported Chiang Kai-shek as a social and political adviser to Chiang's New Life Movement,[18] he later became impressed by the Communists, befriending Zhou Enlai during China's civil war after 1945. Endicott was critical of Canadians, provoking audiences with criticisms of the Canadian government when he was on furlough in Canada

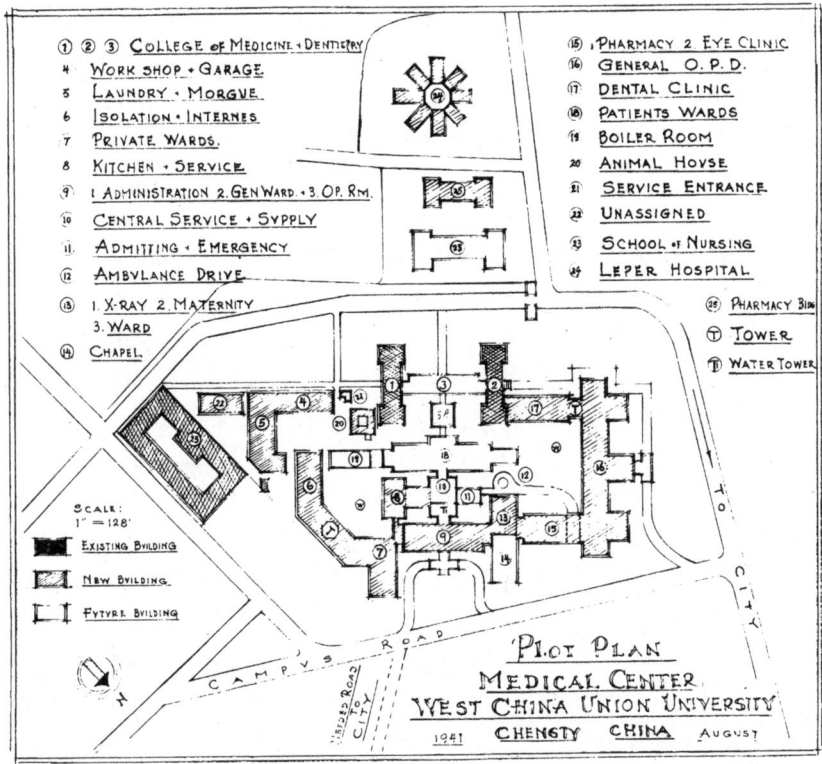

FIGURE 4.1 Plot plan for the University Hospital and Medical Centre, August 1941. |
Courtesy Rockefeller Archive Centre, RAC-CMB_FA065_B158_F1154_001.

between 1942 and 1944: "China's cry for help when the Japanese seized
Manchuria [in 1931] had been a test case of the West's sincerity in up-
holding a new and better world order" – a test which, he contended, the
West had failed.[19] Other Canadian missionaries, including Dr. Robert
McClure, criticized Canada's supply of nickel to Japan, which the Japanese undoubtedly, they argued, used in their weapons against China.
Like Endicott, McClure made numerous provocative public statements
criticizing the government for permitting Canadian nickel to be sold to
Japan at a time when Americans had placed an embargo on the export of
iron and steel scrap to all countries (except Great Britain) outside the
Western hemisphere.[20] Bob McClure also said as much in a face-to-face
meeting with the prime minister of Canada, Mackenzie King – for which
he was required to apologize publicly, or go to jail. McClure apologized.[21]

The authors of the WCUU fundraising brochure also appealed to their readership's sense of justice and fairness by reminding them that Europe was not the only continent experiencing war. They appealed for help by comparing the European and Asian war zones:

> During the past three years there has been a pageant of suffering in China such as the world has seldom seen. Countless millions of people have been driven from their homes, and are trying to build new lives in the far West, under the shadow of Tibet. In addition to some two million battle casualties, perhaps an equal number of those who have been forced to seek refuge in the western provinces has been estimated as surpassing the total populations of Poland, Holland, Norway and Belgium combined.[22]

The brochure praised the spirit of the Chinese, noting that reconstruction continued even while cities were under bombardment, and that "scores of thousands" of orphans were being cared for in the "remote interior."[23] It also noted that "millions of refugees are finding new hope through various organizations in which Christian sympathy finds constructive expression."[24] This was an interesting departure from fundraising appeals a generation earlier, when the Canadian mission hospitals were first built. When the WMS Women's Hospital was built, women's missionary work in China relied on local WMS chapters in Canada to provide regular monetary support. For example, in 1925–26, the WMS in Alberta collected special donations that included $30 from the Westlock Ladies Aid toward the Women's Hospital in Chengdu, and $40 from the Auxiliary of the Calgary Central United Church "in support of a child in China."[25] Canadian churchwomen took such a keen interest in the work in China that one WMS group in Lacombe, Alberta, went so far as to claim that

> China owes a great debt to Christian Missions – for her schools which 236,000 of Chinese children (Protestants) attend, and 100 hospitals besides asylums for Insane, Blind and Lepers of whom China is said to have 400,000 ... Many of these foreigners [i.e., the

Chinese] have lived in poverty, ignorance and dirt in their native countries and have to be educated to need of proper [sic] living conditions, medical care and education. Hospital work provides [the] best "open door" for this instruction and for the gospel teaching.[26]

These earlier fundraising appeals had classified Canadian churchgoers as righteous rescuers of the Chinese, and sharing the Christian gospel as a primary motivator for medical missions. In contrast, the authors of the 1941 brochure – that is, the WCUU board of governors – implicated Canadians as accomplices in China's pain, appealing to their Christian sensibilities to make amends by donating to this worthy cause. It was a novel but insightful approach, given the growing criticism of missions *by* churchgoers themselves (for example, as demonstrated by the Commission of Appraisal on missions chaired by William Ernest Hocking in 1932).[27] By directly naming current controversies associated with Canada's role in China, the WCUU fundraising appeal found a new angle to reflect (and gain from) churchgoers' growing reluctance to be involved in Christian missions in general, and in China in particular. That is not to say, however, that the church at large no longer saw a purpose in missions; rather, the focus of missions had changed.

The original emphasis of missions – including missionary nursing – had been the conversion of Chinese to Christianity. However, by the 1920s, this had shifted to an emphasis on simply caring for those who were suffering. Similarly, although the primary purpose of the WCUU was to provide a Christian education, missionary nurses themselves were inclined to see their primary purpose as serving God not through "bringing people to Christ" per se, but through simply caring for their suffering, and teaching others to do likewise.[28] Still, they did view Christianity as a civilizing religion. Insofar as China's leaders were Christian, China would flourish. This ideal is also reflected in the WCUU University Hospital fundraising brochure:

The leadership of China today is predominantly Christian. Not only are the heads of the State, the Generalissimo and Madame Chiang, ardent followers of the Christian way of life, but thousands of lesser leaders at home and abroad are Christians. This is largely a result of the educational leadership which has been provided by hundreds of Christian schools, and by the thirteen Christian Colleges of China.[29]

It is interesting to see this emphasis on the significance of Christian colleges when, according to British missionary William G. Sewell, "at present not more than 5% of the students attend services in various city churches, and there is need for some organization in the university itself which will serve as a focus for religious activities."[30] This emphasis on how Christianity was influencing China may have been, in part, due to increasing criticism from the government. For example, Sewell also noted that, "for years Christianity has been driven from our public cere-monies [such as graduation] for fear of Government criticism."[31] For that reason, Sewell was "amazed" when the governor of Sichuan, Chang Chuin, gave an address that incorporated Christian ideas. In other words, just as churchgoers in Canada were shifting away from a focus on evangelism for internal reasons (i.e., changing mores within the United Church of Canada), the WCUU was shifting away from public expres-sions of Christian faith for external reasons (i.e., changing political pressures).

The new director of the West China Union University Hospital, Dr. Robert E. Brown, also appealed to the Rockefeller Foundation (RF) for financial support to build the hospital, requesting US$75,000.[32] In his ap-peal, Brown seemed to be pushing against assumptions that the RF might have regarding the limited size of the medical enterprise at the WCUU. He noted that the population served was as numerous as the whole popu-lation of the United States, and that Chengdu, though far removed from the war zone, received the "back wash of the struggle and occasionally bombings also."[33] Brown seemed to be downplaying the air raids, which by all other reports were not "occasional" but rather incessant in Free China. But he may have guessed that the RF would not wish to invest in a building that would likely be destroyed by bombing. As he described it, Chengdu city was at a "safe distance" of 1,200 miles from the Japan-ese occupation.[34] Even if Chengdu city were bombed, he reasoned, the new hospital was located outside of the city, on the WCUU campus, and would therefore be relatively safe. Concerns about bombing, in any case, should not stop the RF from financially supporting a new hospital. "It would be very timid," he reasoned, "to stop such work [i.e., medical and nurses' training] when already begun in the center of 'Free China' among people fighting for life and the freedom of their nation and the survival of democracy."[35]

At the time of Robert Brown's appeal, ten buildings had already been constructed. The real need was equipping the hospital. Of the $75,000 sought from the RF, $50,000 was needed for hospital equipment and supplies, and $25,000 for operating costs due to "unfavorable war exchange and for additional equipment during the first five years."[36] Wrote Brown, "I trust that you will be able to view the matter in this manner and see in the aid here being solicited a supreme opportunity to succor China and its battling, suffering population ... The need is urgent, while the Pacific Ocean is open for shipment and it is dry season on the Burma Road."[37]

On 15 March 1941, Brown wrote to update Dr. Alan Gregg, the director of the RF Medical Sciences Division, on the need and opportunity to support the new University Hospital. Brown was in the United States on a fundraising visit and had raised $5,000 toward his goal of $15,000 to purchase medical equpment from the Red Cross and other sources in Shanghai. The equipment would then be shipped to Sichuan via the Burma Road – a 717-mile route built through Myanmar during wartime to bring supplies from Allied supporters into West China, thus circumventing the Japanese. Brown was requesting that the RF provide the additional $10,000, which would make the shipment effort from Shanghai to Chengdu worthwhile. "This new hospital," he explained, "is like an adopted child and a war orphan. Being a new child, it is not yet on the family budget of the West China Union University, so cannot share in the funds being raised for the Christian colleges at present here in America."[38] Furthermore, "it is a war orphan in that war conditions have prevented the expected British assistance for these equipment funds."[39] For the three medical schools sharing the WCUU campus (WCUU; Qilu; National Central), which had pooled their students, faculty, and equipment, the opening of the new University Hospital at

Chengdu was their greatest priority. "It would be a tragic neglect of an opportunity to serve the Chinese," Brown continued, "with these buildings standing empty and useless."[40] "It would be a great source of relief and encouragement if we could receive further help from [the RF]," he wrote.[41]

Alan Gregg responded with a non-committal letter, noting that he would be glad to have word again from Brown once Brown studied the market for equipment available in Shanghai. Gregg was not convinced of the wisdom of shipping supplies via the Burma Road, since this would mean "more than starting an extremely hard series of tasks and uncertainties, since this is only the first stage."[42] Still, in an entry in his diary dated 24 March 1941, Gregg seemed a bit more positive.[43] In a conversation with Joseph Beech, chancellor of the WCUU, Gregg had obtained more details about how, precisely, supplies would be transported once in Burma. The Red Cross in Burma had ten trucks and was awaiting twenty-eight more. This would improve their ability to move along supplies. In terms of the grant requested ($10,000 for medical instruments plus apparently an additional $25,000 for installation of equipment), Gregg was open to the idea, but wanted first to review the list of requested equipment in light of the RF's preference to contribute to teaching expenses rather than "ordinary hospital care of the sick."[44] Ultimately, Brown's appeals were successful. In addition to support from church-going donors and the Rockefeller Foundation, the WCUU also received $100,000 (in Chinese dollars) from the "China Foundation" for equipment only available locally, and $75,000 (in Chinese dollars) from the British Boxer Indemnity Board of Trustees.[45]

The negotiations continued. In June 1942, the Woman's Missionary Society in Chengdu noted that there was a possibility of purchasing, from the American Baptist Mission, some property that adjoined the new University Hospital, and that "our medical workers" considered an ideal location for the future nurses' training school.[46] At the same time, bed space in the General Hospital had been increased by adding a sanatorium of forty beds. The China Foundation had provided grants toward salaries and laboratory expenses; the WCUU had provided funds for the maintenance of free beds (i.e., where patients did not pay) in the hospital. The University Hospital and the General Hospital were now overseen together as a single United Hospital, although they retained their names.

PUMC WAITING

The uncertainty and turmoil of wartime was by no means limited to West China. In Beijing, which had been occupied since July 1937, the PUMC was also struggling with several challenges, one of which concerned recruiting and retaining foreign (Western) nurses. In 1938, PUMC dean of nursing, Gertrude Hodgman, wrote to a nurse-placement service in Chicago to try to find potential nursing faculty. She noted that, "in the next few years the foreign staff here will be reduced to not more than 4 or 5, and possibly as few as 2 or 3."[47] Hodgman was exploring the possibility of having American nurses come to help for short periods – a strategy that the Canadian mission had also (successfully) used in 1938 to try to attract new missionary nurses.[48] Hodgman was clear on the quality required: "we are exceedingly anxious that any foreign appointment which is made should be of an outstanding person."[49] But it was difficult to find people, outstanding or otherwise. "It is a matter of disappointment to us," the placement service responded three months later, "that we have no nurses to present to you at this time."[50]

On 23 November 1939, almost a year after the first request, Hodgman wrote again with an update. Instead of taking someone from the service, they decided to offer the position to a nurse who was already in China. "We have decided to offer Miss [Margaret] Wyne a position here," Hodgman noted, suggesting that, in so doing, she was turning down a recommendation of someone else by the placement service in Chicago. "Miss Wyne is very much liked here," Hodgman noted, "and that, of course, especially under present conditions, is important."[51] Although Hodgman did not consider the appointment ideal – given that they were looking for someone as a surgical instructor and Wyne did not have much experience in that area – wartime conditions made movement between China and America difficult. "Under the present circumstances here and in America," Hodgman noted, "we feel this is the safer thing to do rather than to attempt to get someone out [from the United States]."[52] As part of their propaganda to the Chinese, Japan was positioning itself as a pro-Asian nation fighting against Western imperialism. Japan's attempt to align themselves with the Chinese against a common enemy (Westerners) incited pockets of anti-Western sentiment, which worried the Americans at the PUMC. "As you can imagine," Gertrude Hodgman wrote, "we have not enjoyed the anti-[Westerner] campaigns that have been going on. Now we are expecting the guns turned against us."[53] Given all these challenges, it is not surprising that, as Gertrude Hodgman had predicted, there were only three foreign nurses on faculty at the PUMC when she left for a furlough in September 1940.

Mary Ferguson, a long-serving PUMC secretary, later described the social and political context for PUMC faculty and students in 1940. Almost every family in the PUMC, she noted, Chinese and foreign, had been separated by circumstances or was facing separation for an indefinite future because of the Japanese military occupation of North China and most of the eastern seaboard.[54] There was rampant inflation, and the Japanese were tightening their control over every aspect of life – censorship and surveillance were ever present. Perhaps most disturbingly, "friends and colleagues suddenly disappeared – one dared not inquire what had happened to them, but the grapevine placed them in Japanese jails, held without charges or trial"[55] (see Figure 4.2). The Rockefeller Foundation's China Medical Board (CMB) wondered how long the funds to support the PUMC could be safely remitted. Both the British Consulate and the US State Department urged women and children to evacuate China while sea routes were still open. "Small wonder," Ferguson wrote, "that there were frayed tempers, misunderstandings, criticisms [and] unreasonableness."[56]

In 1940, PUMC leaders grappled with the idea of evacuating families of American staff and of relocating the college itself to West China. In February 1940, Henry Houghton, acting director of the PUMC, travelled to West China to gather information about medical activities in the interior and to renew contacts with PUMC graduates and former staff who now resided in Chongqing. The next month, he reported on the "splendid work" being done by PUMC nursing and medical graduates and former staff at Chongqing.[57] In November 1940, the wives and children of two American faculty members left Beijing to sail on the first of several special evacuation ships sponsored by the United States.[58] The next month, foreign women and children, "with the exception of women in staff positions the terms of whose appointments include specific insurance provision," were urged to leave China.[59] Despite the warning, all three foreign nurses at the PUMC decided to stay. Margaret Wyne, an American, had been appointed assistant superintendent of nurses in July 1939.[60] Faye Whiteside, also an American, had been at the PUMC since 1919.[61] Ethel Robinson, a Canadian, had been there since 1920.[62]

In December 1940, the deepening threat of expanding Japanese military occupation was foremost in the minds of the PUMC board of trustees. However, while other institutions had moved to West China, the trustees believed that relocating would "cause misgiving and imply that the area is finished with China."[63] They also felt that the "transient situation in West China" was not "worthy of serious consideration for the establishment of permanent medical work."[64] Over the next two months, five families departed for home. Six others decided to stay together in Beijing – with the understanding that they would take full responsibility for any dangers this might place them in. The trustees, in May 1941, moved forward with teaching plans, rehiring staff, and admitting new students for the fall term. A larger than average nursing class was expected, and all preparations for a normal year were underway.[65] The PUMC hospital and outpatient clinics, in the meantime, were busy, even overwhelmed with patients.

Minutes of the college's Nursing Faculty Committee from 1941 give a snapshot of the faculty priorities and concerns. On 27 February of that year, there were thirty faculty members, including dean of nursing Vera Nieh, foreign nurses Faye Whiteside, Ethel Robinson, and Margaret Wyne, and twenty-five Chinese faculty, two of whom were "on leave abroad" – likely as Rockefeller fellows or otherwise sponsored by the RF.[66] Besides discussion of typical faculty concerns such as "how to write up a student's efficiency record" and "how to reduce the heavy teaching load of supervisors," the group discussed "which method (military or democratic) is better in disciplining students?"[67] It was agreed that "both methods are acceptable" and should be used according to the individual situation. When Vera Nieh raised the question of whether teaching should be conducted in English, the group decided that "all formal and informal discussion should be given in English" and that all instructors and students "are to speak English to each other during duty hours."[68] Questions about the use of democratic versus military discipline and English versus Chinese language are the first hint of PUMC nursing faculty challenging tacit (Western) PUMC values and practices; the question of using English for teaching would be raised again after the PUMC School of Nursing relocated to Chengdu. In the meantime, the school reported an entering class of twenty students in 1941. The hospital was still crowded, and, in anticipation of ongoing difficulties, coal stocks were being maintained and a six-month supply of staples reserved.

BERNICE CHU CHEN'S PROPOSAL FOR WEST CHINA

By 1940, a number of individual PUMC nursing alumnae had relocated to Free China and were starting to give thought as to how they might collectively support the nursing work there. PUMC alumnus Bernice Chu Chen, for example, was working in Chongqing as the Ministry of Education's secretary of the Commission on Nursing Education. In October 1940, she prepared a confidential report on aims the Commission hoped to accomplish regarding nursing education between 1940 and 1943, which Chu Chen sent to Mary Tennant, acting director of the International Health Division of the Rockefeller Foundation (IHD).[69] In it, Chu Chen urged the need for nursing education in China to pick up the pace. Over the previous five decades, she argued, the priority had been the training of bedside nurses, with an emphasis on "quantity rather than quality."[70] While acknowledging that "the majority" of the nurses were doing good work, Chu Chen argued that there were simply not enough of them.[71] In order to meet the demand for better-trained nurses, she posited that the priority should be to "make an effort to [first] produce a group of satisfactory teachers and administrators."[72] Following this principle, she noted, the central government was stressing the training of graduate nurses, preparing them for teaching and administrative positions "in the most needed nursing schools in the country."[73] In other words, Chu Chen was looking to initiate a nursing education project undergirded by PUMC principles.

The report proposed that the RF support the commission in its aim to train a small group of graduate nurses, approximately twenty every year. The idea would be to select a school of nursing in Free China for the training of graduate nurses in institutional (as opposed to public health) nursing.[74] The plan proposed five methods to meet the objective of training graduate nurses: select the National Central University School of Nursing as the centre of training; select prospective graduate nurses; send student records on didactic and practical nursing teaching and administration to the Technical Committee on Nursing Education for approval; upon graduation, require nurses to work for two years at the institution where they received their initial training; and have students spend their first year at the National School of Nursing and the second year practising teaching and administration in their original schools.

One of the most interesting aspects of Bernice Chu Chen's report is her perspective on mission nursing schools in Free China, including those associated with the Canadian mission. In her view, nursing education at mission schools was inferior. "The drawback of the majority [of] missionary nursing schools," she noted, "is that most of the scheduled [hours] for various subjects are not strictly given by the teachers."[75] This was because schools typically only had one or two full-time instructors, the rest being "honorary" teachers – typically physicians. Most of these honorary teachers felt that teaching nursing students was "extra baggage," and, as a result, their teaching was not thorough, and the students were poorly trained. To address the problem of poorly trained nurses, Chu Chen suggested that, rather than the Ministry of Education continuing to allocate the same, small sum of money to a number of schools, to invest instead into the better schools. In this scheme, schools considered as "grade A" would receive $4000 each, whereas "grade B" schools would receive $2000 each.[76] The Canadian mission school in Chengdu was listed as one of the two "grade A" schools; the Canadian mission schools at Chongqing and Ziliujing were listed as two of the four "grade

B" schools.[77] The total cost of the proposal, which Bernice Chu Chen hoped the RF would fund, would be $48,000 over three years, a quarter of which would likely be used as salary stipends.

The initial response of the RF to Chu Chen's proposal was lukewarm. In a letter dated 15 January 1941, Marshall C. Balfour, the IHD director, disagreed with Chu Chen's perspective that there was a need for a program for graduate nurses.[78] He suggested that this need was already being met by the PUMC. Furthermore, he stated, what Chu Chen was proposing as a two-year postgraduate program would repeat much that "should have been done in an effective undergraduate" program.[79] Regarding Chu Chen's second proposal, Balfour doubted that the RF could contribute any subsidies for "grade A" or "grade B" schools – with the possible exception of one school. He supported, in principle, the idea of developing one first-class school in the southwest, either at the National Central School of Nursing in Chongqing or the Canadian Mission School of Nursing in Chengdu.[80] However, in terms of stipends, he believed that these were the responsibility of "official agencies, such as the Ministry of Education."[81]

Although Balfour did not warm to Chu Chen's recommendations regarding a postgraduate program or subsidies for schools in Free China, he did seem aware of the need and opportunity to support nursing work in Sichuan. In a letter dated 1 May 1941, Balfour wrote to Dr. Y.C. Wang, secretary of the Commission on Medical Education, that now was not an opportune time to put Chu Chen's plan in place.[82] Balfour's primary concern was the lack of nursing leaders to take up the necessary tasks. "To speak quite frankly about the matter," he wrote, "there are perhaps four nurses in the Interior who, by training and experience would be capable to undertake such a task" – namely, Bernice Chu Chen, Hsu Ai-Chu, Chou Meiyu, and Pao Ai-ching.[83] Of these, Chu Chen had a full-time job and family responsibilities, Hsu Ai-Chu was fully occupied in her present service at Wei Sheng Shu, Chou Meiyu was expected to continue working with the Red Cross, and Pao Ai-ching, "the one who has perhaps accomplished the most in nursing education and whose school has produced the best trained graduates of any in the Southwest, has, I understand, been removed from her position as Directrix of the Central School, by the Ministry of Education." Consequently, until there were a greater number of trained and qualified personnel from Beijing, or until younger nurses could be trained through preparation abroad, "it seems logical to adjourn the plan as contemplated."[84]

Although Balfour did not take up Chu Chen's proposal, it did plant a seed for the idea of the RF being involved at some level in the support of nursing education in Free China. On 27 October 1941, having identified a lack of well-qualified nursing leaders to take up a nursing education project in Free China, Balfour sent a note to Mary Tennant with copies of curriculum vitae of three prospective fellowship candidates who "may come up for consideration at some future time." The idea was "preparatory thinking and planning with respect to the possible establishment or improvement of one good nursing school in Southwest China in the future."[85] Thus, while Bernice Chu Chen's proposal was not directly accepted, it may still have influenced later decisions to support the reopening of the PUMC at the WCUU in Chengdu – which would have the de facto effect of "raising one of the existing schools to a higher standard."[86]

In the meantime, a question mark still hung over the future of the PUMC School of Nursing in Beijing. By the end of June 1941, the recent outbreak of German-Soviet hostilities was impacting the number of steamliners available to passengers wishing to leave China. All boat reservations after July 1941 were cancelled.[87] The window was closing for Americans and Candians to return home, as well as for Chinese fellows abroad to get passage back to China. It was also becoming more difficult (and expensive) to evacuate to West China. In August 1941, the Rockefeller Foundation offered financial help to staff wanting to get to West China. However, a new barrier had arisen: the Japanese were enforcing new regulations that would make it difficult to leave Beijing.

During the fall of 1941, the RF China Medical Board warmed up to the idea of temporarily moving medical personnel to West China and offered to pay the necessary transportation and maintenance costs. Henry Houghton at the PUMC declined, replying that the "entire program" was going on "normally" and there was "no occasion for alarm."[88] This was a surprising response, and it is possible that Houghton was downplaying the situation for the Japanese censors. After all, the PUMC trustees had been considering the possibility of a move for the past year. As wartime conditions worsened, it was also not clear whether any considerable number of faculty could get out safely. If anything was to be done, it would have to be "arranged with the utmost discretion," since, as Houghton noted, "the College itself cannot appear as party to such a scheme, for the military high command would deal with us instantly."[89] Besides, the journey west would be long, rough, and hazardous and, the trustees determined, could only be done "furtively" and only by men, which meant no nurses, since all were female. Closing the PUMC in order to move faculty to West China would be difficult and delicate; every important staff member would be a "marked man."[90] There was no plan, therefore, to relocate the medical school. Instead, the most ambitious plan that could be realized was the attachment of medical (and presumably nursing) faculty to other schools and hospitals in West China.

In November 1941, rumours started circulating that the PUMC was about to close.[91] In response, the trustees sent out a notice on 12 November 1941 to all medical staff and students, stating that it was the board's desire and expectation that "this normal state of affairs will continue" and that no change in the program would be contemplated unless necessitated by circumstances beyond the college's control.[92] Three weeks later the Japanese military bombed Pearl Harbor. It changed everything.

THE BOMB THAT CHANGED EVERYTHING: REVERBERATIONS
FROM PEARL HARBOR

On 8 December, senior nursing students at the PUMC gathered nervously in hospital classrooms to start the first of a few days of national examinations set by the Nurses Association of China (NAC). This was an extremely significant event. As Vera Nieh later recalled, "besides the examination of your own school, all the nurses had to take the examination by the Nurses Association of China. It's a worldwide examination; it's very strict."[93] These final exams, in which the students would demonstrate their practical nursing skills and knowledge according to standardized questions, and which were necessary for graduation, were set for 8:00 a.m. The two external examiners – American missionary

Margaret May Prentice, director of the Isabella Fisher Hospital nursing school in Tianjin, and Chao Pei-chen, director of the Douw Hospital nursing school – had travelled to the college for the occasion.[94] Awaiting their arrival were Vera Nieh, dean of the PUMC School of Nursing, and Faye Whiteside, superintendent of nurses.[95] Arriving by rickshaw, Prentice was warmly greeted by Nieh and Whiteside. Shortly afterwards, Chao, arrived. Unaware of the catastrophic attack on Pearl Harbor just hours earlier, Prentice and Nieh were shocked to hear from Chao that she had just seen large truckloads of armed Japanese soldiers "racing through the streets in all directions," with soldiers "running to the gates" of the PUMC.[96] Within minutes, the Japanese had closed and stood guard at the gates, effectively locking the nursing faculty and students inside, and the rest of the hospital staff out. Although staff arriving for duty initially crowded at the gate, "making vain attempts to get in," gradually they scattered, "under great apprehension," as large posters started going up in the streets announcing the declaration of war between Japan and the United States. Within the hour, Japanese soldiers were wandering all over the PUMC premises, including inside the PUMC Hospital, and guarding every hallway.[97]

Nieh later recalled, "I telephoned to the Director [Henry Houghton] immediately – that was at seven o'clock in the morning; you know nurses work early in the morning!" However, "the phone was cut; the line was cut entirely. And then when I went to the corridor I saw the Japanese soldiers coming in with their guns, and I immediately thought, my, if they go to the classroom my students would be so [nervous] that they [would not be able to] pass their examination." So Nieh went into the examination room and told the students, "we have the Japanese soldiers [here to] visit the PUMC Hospital. They may come to the classroom, but don't be disturbed ... They won't bother you."[98]

Faced with the dilemma of whether to cancel an exam necessary for graduates to be employed as nurses, Chao Pei-chen urged the others to "hurry with the examinations, make them short, and get them over with so the students can have their grades and I can get back to my hospital."[99] They would shield the students from the full truth while Vera Nieh scouted the building. "Unless you feel it would be best to hide the students some where in the Hospital," Margaret Prentice recalled telling Vera Nieh, "or try to get them off to their own homes, we might be able to hurry the examinations through, giving each nurse an opportunity of explaining the bare essentials in each of her four questions, and finish everything before whatever is brewing, boils over."[100]

Opening the sealed envelope that contained the NAC exam, Prentice and Chao chose four questions "which would require the least time for demonstration of nursing treatment and care."[101] According to Prentice's recollection, Vera Nieh returned with the dire news: although she did not see any immediate threat to the students, there *was* a threat to Margaret Prentice, as an American. "If you wish to try to escape to West China, feel free to do so now," Nieh told her.[102] Convinced that it would be impossible to evade Japanese guards in any case, Prentice decided to stay and oversee the exams.

Having told the students that Japanese students were visiting the PUMC, Vera Nieh waited in the examination room. "The soldiers came in," she recalled, "[but] they didn't do much; they just talked to everybody doing [their practical exams], the examiners and the students, [and then] the soldiers went away."[103] When any of the occupying troops looked into the classroom, the students paid them no heed but kept focused on their exams.[104] However, as Japanese soldiers continue to stream in, it was impossible to keep the real situation from the students. Nieh and the others decided to give them the full story, including announcements in the street that America was at war with Japan.[105] Margaret Prentice recalled telling the students to speak only Chinese during the exams, noting "the Japanese seem to have a jealous streak about Chinese speaking English."[106]

Japanese guards had taken over the superintendent's office.[107] They were stationed in every ward and in every corner of the PUMC Hospital. A large number of soldiers were required to guard the whole hospital. "It was fun from the first," recalled Dr. Stephen Chang, "to see the soldiers completely lost over the maze of the place."[108]

According to a report by PUMC secretary Mary Ferguson, the "burden of meeting the situation as the occupation took place fell on the nursing service [i.e., nursing staff] and resident doctors of the hospital, who all remained at their regular work and kept themselves calm in a way that deserves the highest praise."[109] Fortunately, Faye Whiteside, the superintendent of nurses, had come on duty early that morning and was in the hospital before the soldiers came in. "The presence of so responsible and senior [sic] a person as she," wrote Ferguson, "helped greatly to prevent any panic."[110] Ferguson also credited Dr. S.T. Wang for finding a way into the hospital, even though it was closed off, and subsequently serving as a liaison officer between staff and the Japanese unit of occupation. "Thanks to his tireless efforts and patience," Ferguson wrote, "at no time did the situation get out of control."[111]

Vera Nieh later wrote that the nursing students performed beautifully in terms of being able to complete their exam even while the PUMC was being taken over by Japanese troops. "Under such a state of chaos," Nieh recalled, "the students managed to complete all their graduation examinations satisfactorily."[112] In Nieh's view, the students had "acquired the 'inner equilibrium' from their training as nurses!"[113] Mary Ferguson specifically credited the students' PUMC training. For her, this incident and the response of PUMC nursing students and staff were "characteristic of the imperturbability with which the whole student body and staff throughout the institution met the crisis."[114]

While the exams continued for three days, it appears that Margaret Prentice and Chao Pei-chen were required only for the first day. After having tea with Faye Whiteside, Prentice left – only to be arrested when she returned to Tianjin. She was placed in prison in Tianjin for thirty-five days, after which she was placed under house arrest. On 28 March 1942, she was sent to the Weixian Internment Camp. She was repatriated back to the United States on the MS *Gripsholm* on 15 September 1943. The three foreign nurses on the PUMC staff were also arrested and interned: Faye Whiteside at Weixian Camp and Margaret Wyne and Ethel Robinson at Chapei Camp.[115]

ENEMY ALIENS

By the time of the attack on Pearl Harbor, it had been four years since universities and colleges started to evacuate from Japanese-occupied regions, fearing Japanese bombs and the physical takeover of the institutions. However, it was not until the United States entered the war with Japan that the Japanese military had the pretext it sought to "legitimately" take over foreign universities and other institution; Americans, the British, and citizens of British dominions (like Canada) were now "enemy aliens."[116] In Jinan, nursing students at the Shandong Christian University (Qilu) were also in the middle of writing NAC exams when Japanese soldiers streamed onto campus and locked the gates.[117] In Tianjin, armed Japanese soldiers took over the Douw Presbyterian Hospital, after searching for any American workers on site.[118] They even took over small sites, such as St. Paul's Anglican Hospital in Sanqui, Henan.[119] The swiftness of the move took staff and students (and patients) everywhere by surprise. It also highlighted how highly coordinated the Japanese occupiers were.

A series of foreshadowing events described by Margaret Prentice in her recollection of the days leading up to the PUMC exams confirmed this sense of Japanese readiness to extend its control in the immediate aftermath of the bombing of Pearl Habor.[120] Preparing to travel by train from Tianjin to Beijing a couple of days before the exams, Prentice went to the Japanese police station to seek a travel permit. As she later recalled, the officer had difficulty concealing his surprise when she stated her intention to be at Beijing by 8:00 a.m. on 8 December. He also asked the unusual question of how many Americans worked at her hospital in Tianjin (she was the only one). When she returned the next day to pick up the permit, she hesitated in front of the officer, who gave what she recalled as an "icy, hateful stare." By premonition, she decided to take "plenty of money" – two hundred dollars – along on her trip.[121] Arriving at the train station on Saturday, Prentice was initially refused admission to the platform; she did not have an "emergency" vaccination certificate recently ordered by the Japanese. She described a chaotic scene of Chinese officers beating and yelling at passengers as they tried to push through turnstiles without showing the necessary certificate. Avoiding the vaccination units set up along the street, Prentice rushed back to the hospital for assistance from colleagues. One nurse, a Miss Chu-Ke, quickly "vaccinated me on my lower arm because my sleeve was too tight to raise higher," while another, a Miss Ku, "filled out the blanks required for vaccination."[122] Prentice made it back to the train on time. She found a vacant seat opposite a middle-aged Japanese man, who "stealthily" asked her what Americans thought of the "unsolved American-Japanese problems." Not knowing how to respond, she stated that she thought Americans hoped the problems would soon be settled satisfactorily to all concerned. As she later recalled, the atmosphere, re-marks, and actions of the Japanese all around were unsettling: "There was something eerie in our midst," she wrote.[123]

The main aim of the Japanese when they marched into the PUMC and other foreign institutions on 8 December 1941 was to identify and arrest enemy aliens working on site. Initially imprisoned or placed under house arrest, American, British, Canadian, and other (mostly European) staff were eventually interned in camps set up around China for that purpose (see Appendix 3, "List of Interned Nurses in China"). As soldiers en-tered the PUMC, others simultaneously went to the director's residence, where Henry Houghton, Trevor Pryse Bowen, and Hamilton H. Anderson were having breakfast. Houghton and Bowen were taken into custody, first to Lockhart Hall, where the Japanese had installed their general headquarters for the gendarmerie.[124] Then they were taken to the barracks of the United States Marines, where they were held for a month with a mixed group of enemy aliens.[125] While the three men remained in custody, all of their companions were released on 8 January 1942, except Dr. I. Snapper, the Dutch professor of medicine at the PUMC, and John Leighton Stuart, president of Yenching University. The men were taken to the Ying Compound (Houghton's home), still under guard.[126] Snapper was a department head of medicine, which, to the Japanese, meant he was dean of medicine – they thus had mistaken him for someone else. However, when they realized their mistake, they did not release him.[127]

In a censored report, Mary Ferguson later outlined a few more de-tails about the broader implications and events surrounding the Japanese invasion after Pearl Harbor. See Figure 4.2 Report by Mary Ferguson provided to the US State Department, from the MS *Gripsholm*, 1943. "News of the outbreak of war reached most people in Peking [Beijing], Chinese as well as foreign, through a Shanghai broadcast at 8 a.m. on

PEKING, CHINA
December 8, 1941 - September 15, 1943

News of the outbreak of war reached most people
in Peking, Chinese as well as foreign, through a
Shanghai broadcast at 8 a.m. on December 8th which
gave the bald statement of fact only. American and
British broadcasts picked up later told of the attacks
on Pearl Harbor, Manila and other places.

Large placards appeared throughout the city, hasti-
ly written by hand in English, Russian and Chinese, in-
structing "enemy nationals" to register at the Japanese
Embassy without delay giving detailed information about
their property, movable and immovable, funds on hand and
in local banks, limiting their movements to a radius of
six kilometers from their residence, and forbidding
assembly of groups of more than three persons.

Early in the morning and in some cases before word
of the outbreak of war had been received, Japanese military occupied such "enemy" institutions as banks,
schools, hospitals and mission compounds. Prominent
among these were the National City Bank of N.Y., Yenching University, and the Peiping Union Medical College,
the two latter being cordoned off so that no one could
get in or out on December 8th. The following day persons identified as being on the staff were allowed to
pass the sentries and thus reestablish contact between
the inside and outside. The degree of isolation varied
in different cases, seeming to depend on the officer in
charge at each individual place. Most "enemy" telephones were cut on December 8th but a few seem to have
been overlooked so that it was possible for some of the
isolated groups to communicate with each other.

Immediate internment was the expectation of most
"enemy nationals" many of whom packed suitcases in

FIGURE 4.2 Report by Mary Ferguson provided to the US State Department, from
the MS *Gripsholm*, 1943. | Courtesy Rockefeller Archive Centre, RAC-CMB_FA065_B57_
F397_001.

December 8th which gave the bald statement of fact only," she recalled.[128]
Only later did American and British broadcasts report the attacks on
Pearl Harbor and other places.

> Large placards appeared throughout the city, hastily written by
> hand in English, Russian and Chinese, instructing "enemy nation-
> als" to register at the Japanese Embassy without delay giving de-
> tailed information about their property, movable and immovable,
> funds on hand and in local banks, limiting their movements to a
> radius of six kilometers from their residence, and forbidding as-
> sembly of more than three persons.[129]

Early that morning, the Japanese military "occupied such 'enemy' institutions as banks, schools, hospitals and mission compounds."[130] This included Yenching University and the PUMC, both of which were
cordoned off so that no one could get in or out until the next day, when
persons identified as staff were allowed in.

The PUMC, Occupied

After the Japanese army – specifically, the Army Medical Service – took
over the PUMC, the hospital outpatient department never reopened.
And, after 8 December 1941, no new inpatients were admitted, with the
exception of "a handful of emergency cases" when the commanding officer gave special permission.[131] During that time, a Mrs. J.H. Ingram
died of typhus fever. The Japanese occupiers "evidently had no specific
information or instruction as to the plans of the higher authorities" in
regards to the PUMC, so the Army Medical Service aimed to keep things
"running normally as far as possible" and to prevent the pilfering of
PUMC property and equipment. At first, discharge of patients was not
encouraged, "since this would eventually empty the hospital."[132] All
members of the staff were subjected to bodily searches going in and out
of the property gates. At first, the Japanese slept in the corridors. However, after a few days, they turned one of the wards into a dormitory for
the soldiers.

During the first week of occupation, there were no classes. However, PUMC students (medical and nursing) remained in their dormitories. All of the gates to the hospital compound were closed except the west gate, which the Japanese used themselves, and the north gate – the hospital service entrance – through which everyone else had to pass, and where they were subject to the "most thorough" inspections.[133] Those entering had to take off their hats, bow, and present their identification cards. "The nurses had the hardest time," recalled Dr. Stephen Chang. "How the soldiers gloated over the examinations." In one case, a nurse was wearing a menstrual pad, and a sentry insisted on displaying it. The woman screamed, bringing an officer to the scene. The officer slapped the sentry, Chang reported, "and I heard the fellow was severely punished." After that, the inspections of the nurses "never became so bad, but [was] often bad enough."[134]

At first, it seemed that the Japanese might allow the PUMC to remain open.[135] A faculty meeting was called and was attended by all faculty. Dr. Fortuyn insisted that no decisions could be made (or, at least, would be valid) without approval from the CMB headquarters in New York. Dr. Harold Loucks disagreed.[136] The way around the requirement to involve New York was to have only Chinese faculty attend the meetings. "That saved the day," recalled Stephen Chang. "After that all meetings were without foreigners."[137] The (Chinese) faculty discussed whether to keep only the hospital open, or both the hospital and the school. Stephen Chang had heard from Dr. Mashuhashi that there had been "a standing order from Tokyo to close all American and British schools."[138] Officially, the PUMC was in that category, but the hospital was a different issue. Yet, if only the hospital were kept open, staff who were not connected with the hospital would be without salaries. Dr. S.T. Wang, superintendent of the PUMC Hospital (and the only senior administrator still functioning in their role), did not want to have to ask the non-hospital staff to sacrifice themselves while he continued somehow to run the hospital. Accordingly, the Chinese faculty group decided to "swim or sink together."[139] All the plans from there were to include both the medical and nursing schools.

The faculty's first recommendation to the Japanese was not accepted, so they kept revising the drafts.[140] In the meantime, they obtained permission from Major Suzuki, the Japanese commanding officer, to carry on classes and allow students into the hospital again. Regular class work continued from 15 December until 19 January 1942. Although no new inpatients were received at the hospital, students were able to continue their clinical work with the patients who remained. However, with everyone under so much pressure – and with the place rife with rumours – work was at a virtual standstill. Patients were now encouraged to leave.

Soldiers slept anywhere they liked, "but mostly on the floor around the information desk." As Stephen Chang recalled, "I always had the impression that [the information desk] was the only place they were sure they would know when they woke up so that they [wouldn't] be late for duty."[141] The Japanese paid the staff salary for December. This made the staff hopeful that the hospital would remain open. Members of a faculty committee "worked continuously" on a plan for the hospital, various versions were "disapproved continuously." Chang was told "again and again" that it was "hopeless" to include the school with the hospital.[142]

On 19 January 1942, Dr. S.T. Wang was notified by the Japanese commanding officer that "classes must be discontinued that day, that the preclinical departments should be closed by the end of the week, and that all students must leave the main buildings within two days – staying in the dormitories only until arrangements for departure could be made."[143] Students would be "allowed to take away any books and instruments which were their personal property."[144] It came as a "great blow" to be "suddenly told that the local Japanese Headquarters had decided to close the PUMC [education work] and to take over the hospital for a base hospital."[145] "You can imagine the effect of this tragic news," Dr. Stephen Chang wrote Dr. Claude Forkner. "There we were trying to keep up for over a month and were always given hope, but actually we were only be[ing] strangled slowly."[146] Wang called a meeting with all senior staff of the PUMC, noting that the house staff would soon, like the students, be dispersed. The number of patients had decreased to about 130. The commanding officer was willing to allow patients who were seriously ill to remain as long as necessary, with as many members of the medical and nursing staff as would be needed to care for them. However, Wang noted, "no new patients would be admitted for the duration of the war."[147] After much discussion, it was unanimously agreed that it would be best for all concerned to close the whole institution – including the hospital – on 31 January 1942, and that "it should be possible to discharge or transfer all patients from the hospital by that date."[148]

As Stephen Chang later remembered, rumours spread that the reason the Japanese closed the hospital was because people like I.C. Yuan and Hsien Wu "and others of the non-clinical staff" had insisted on "swimming or dying together."[149] The general opinion was that, if the faculty had petitioned for the continuation of only the hospital, it would have been allowed to stay open. "The closure of the hospital of course affected the employees [sic] class most and many of them wanted to beat up the above mentioned professors [i.e., Yuan and Wu]." Chang himself believed that the hospital would have been taken over by the Japanese eventually in any case. "It would have been much worse if we [PUMC faculty] had been kept and forced to work for [the Japanese]," he noted. "A slow death is always a more painful death."[150]

On 19 January 1942, the day that Major Suzuki informed faculty that the PUMC would be closing – the Education Division of the PUMC Governing Council held an extraordinary meeting at which members of the two senior classes in medicine and nursing were granted degrees and diplomas normally given in June.[151] Undergraduate students also received a transcript of their academic record. Suzuki allowed Henry Houghton, then under house arrest, to sign the makeshift diplomas, and the graduating students to take a class picture.[152] "There were no graduation exercises held," Mary Ferguson wrote, "but the graduates were happy because it was possible to have Dr. Houghton's signature on their diplomas, and a class picture was taken in cap and gown."[153]

According to Stephen Chang, a Mrs. Thurmer worked very hard to get permission for Mary Ferguson to see Henry Houghton and have him sign all the diplomas. Dr. Mashuhashi, who had been surreptitiously supporting the Chinese faculty up to that point, was of such help "that at one time he was given severe warning by the [Japanese] Headquarters that he might be court-marshalled if he helped the Chinese too much."[154] Chang was both impressed and grateful. "If when the war is over and [Mashuhashi] is still alive I hope the PUMC will do the magnanimous act and thank him officially for what he did while we were in trouble." Mashuhashi ensured that he himself did the inspection at the South Gate when the students made their final departure. Mary Ferguson was also at the gate to say goodbye to each one of the students. "It was a very sad day indeed for her and I think she was great not to have broken down," Chang recalled. The students passed in a single file and went out "like a funeral procession."[155]

Dr. S.T. Wang was in charge of closing the hospital.[156] Vera Nieh was in charge of closing the nursing school. Stephen Chang noted that Nieh "not only closed the school smoothly, but even arranged for the students to finish their work in some other hospitals. She was great all through these days."[157] To Nieh, it was important to ensure that the nursing students were looked after. "After getting the order from the Japanese," she later recalled, "my students, they were all excited and they cried, and I told them I would do my best [to help]."[158] She made arrangements according to the students' wishes. For those who wanted to return home, she arranged for them to be sent home safely. For those who wanted to complete their studies, "[I] tried my best to arrange it to the different hospital nursing schools ... I asked the [nursing service] to type up [for] each student what more theory they need[ed], and how many hours, and what kind of [nursing] service they need[ed] to practice before they can graduate."[159] She found placements for all of the senior students, in Beijing, Tianjin, or Shanghai, to complete their practical experience.[160] By all accounts, Nieh and her colleagues made suitable alternate arrangements for all of the nursing students – something that would be considered extraordinary by any standards.

On 31 January, all staff were paid, including an additional one-month salary. As each received their pay, they turned in their identification pass and left the building, carrying their personal property with them. Women's dormitories, including those for nurses, were closed on that same date. "When the nurses left Oliver Hall," Stephen Chang recalled, "they left the place in a mess and the Japs were mad."[161] Chang and Mary Ferguson subsequently went through the medical student dorms themselves, ensuring everything was in order. The Japanese now had complete control of the PUMC.[162]

SCATTERED LIVES

After the PUMC was closed, staff and students were "scattered to the four corners of the country."[163] They picked up work wherever they could find it. Most medical staff went into private practice. For a short period, it was thought that perhaps the PUMC could take over the Central Hospital ("as badly run as any hospital could be") from a group of French Catholic nuns.[164] However, the Japanese would not allow it. Still, the Chinese managed to "infiltrate" the Central Hospital: "Instead of getting ... many PUMC people in at one stroke, they now resorted to the infiltration method and now the whole of the Central Hospital is manned by PUMC staff, down to the telephone operator and messenger boys." While a much smaller hospital than the PUMC, the Central Hospital worked well as a PUMC alternative, since there were "no Japanese doctors or nurses or advisors there."[165] One group of graduates went to Tianjin, rented a hotel, and changed it into a hospital; PUMC alumnus Wang Loh Loh (Wang Yi) was the nursing superintendent there before she moved to Free China. By July 1943, Dr. Stephen Chang, who was by then also in Free China, noted that all the PUMC students who had gone to Shanghai and other places "turned to Free China, and many have managed to cross [the border to get there]."[166]

The Chinese populace was upset by the closure of the PUMC, which they saw as an "inhumane act."[167] According to Stephen Chang, the Japanese therefore tried to justify its closure by "proving to the people what an inhumane and rascally institution PUMC was." First, they asserted that the PUMC "cut open the dead Father of the Chinese Republic and stole all the insides and kept them in bottles." In order to prove their point, they had a "very impressive" memorial service in the room where Sun Yat-sen was supposed to have died "and a bottle containing his carcinoma of liver was displayed and worshipped." Journalists and "important people" were invited, and pictures filled the newspapers for days. The "carcinoma finally went down in state to [Nanjing] to lie with the mummy."[168] Second, the Japanese claimed that the PUMC had destroyed or stolen the "Peking Man," a famous fossil skull of *Homo erectus* discovered in 1923–27 during excavations near Beijing. They pledged to "leave no stone unturned until this rare specimen of archeology was returned to the Chinese people." Henry Houghton and Trevor Bowen were interrogated about the Peking Man. Archeologists came from Japan to check over the skulls in the anatomy department. Newspapers were full of the theft of Peking Man for weeks, until they finally died out after they failed to find the skull. "The skull was, of course, no more in PUMC," noted Stephen Chang, in a letter to Dr. Claude Forkner, mysteriously adding, "I think you know where it might be."[169]

After the PUMC closed, former administrators attempted to transfer a contingent of Chinese staff, including nurses, to another hospital, but the Japanese did not favour the idea of the PUMC carrying on its tradition elsewhere.[170] Some former staff managed to slip through the lines to West China, but this was not possible for many.[171] As far as students were concerned, most were from the South and wished to go to Shanghai, but no one could travel in occupied areas without travel passes issued by the Special Police (Chinese forces working for the Japanese).[172] Normally, a person had to apply for a pass and then wait until they were summoned and questioned. The PUMC was given only two weeks to get the passes, and there were at least fifty students, a hundred nurses, and some other fellowship students who wanted to go to Shanghai.[173] Stephen Chang asked Dr. Mashuhashi for help, and he got Dr. Yokomini, the new superintendent, to provide a guarantee for all of the applications. Chang wrote up the applications and got Yokomini's seal on all of them. Now the Special Police had to approve the applications. "The Chinese traitor in charge of traveling passes," Chang noted, "was a very nasty chap." He slapped the first student and said, "before you PUMC people were running dogs to the Americans, and now you're running dogs to the Japanese." He refused to issue the passes. That meant, "of course, that Yokomini lost face," Chang continued, "and it was in no time after that that all passes came out all right."[174]

Nursing students who went to Shanghai were absorbed into various hospitals.[175] In Beijing, Vera Nieh had arranged for first- and second-year nursing students "who were interested in continuing their nursing [program]" to transfer to the nurses' training school of the Presbyterian Douw Hospital.[176] Since most of the PUMC faculty were still in Beijing, all the class instruction for PUMC students at the Douw Hospital was provided by former PUMC staff. Students gained clinical experience in the Douw Hospital as well as at the Health Station in Beijing. Arrangements were also made for third-year students to complete their practical training in hospitals in Beijing and Tianjin.[177] The PUMC diploma of nursing was awarded to eighteen students who completed their course of study in the middle of June 1942. Nieh later noted that, "since no open meetings of any kind were allowed, a quiet graduation party was given for them at the YWCA."[178] Three first-year and seven second-year students eventually completed their nursing program by "grafting" onto clinical experiences at the Douw Hospital and the Health Station, passing the NAC exams in 1943 and 1944, respectively. They were not, however, allowed a PUMC diploma until they completed additional practical work. The 1943 students were required to undertake six more months at the PUMC Hospital, or at some hospital abroad (by 1948, several of these nurses had gone to the United States). The graduates from 1944 were required to do one more year of practical work as well as class work at the PUMC. Of the ten students who passed their NAC exams in 1943 or 1944, eight were doing "this make up work here and abroad" in 1948.[179]

To Stephen Chang, who was intimately involved with the closing of the PUMC, "those were the days when the real character of the man came out."[180] Dr. Mashuhashi proved himself loyal to the PUMC beyond anything Chang would have expected of a Japanese national. Vera Nieh proved her excellent organizational skills and did not leave until every student's plans were attended to. He also credited students, whom he characterized as cooperation personified, with the smoothness of the closure of the school: "They stuck around me and helped me at every turn. It was really a joy to see that while many of the older fellows of the college proved unworthy of their high calling, the students rose to the situation magnificently."[181] Some students arranged for others to have travel funds to return home. Chang rented a house and boarded as many students as he could. Dr. C.H. Chu took in three students until they could get away. Dr. S.T. Wang stayed on at the PUMC Hospital for an additional month after the students left to complete the transfer to the Japanese military.

STEPHEN CHANG: NOTES FROM THE INSIDE

Having taken over the PUMC Hospital and campus, the Japanese military retained a skeleton staff of PUMC employees to assist them. They included the former secretary to the PUMC director (Mrs. Thurmer), the librarian (Dr. Mashuhashi), the supervisor of buildings and grounds (Mr. Yang), an assistant engineer (Archie Chang), and the custodian of keys (James Chen).[182] In addition, sixty servants were retained to keep the buildings in order, including a contingent of approximately twenty laundrymen, a dozen janitors, and others with roles such as electrician, gardener, and carpenter.[183] Dr. Stephen Chang was also retained to help.

In a fourteen-page, single-spaced report written from the safety of West China in July 1943, Chang detailed for Claude Forkner, the director of the China Medical Board, behind-the-scene events in the PUMC before and after the takeover. Although he prefaced his report with the disclaimer that "I'm afraid I cannot call this an official scientific report as the thing happened one and a half years ago and the whole thing was a nightmare anyway," what he wrote was a clear and remarkable indictment of the Japanese.[184] To Chang, the events of 8 December 1941 were simply the culmination of what the PUMC had had to put up with in the preceding months. Although he was employed by the PUMC as a physician, Chang had also been appointed by the Japanese as the proctor of the men's dormitory and, unofficially, their "assistant recorder." In his roles, Chang had many opportunities to visit the local, special, and Japanese police, to whom he was required to report on the various activities of the school. This included reporting on suspected espionage by American citizens of Chinese descent. On one occasion, a student was not in his bed during the nightly head count. He had disappeared. After four days of inquiry, they found that he had been taken to the Japanese gendarmerie, where he had been "put through the third degree and suffered much ill-treatment." The student had been taken from the steps of the YMCA, where he had a cup of coffee every night; the Japanese thought he was going there regularly to provide espionage reports.

To Chang, "the servant class" at the PUMC caused "great trouble" in the months leading up to Pearl Harbor. They were backed, he asserted, by Japanese-controlled Chinese police. In one case, a Miss Hirst, the chief of housekeeping services, caught a servant smoking during office hours "and fired him on the spot." The man slapped her in the face, breaking her glasses. He was taken to the police, but, instead of punishing him, they fined Miss Hirst $300 "for being impolite to the servant." In another instance, the PUMC Dietary Department started a sit-down strike after a staff member had been dismissed. PUMC comptroller Trevor Bowen went downstairs to meet with the striking workers, where he was subsequently "beaten up." Those involved decided it was no use to call the police. "Such things never happened before in the annals of the PUMC," wrote Chang – and, were it not for Chang's report, it is unlikely they ever would have been recorded.

On 8 December 1941, Stephen Chang was listening to a Shanghai radio station when he heard the words, "Ladies and Gentlemen, I have only one announcement to make. Japan has declared war on Great Britain and America. All Americans and British are requested to stay home and keep tuned for further news and instructions. This is probably my last announcement." And it was. Chang called the hospital information desk and received the news that Japanese soldiers were at that moment entering the gates and encircling the whole hospital. Dr. Harold Loucks, who lived in a residence across from Chang, called up the Ying Compound where Trevor Bowen was staying. Bowen answered the phone only to tell Loucks that, "at that very moment the Japs were walking towards him to arrest him." It was the first day of classes after winter break, and students had just returned to the dormitories. Chang pulled the dormitory fire alarm and, when everyone was assembled in the dining room, announced the tragic news. All students who had homes to go to in the city should move home immediately, he stated, and those who had no home close by should at least, and immediately, find a place to move their belongings to. Those who wanted to stay, could, but those who wanted to "beat it" should do so. "Within a half hour," Chang wrote, "the whole Wenham Hall was empty." When the Japanese soldiers arrived shortly thereafter, Chang took them around to the dormitory and told them that "many students had not come back after winter recess." The soldiers took the keys from Chang and told him that if anybody took anything from the dormitory, he would be shot.

For the next few days, the dormitory was disconnected from the hospital. This was significant, since the hospital kitchen normally brought over food and coal. However, according to Chang, the hospital was commanded by the Japanese army, whereas the dormitory was commanded by the gendarmerie. Chang and the students kept up the heating in the dormitory by burning "enemy propaganda material." Chang was given four hours to list every item in the dormitory and provide a price for each. Thinking that the list might be used for reparations after the war, Chang gave high estimates. However, after he submitted the list, the Japanese informed him that, if anything from the list were broken or stolen, Chang would be personally responsible to pay for it. He had to sign papers promising to act for the Japanese in guarding the property against sabotage. He also had to go to the Special Police to promise he would spy on American citizens of Chinese descent and the one German Jew who was living at the PUMC.

Chang noted that, on 8 December, practically every staff member living at the North Compound "ran away" but almost none from the South Compound. He was angry with I.C. Yuan, who had departed immediately without helping the female students in the women's dormitory in the North Compound. Things were so frantic that "one assistant professor in his haste to beat it," Chang recalled, "forgot to take away his baby sleeping upstairs." The baby was eventually retrieved. To Chang, those who panicked and left without considering others were, simply, selfish.

Japanese sentries stood guard throughout the dorms. The Chinese staff and students were required to keep them supplied with whiskey and beer, and peanuts to go with the drinks. If the Chinese wished to smuggle something in or out of the dorms, they would give the sentries "an unusually liberal dose" of alcohol and the sentries "would doze off into oblivion." The Japanese went through the offices of the director (Henry Houghton) and comptroller (Trevor Bowen) and recorder but, as Dr. Mashuhashi later told Stephen Chang, since they were "not gifted with the knowledge of the English language, they left in disgust." Nor did the Japanese force open the safe in Houghton's office, which was a "lucky carelessness," since it contained many personal documents. (Mary Ferguson later secretly emptied the safe.) Instead, the Japanese left his office with cigarettes that Houghton kept for guests.

On about day three or four, the Japanese asked Chang to remove some band instruments from storage. Since the United States Marine Band had recently played a farewell concert at the PUMC, the Japanese believed the instruments had been left behind. Chang could not find the instruments, and "for days I had to go with them through the basement rooms to look for the ghost band." Eventually, the Japanese gave up on the band instruments, instead insisting that Chang entertain them "most every other day" on the pipe organ. Curiously, they kept requesting the hymn "Nearer My God to Thee." Eventually Chang asked why they kept insisting on that song. The Japanese soldiers responded that they had heard that, when an American ship sank, those aboard always played or sang this hymn. "They like to hear it," Chang wrote, "because they believed all the American warships were being sunk."

The PUMC property was used for a variety of purposes: a military hospital, a serological institute, gendarmerie headquarters, a hotel (in the men's dormitories), and general residence.[185] Immediate plans were made to accommodate some 1,000 wounded soldiers in the hospital, now under "the Suzuki unit." The college buildings went to the unit in charge of epidemic prevention. The compounds went to the army headquarters for the officers. Oliver Jones Hall and Lockhard Hall (dormitories) went to the gendarmerie. Wenham Hall was slated to be an army dormitory. Some 900 wounded arrived the first week. They "all came in at midnight and streets were put under martial law to prevent people seeing them come in." After a few days, the Japanese came up with an idea. They "roped off the street in front of the hospital gate with a sign, 'Smallpox.'" This is when Stephen Chang was secured to entertain the patients by playing the pipe organ. Deciding that the instruments and supplies were not suitable to care for Japanese patients, the soldiers removed basins, inhalation pots, infusion sets, enema cans, and bedpans, ostensibly to burn them in a bonfire. "Grand scale looting by the soldiers soon followed," wrote Chang, and "one could buy anything from the streets from the PUMC." Even organ pipes were taken down and "blown by the soldiers up and down the streets." There were only two medical officers in the hospital to care for all the wounded. The pharmacy "was pitiful," wrote Chang: "The soldiers chose the beautiful bottles and poured off the contents and took the bottles away to play with."

As time went on, the Japanese found it more and more difficult financially to keep up the hospital. Eventually they discharged everyone except Archie Chang, who had to look after the electric generators and other electric appliances. Machinery, steam-pipes, stoves, and scraps (including wire from animal cages) began to disappear, "probably on their way to Japan." By the time Stephen Chang left Beijing for Free China, the pharmacy was completely empty, and all of the library books were for sale on the street.

INTERNMENT AND REPATRIATION

There were 300,000 Allied nationals in Japanese hands during the Second World War.[186] Quite apart from military prisoners of war, Japan held 13,544 civilian men, women, and children captive in China and Hong Kong, including 2,610 Americans and 311 Canadians.[187] Missionaries made up only a fraction of the total number of internees: 10 percent of Americans (245 individuals) and 3 percent of Canadians (10 individuals) were missionaries. Nurses constituted an even smaller proportion of internees – 1 percent of the American (25 nurses) and 4 percent of the Canadian internees (13 nurses).[188] Placed in this context, the number of PUMC nurses who were interned is remarkable: they made up 36 percent (5 of 14) of the total of interned PUMC faculty and staff. Three of the interned PUMC nurses were American, one was British, and one was Canadian. None of the Canadian West China missionary nurses were interned, a direct result of living in Free China. Three of the North

TABLE 4.1 Interned PUMC staff and faculty

Surname	Given name	Nationality	Place	Occupation	Camp	Dates interned
Anderson	Hamilton H.	American	PUMC	Professor of medicine	Weixian	Mar.–Sep. 43
Alston	William Graham	British	PUMC	Chief engineer	Peking British Embassy	May 43–Aug. 45
Alston	*n/a*	*–*	*–*	*Wife*	*Peking British Embassy*	*May 43–Aug. 45*
Alston	*Ethel M.*	*–*	*–*	*Daughter*	*Peking British Embassy*	*May 43–Aug. 45*
Bowen	Trevor Pryse	American	PUMC	Comptroller	Peking British Embassy	Dec. 41–Aug. 45
Ferguson	Mary Esther	American	PUMC	Secretary	Peking British Embassy	May–Sep. 43
Ferguson	*John Calvin*	*American*	*–*	*Retired*	*Peking British Embassy*	*May–Sep. 43*
Hirst	**Elizabeth H.**	**American**	**PUMC**	**Nurse**	**Weixian**	**Mar.–Sep. 43**
Houghton	Henry Spencer	American	PUMC	Director	Peking British Embassy	Dec. 41–Aug. 45
Loucks	Harold H.	American	PUMC	Professor of surgery	Weixian	Mar.–Sep. 43
McMillan	**Elizabeth**	**British**	**PUMC**	**Nurse**	**Weixian**	**Mar. 43–Aug. 45**
Pratt	Miriam I.	American	PUMC	Dietician	Weixian	Mar.–Sep. 43
Pratt	*Jane*	*American*	*–*	*Daughter*	*Weixian*	*Mar.–Sep. 43*
Pratt	*Nancy*	*American*	*–*	*Daughter*	*Weixian*	*Mar.–Sep. 43*
Pratt	*Margaret*	*American*	*–*	*Daughter*	*Weixian*	*Mar.–Sep. 43*
Robinson	**Ethel E.**	**Canadian**	**PUMC**	**Nurse**	**Chapei**	**Mar.–Sep. 43**
Snapper	Isidore	Dutch	PUMC	Professor of medicine	Marine Barracks	Dec. 41–Aug. 42
Whiteside	**Faye**	**American**	**PUMC**	**Superintendent of nursing**	**Weixian**	**Mar.–Sep. 43**
Wyne	**Margaret**	**American**	**PUMC**	**Nurse**	**Chapei**	**Mar.–Sep. 43**

NOTE: PUMC nurses are in bold; family members of PUMC staff/faculty are in italics.

China Mission nurses (Dorothy Boyd, Margaret Gay, Clara Preston) also avoided internment by evacuating to Free China. Four Canadian nurses who chose to stay in occupied regions (against consular advice) were interned: Susie Kelsey, Mary Boyd Stanley, Betty Thomson Gale, and Georgina Menzies Lewis. Of these, Susie Kelsey was the only one repatriated, in September 1943. The others remained imprisoned until Japan's surrender, in August 1945. Of the five interned PUMC nurses (Elizabeth Hirst, Elizabeth McMillan, Ethel Robinson, Faye Whiteside, and Margaret Wyne), four were repatriated in September 1943; only British nurse Elizabeth McMillan (and the other British PUMC internees) remained interned until August 1945 (see Table 4.1).

When the Japanese military took over the PUMC, one of the immediate orders of the day was to identify and detain "enemy aliens" – that is, citizens of Allied nations, including the United States, Canada, England, Australia, New Zealand, the Netherlands, and other European allied states. The evacuation and later internment of Allied citizens had, of course, an impact on the number of foreign nurses working at the PUMC. The number of American nurses at the PUMC had peaked in the 1920s, steadily declined through the 1930s, and zeroed out after 1942. The number of Chinese nurses rose steadily until 1935, held fairly steady through the second half of the 1930s, and fell precipitously during the

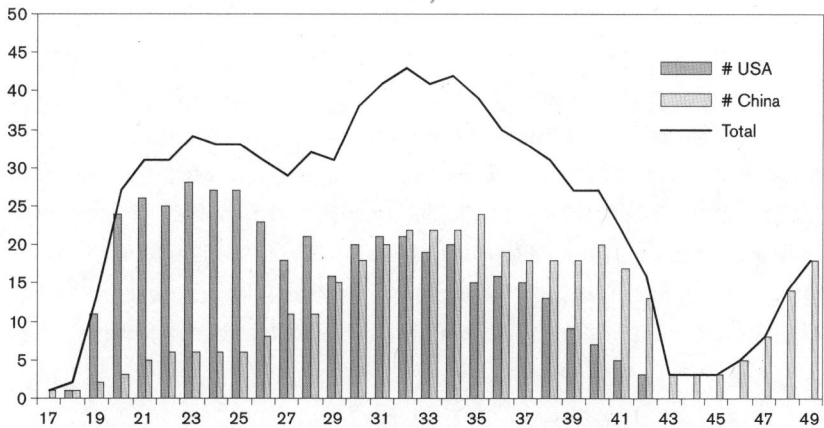

FIGURE 4.3 Number of American and Chinese nursing staff at the PUMC, 1917–49. | Data compiled by author.

refugee PUMC years (1943–46), only to start to rise again following the return to Beijing. During and after the war years, the PUMC staff was predominantly, and then exclusively, Chinese (Figure 4.3).

At the PUMC, most "enemy" telephones were immediately cut once the Japanese took over the campus; the few that were overlooked allowed some of the isolated groups to communicate with each other.[189] Most of the PUMC enemy aliens expected immediate internment and packed their bags expectantly. Yet, initially, only a few were detained. The Japanese gendarmerie set up temporary offices in the PUMC and questioned a group of twenty or twenty-five American and British men ("educators, missionaries, ne'er-do-wells, newspaper men, engineers").[190] After a day of waiting and questioning, they were transferred to the American Marine Barracks. About a month later, all were released, with the exception of Dr. John Leighton Stuart, president of Yenching University; Dr. Henry S. Houghton, director of the PUMC; Dr. Isadore Snapper, a professor of medicine; and Trevor Brown, the comptroller of the PUMC. No specific charges were ever made; the released men had no more idea of the reason for their release than the reason for their arrest.[191]

The four remaining men were held on the third floor of the Marine Barracks in Beijing for a month. They were then held for a month at Henry Houghton's home (Ying Compound on the PUMC campus) before moving into the rear quarters of the residence of a British businessman in Beijing, along with seven guards.[192] In August 1942, Snapper was released, part of a group being repatriated. Approximately 600 expatriates from China would depart Shanghai aboard the Italian steamer *Conte Verde* and sail as far as Lourenço Marques (Maputo), the capital of Mozambique. There they would meet up with 900 expatriates from Japan, sailing aboard the *Asama Maru*. These 1,500-odd passengers would transfer to the *MS Gripsholm*. Repatriation would take ten weeks.[193] The *Gripsholm* served under the International Red Cross with a Swedish captain and crew. It made thirty-three exchange trips through the war, carrying over 27,000 repatriates.[194] Although Snapper was released, the local military refused to allow the other three to go. They were held incommunicado and spent the rest of the war "in detention."[195]

In February 1942, a Japanese-controlled newspaper in China had this headline: "Peking Union Medical College, Yenching University Abolished: Japanese Army Authorities Get Proofs of Their Pro-Chungking [Chongqing] Activities."[196] The article stated that, "since the outbreak of the China Affair, [these universities] had shown indisputably hostile attitudes against Japan."[197] It also asserted that the universities showed pro-British and pro-American activities. "It is much to be congratulated," it concluded, "that many of the teaching staff or students of these two schools have awaken[ed] to the ideal of the construction of the Greater East Asia new order."[198] Those who left the PUMC or Yenching, the article claimed, would be helped to enter other schools or professions.

According to a 15 May 1942 report by Mary Ferguson, foreign staff at the PUMC who were not placed under immediate arrest were confined in their own homes and unrestricted in their movements within the city walls.[199] Two of these, Dr. Harold Loucks and Dr. Hamilton Anderson, moved to a house in the Methodist mission compound so they could continue to practice, by caring for the foreign community, and to advise and support junior members of the PUMC medical staff working at the Methodist and Presbyterian Hospitals.[200] They lived with Professor Davis of Yenching University and Mr. Henson of the Methodist mission.[201] Anderson became the medical officer for Americans and British living in Beijing. Loucks went around the city acting as a consulting surgeon to all the mission and private hospitals, getting around by bicycle.[202] By the winter of 1942, the Japanese decided to take over all mission hospitals, starting with the British Charity Hospital, followed by the Methodist Hospital, the Sleeper Davis Women's Hospital, and finally the Presbyterian Hospital. After this takeover, Loucks could no longer visit the hospitals openly, but the staff would arrange "the big operations at night for him after the Japs had gone home to sleep."[203]

Most of the senior members of the Chinese medical staff found work in private practice in Beijing or Tianjin, with the younger ones establishing practices independently or in groups.[204] The "lowest-paid" group of PUMC employees found work as day labourers, "peddling peanuts and fruit, pulling rickshaws, or operating the new tri-cycle rickshaws."[205] It was the clerical staff who felt the loss of employment most severely.

"Their chief tool, familiarity with the English language," wrote Mary Ferguson, "is now a handicap."[206] There was simply not a demand for English-language skills in Japanese-occupied China, and those who spoke the language were regarded with hostility. Stephen Chang noted that Ferguson, who helped out Dr. Hoeppli, the Swiss consul in Beijing, after the PUMC closure, "lost over 30 pounds these days and she was as near to a nervous breakdown as anybody could be. Poor girl, the stress and strain of it all was really too much for her."[207]

For her part, Ferguson, in a May 1942 report, expressed gratitude to the CMB for the various messages that came to the PUMC via the "Swiss authorities." She noted that the foreign staff of the PUMC were "most appreciative of the efforts being taken in New York for their repatriation."[208] She also noted that Harold Loucks, along with William Alston and his wife and daughter, had decided to stay in China rather than be repatriated. Ferguson herself also preferred to remain in Beijing with her father, retired physician John Calvin Ferguson, who was not applying for repatriation. The rest were hoping to return to the United States and applied for repatriation.

In March 1943, Allied citizens living in Beijing, Tianjin, and Qingdao were interned in Weixian (Weihsien), located about 100 miles northwest of Qingdao. On 24 March 1943, over a year after the Japanese takeover of the PUMC, the first group of enemy aliens – chiefly Americans – was sent to Weixian Camp. This included PUMC surgeon Harold H. Loucks and PUMC nursing faculty Faye Whiteside and Margaret Wyne.[209] The second group – British, Dutch, and Belgians – was sent on 29 March 1943.[210] The Japanese made extensive searches of luggage, and then required each person, irrespective of age or physical condition, to walk from the assembly point at the American Embassy to the railway station, each carrying their own luggage.[211] Gladys Stephenson, the British missionary nurse who collaborated with PUMC nursing after the Shanghai Incident in 1932, was interned in Shanghai from April 1943 to August 1945 at the Lunghwa Internment Camp.[212]

Following the departure of the two groups of internees, life for those remaining in Beijing "settled into a quiet routine that was undisturbed" until 29 April 1943, when Japanese physicians were sent to re-examine those previously exempted due to health reasons to determine how many had improved sufficiently to be interned.[213] Twenty-five more individuals were sent to Weixian Camp on 15 May. At this point, all of the PUMC staff were interned at the Weixian Camp in Shandong except Ethel Robinson and Margaret Wyne, who were interned at Chapei Camp, and Houghton, Bowen, and Stuart, now interned at the Peking British Embassy Camp. The latter three men were not provided with food or an allowance for maintenance; a small monthly allowance was given to the two servants who cared for their needs, and in the winter of 1942 they were provided coal. Their maintenance was first covered by ample funds on hand, and later by money smuggled in by foreign friends, to whom it had "been supplied by loyal Chinese friends." They were allowed to write and receive letters after censoring by the gendarmerie, and to receive books and gift parcels of food and toiletries that were left at the gate. "As far as is known," Mary Ferguson wrote in 1943, "no specific charges have ever been laid against these three men, nor have they had a judicial trial."[214] Henry Houghton and Trevor Bowen were questioned "as to the whereabouts of the skull of the Peking Man" (which, as discussed above, had disappeared in December 1941), with Bowen being kept at gendarmerie headquarters for several days of intensive questioning on the subject.[215] Neither of the men was in vigorous health. Henry Houghton suffering from sprue and a hernia, while Trevor Bowen was reportedly "highly strung and subject to periods of serious depression."[216]

Compared with other internment camps, the Peking British Embassy Camp was small: it held prisoners over the four years of its existence, compared with, for example, Pudong Camp, which held over 1,200 prisoners.[217] Of the fifty-four prisoners, half were still there in August 1945. Most of the others had been moved or repatriated, although seven had died. The camp housed both men and women, ranging in age from twenty-seven to eighty-two; there was also one infant. Nineteen were British; thirty-three were American; two were Dutch. It was unusual (and unusually cruel) for Houghton, Stuart, and Bowen to be held in detention.[218] According to Dr. Stephen Chang, the Japanese considered the three to be "political prisoners." Therefore, they were directly under the authority of the Japanese army; the Swiss consul had no opportunity to oversee living conditions, as they did with other civilian internees.[219] The three stayed locked in the servants' quarters. One night a business nearby caught fire. The Japanese sentry just locked the door where the three were kept. Fortunately, the fire was brought under control.[220] Although none of the remaining Chinese PUMC staff had access to the men, Dr. Mashuhashi did get to see them and told Dr. Stephen Chang that they "look all right" – perhaps with the exception of Trevor Bowen, who "has gone native and basks in the sun every day without anything between him and his Creator." Houghton described his four years of imprisonment as "an infinity of bleak silence."[221]

In September 1943, all PUMC Americans (except for political prisoners and Americans of Chinese descent, whom the Japanese did not consider American citizens) and a few others who chose to stay with friends at Weixian Camp were repatriated.[222] This included nine of the fourteen interned PUMC staff and faculty and their families – totalling twenty individuals. Houghton and Bowen were originally slated to be repatriated, but their names were removed by the local Japanese high command – without explanation.[223] The Japanese had no intention to repatriate them.[224] Asked later why the three were held separately and treated differently, Houghton surmised that "the only tenable theory seemed to be that the Japanese military mind simply could not conceive of institutions like Peking Union Medical College or Yenching having been created by private philanthropy or religious zeal. They must be instruments of the American government for winning the hearts of Chinese youth and thus thwarting their own imperialistic designs."[225]

Although most records have the PUMC internees departing in September 1943, it seems that some of them attempted to evacuate earlier, before the war broke out. They included nurses Faye Whiteside, Margaret Wyne, and Elizabeth McMillan,[226] along with Mr. Ballou (trustee), Mr. Griffiths (chaplain), Dr. Boots (professor of dentistry), Dr. Whitaker (professor of obstetrics and gynecology), and Mrs. Loucks and her son. According to a letter from Stephen Chang to Claude Forkner in July 1943, these nine had left China on "the last boat back to America."[227] They were caught in Manila when the war broke out, in December 1941. In Manila, they were all forced to enter concentration camps, "except Mrs. Loucks because she had sense enough to wear a Red Cross uniform and the Japs allowed her to live outside doing her errands of mercy." Finally, when it was decided that they were to be repatriated, the three single women (Whiteside, Wyne, McMillan) and Boots were sent up to Shanghai to catch the boat and the rest were left behind to wait for the same boat (likely the *Gripsholm*) to pick them up in Manila.[228] The four in Shanghai had all been sick in Manila. Dr. Stephen Chang saw them a few times in Shanghai, "and they were all thin and sickly." "What they went through," Chang remarked, "was something terrible, but scarcely had they settled down in Shanghai when they were ordered to enter [a] Concentration Camp there again." Elizabeth McMillan went to the county hospital instead since she was suffering from beri beri. Ultimately, Wyne was interned at Chapei in March 1943, at which time Whiteside, McMillan, and Harold Loucks were interned, with 2,500 others, at Weixian. It is not clear what happened to the others in the Manila party. After the internees departed Beijing and Shanghai, anyone, "Chinese or Japanese," who had helped them was "arrested by the Japanese and punished as traitors."[229]

In apparent anticipation of heading to the Weixian Internment Camp themselves, Harold Loucks and Hamilton Anderson had, for weeks, been collecting surgical instruments and supplies for use in the camp. When Stephen Chang decided to migrate to Free China, he was able to donate or sell a lot of supplies to them (presumably from the PUMC). "Undoubtedly," wrote Chang, "Dr. Harold Loucks became the moving spirit of the camps."[230] His services would have been welcome; a week after they arrived in Weixian Camp there was a typhus outbreak.

By July 1943, Mary Ferguson and her father were still exempted from the internment camp because of the father's old age, which allowed Mary to keep track of what was happening in China and, on occasion, to smuggle this information out to the United States (see Figure 4.4). "Old Dr. Hopkins" was also exempted (he had lived in China for fifty-five years). However, all three did have to move into the embassies. William Alston was made the custodian of the British Embassy and Dr. James Yee, "one of our American Chinese housestaffs," became custodian of the American Embassy. Three American staff of Chinese descent and

March 7, 1945

Dear MCB - Just a note to tell you how things are with us in this part of the country, and to say how much we envy you where you have the chance to be! HSH, TB, and JLS are still in the same residence which has been their home ever since they moved from Ying last May. They have all kept well, are in surprisingly good spirits if one may judge from the letters which they mail to their friends, and are hoping that the various efforts (about which they have unofficial tidings, there being ways and ways for such communications) to make certain that they are on the next sailing home will have the desired effect. They have had and still have sufficient funds to keep to their normal standard of diet, rising prices notwithstanding, and we have made arrangements to ensure the continued supply irrespective of the presence or absence in this city of any or all of their friends. This information should be a satisfaction to their families at home.

To supplement the general information you will be getting about happenings elsewhere, you will be interested to know that since February 15th CGC has joined a lot of men who are living across the Whangpoo in some mill premises; with him is young Bill Alston; Miss Robinson and Miss Wyne are with a large group of Americans in some university buildings several miles beyond stjohns; Miss Macmillan is in Country Hospital having treatment for polyneuritis and we hope her stay there can be indefinitely prolonged; also in Country Hospital is Dr. Dunlap making a protracted convalescence from a prostatectomy last November, but his family are this week joining Miss Robinson and Miss Wyne; BERead is to be at Lunghwa with another group. No one quite know the why of this general moving around, but it seems all-inclusive. It hasn't hit us here yet, and until it does we still hope for the best, but no one will be surprised if some fine morning we find ourselves on a train bound for Shantung. We've been most fortunate in many respects thus far and ought to be able to "take it" with a good grace if it comes our way.

We gather enough bits of information from one source or another to have some idea of the things that you and our former colleagues and bosses are doing in your bailiwick, and we are all happy that so much is possible. Our only regret is not to have a share in carrying things on - but to have the m go on is after all the important thing, and that we are thankful for. Blessings and the best of luck to you all!

You will know we all will be interested in this bit of direct word, both where you are now and at home. Perhaps some time you might even get some message back to us - the bearer of this note will have ideas on the subject. With best greetings, yours as always -

MEF

FIGURE 4.4 Mary Ferguson's March 1945 letter, smuggled out of China. | Courtesy Rockefeller Archive Centre, RAC-CMB-B162-F10.

two students were also exempted from camps. In addition to PUMC faculty, a number of Yenching professors were also arrested and imprisoned for months. Before he fled to West China, Dr. Stephen Chang was arrested (he called that an "honour") and was held for seventeen days. The others were kept for between seventeen and fifty days. The Japanese were keeping a close eye on PUMC and Yenching staff; as

Chang characterized it, ("any slip would mean trouble."[231] All of the Christian churches (Western and Chinese) had to have Japanese advisers, and the sermons each Sunday had to be approved by the Japanese Special Police before they could be delivered from the pulpit.

* * *

Although they did not realize it at the time, the WCUU and PUMC were making preparations that would set the stage for the PUMC School of Nursing to move to West China. In West China itself, the construction and equipping of the new University Hospital meant that a new space would be available on the WCUU campus that would be suitable for hosting an elite nursing school. Missionaries, including those on the WCUU board of governors, were feeling an increased sense of responsibility toward China, expressing guilt and shame over their own countries' indirect support of Japan's ambition by selling the empire material with which to make bombs. Missionary nurses were slowly evacuating, leaving a gap in both nursing education and practice. At the PUMC, rumours bubbled about increasing danger. Although PUMC administrators downplayed the sense of urgency, they did take the time to check out the possibility and impact of moving to Free China. In addition, PUMC alumna Bernice Chu Chen laid the groundwork to consider how the development of a PUMC-style nursing school in West China could contribute to the war effort. Thus, by the time the Japanese attack on Pearl Harbor triggered the Allies' declaration of war against Japan, both the PUMC and WCUU were primed for what would become the refugee PUMC in Chengdu.

The swiftness with which the Japanese military moved once war was declared is stunning. Clearly, the entire episode was carefully calculated. Within hours of the initial attack, Western institutions all over China were taken over, and Westerners arrested. If, as Dr. Stephen Chang noted, a crisis of this amplitude brings out a person's true nature, the responses by members of both the WCUU and PUMC show a depth of courage and integrity that legends are (and were) made of. Vera Nieh shone in her calm and courageous approach to the Japanese takeover of classrooms while nursing students were taking the most important examination of their lives. Nurses Faye Whiteside and Margaret Prentice, PUMC administrators Mary Ferguson, Harry Houghton, and Trevor Brown, and Yenching university president John Leighton Stuart demonstrated grace under fire; ultimately, the women were interned and the men imprisoned. Dr. S.T. Wang and Dr. Stephen Chang, among those left behind to provide support to the Japanese, showed a selfless regard for the good of the PUMC, finding ways to meet the demands of the Japanese while also protecting students, staff, and property. Each was willing to take risks for the institution and what it represented. That they seemed, at the same time, to accept their fate showed a remarkable level of commitment to their work. Perhaps most remarkable, however, was Dr. Mashuhashi, whose willingness to resist and subtly disrupt the work of his own Japanese countrymen showed courage deserving, as Stephen Chang suggested, official thanks when the war was over. It is not clear that this ever happened.

Part 2

After the Closure of the Peking Union Medical College

CHAPTER FIVE

Starting Over in West China (1943–45)

Displacement and Reimagining Elite Nursing in Free China

Despite present disasters, I wish to assure you that West China will stand ready to render every service of which they are capable. Just what can be done, I do not know, but whatever it may be, I want you to know that you can count upon us, as in the past we have counted upon you.

> — *Joseph Beech, WCUU chancellor, hand-written note to Dr. Alan Gregg, director of the Rockefeller Foundation's Division of Medical Education, 11 December 1941*

It is our great hope that before long we would be going back [to Beijing] to pick up the broken string and build a better and nobler PUMC.

> — *Dr. Stephen Chang, Chengdu, July 1943*

According to the *Chinese News Service* printed and distributed in New York, in 1943 there were 133 colleges in China, 25 more than before the war.[1] Of China's prewar colleges, 91 were reportedly destroyed or occupied by the Japanese, but only 19 institutions closed because of the war. "Most of the others have joined in the mass migration of colleges, and reestablished themselves in temporary sites in unoccupied China," the news service noted.[2] Forty-three new colleges had opened since the war, including teachers' colleges and medical and other professional or technical schools. In April 1943, the Chongqing University Medical College, in an appeal to the Rockefeller Foundation (RF) for funds, noted that there were five refugee medical schools in Sichuan at that time: Shanghai Medical College, the Kiangsu Medical College, the Tung Chi Medical College, the Qilu Medical College, and the National Central University Medical College.[3] Two of these – Qilu and National Central

– were among the five universities being hosted by the West China Union University (WCUU) in Chengdu. The idea that the WCUU would be the premier medical university in Sichuan after the war – that is, after the medical schools returned to their home sites – was galling to some in China. The April 1943 memo to the RF from the Chongqing University Medical College exemplified the opinion that mission universities like the WCUU should not be supported: "It is just a matter of time that these [refugee] schools will one by one move out of this province. What would be left to lead the province in the field of medical education will be the West China Missionary Medical College [i.e., the WCUU]. Its history is almost thirty years long *and has failed to produce leadership*. It is for various reasons very doubtful that the Government of [Sichuan] will call upon the missionary school to develop basic personnel in medicine and public health."[4]

Such negative opinions of the WCUU were particularly pronounced during the period when the elite Peking Union Medical College (PUMC) School of Nursing was hosted by the Canadian West China Mission (WCM) and the union university it was part of, the WCUU. Educators in the interior were well aware of the prestige (and funding) that hosting the PUMC would bring to their schools, and there were other institutions besides the WCUU that hoped to be chosen as the refugee site for the Beijing college. That a "backwater" missionary institution would be chosen was surprising and caused consternation among other institutions. Yet that was only part of the conflict. The three years during which the refugee PUMC was housed at the WCUU were rife with interpersonal, interdisciplinary, and inter-institutional strife. Six years into the War of Resistance against Japan, reserves – physical, emotional, and financial – were almost depleted. Leadership by Western nurses was almost non-existent, and missionary nursing had almost completely disappeared. That left Chinese nurses – the protégées of two very different institutions, the PUMC and the West China Mission – to sort through how best to maintain the momentum of nursing education. This was the first time in China's history that nursing was widely viewed as an indispensable national resource; what happened locally, then, also had a national effect. After providing context about the nursing situation at

Chengdu prior to the arrival of the PUMC nurses, this chapter will examine ways in which the refugee PUMC continued to unsettle nursing norms, disrupting the traditional (missionary) approach to nursing by spreading the gospel of the PUMC.

NURSING EDUCATION IN WEST CHINA, 1942-43

In her book on wartime health care in China, Nicole Elizabeth Barnes notes that young women had a great incentive to study nursing, including a patriotic opportunity to contribute to their country during a time of need.[5] Sichuan and its wartime capital, Chongqing, had become a hub for nursing education. Whereas, prior to the war, virtually all of the nursing students at the Canadian mission hospital schools of nursing in Chongqing came from Sichuan, by 1943, 50 of the approximately 100 students at that nursing school came from provinces other than Sichuan.[6] Although there were a number of nursing programs in Sichuan, this section focuses primarily on the two in Chengdu: the Canadian Mission School of Nursing (Renji) and the new University Hospital School of Nursing. Both were associated with the WCUU, albeit in different buildings.

By 1941 plans for the new University Hospital and associated Nursing School at the WCUU were well underway, with one critical exception; no one wanted to take responsibility for running it. The WCUU Women's College was willing to support the establishment of a degree (baccalaureate) program in nursing at the WCUU, but not to take responsibility for the School of Nursing itself. The Canadian Woman's Missionary Society (WMS) also refused. It was operating the Renji School of Nursing, and had plans to rebuild the WMS Hospital that had burned down in 1940 and had no desire to take on the second school at the University Hospital. The WMS would be willing to donate some of its insurance money from the fire but did not want to take on responsibility for the School of Nursing unless it was approached as a joint venture with another group.

The situation remained at a stalemate through 1941. This left the WCUU in limbo, and particularly the Medical College, which depended on a functioning nursing school to run and staff the hospital where its medical students would train. Time was of the essence; the University Hospital was set to open some of its wards in the fall of 1942. In the meantime, in June 1942, the WCUU prepared to make alternative plans in case Renji was not operational in the University Hospital by the time the hospital opened: in such a circumstance, the Medical College would itself arrange for "nursing service" to be provided by graduate nurses and nurse's aides.[7]

Finally, by the fall of 1942, things fell partially into place: Renji had *partially* moved over into the university, which was only *partially* opened. The stress of the situation was captured by Canadian missionary nurse Margaret Lee in October 1942:

> The situation is much better than it was when Miss Wellwood started the hospital and nurses' taining [sic] school, but the standards are still comparatively low. Both the graduate staff and the students seem to be able to think of more ways of doing things incorrectly than I could think of in a year. Everything requires close checking. Though the standards are low we cannot blame them entirely for we lack many of the necessary thing[s] which would help them. Our equipment has run low. A situation like this makes the new class of probationers practice the right procedures in the best way. The students say, "Miss Lee, what shall we do; there are no rubber sheets nor draw sheets on some of the beds in the wards?" Such is the situation in which we find ourselves in a war-torn world and country.[8]

The new University Hospital, with its up-to-date facilities (see Figure 5.1) officially opened on 23 February 1943.[9] The Renji School of Nursing would operate out of both the University Hospital and the General Hospital. However, there were no accommodations for the additional students who were now training at the University Hospital.[10] Since there were only about forty inpatients in the University Hospital, the nursing students used the empty wards for their accommodations.[11]

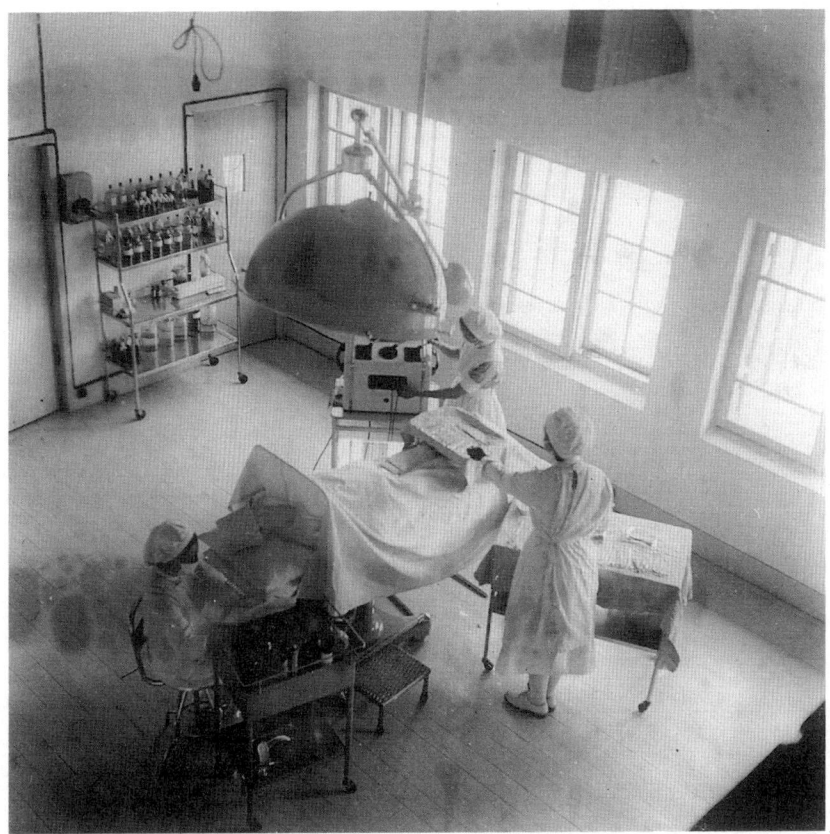

FIGURE 5.1 Operating theatre at the WCUU University Hospital, ca. 1943. | Courtesy Rockefeller Archive Center, RAC- CMB_FA065_B1144_F1042_010.

The Renji School of Nursing faced the "triple difficulties" of organizing adequate housing, teaching, and practice for students at both the University Hospital and the General Hospital. Eva Chen, a graduate nurse, was superintendent of nurses and had been "managing in the face of great difficulties."[12] The pressure was great to graduate as many nurses as possible. Although Renji was graduating about thirty nurses each year, "the demand during these war-torn days is greater than the supply."[13] Furthermore, the number of missionary nurses in West China had decreased from eleven in 1940 to six in 1942 (Table 5.1). The number would continue to decline, to a low of two in 1945.

TABLE 5.1 Nurses at the WCM, 1941–46

Name	Year Arrival	Departure	Notes	1941	1942	1943	1944	1945	1946
Caroline Wellwood	1906	1944	Resigned 1942	×	×				
Irene Harris	1921	1945			×	×	×	×	×
Alma Tallman	1924	1945	On furlough 1941, 1945		×	×	×		
Cora Kilborn	1927	1950	On leave 1938–44				×	×	×
Mary Crawley	1929	1942	Resigned 1941	×					
Dorothy Fox	1939	1943		×	×	×			
Margaret Lee	1939	1944		×	×	×	×		
Clara Preston	1940	1943	Seconded from NCM	×	×				
Total number of nurses at WCM				5	6	4	4	2	2

WEST CHINA TURNOVER

In November 1942, veteran nurse Caroline Wellwood decided to retire. She had been working as a missionary nurse in China since 1906. The ongoing war, compounded by the destruction of the Women's Hospital and the reconstitution of the Renji School of Nursing, which she had founded, had taken a toll. Wellwood sold her belongings and headed back to Canada.[14] At about the same time, Dr. Retta Gifford Kilborn, who had started the WMS Women's Hospital with Wellwood, died in Canada, on 1 December 1942. Kilborn had been gradually going blind "from paralysis" and became "such that she was helpless. Latterly she could scarcely speak."[15] Kilborn's daughter, Canadian missionary nurse Cora Kilborn, had been in Canada caring for her mother since 1938.[16] The hope within the WMS was that Cora might now return to China.[17]

> A cable telling of the death of Dr. Gifford Kilborn came a few days ago. It is a happy release for her, but Cora will be very lonely. Having had the care of her for some many years, the loneliness will be all the greater. I wonder if Cora will consider coming back to China now. We certainly would welcome her with open arms. The

need for nurses is as great as ever, and especially for one of her experience and qualifications.[18]

Travelling between Canada and China had become extremely difficult. Caroline Wellwood got as far as Bombay and was not able to secure transportation further. Four months later, in March 1943, she was still there, reporting that "this stay in India has been quite a delightful experience apart from the anxiety of getting a passage home."[19] It was not until July that she was back in Canada.[20] Dorothy Fox took over from Wellwood as the superintendent of nurses at the General Hospital.[21] Margaret Lee also worked at the General Hospital, as the operating room supervisor.[22] In February 1943, Lee assisted as the obstetrics and gynecology services were moved to a unit of the new University Hospital.[23]

In January 1943, Clara Preston was reportedly ill. She had not been well for a long time, but the WCM had hoped that giving her an extended holiday the previous summer would help her to "pick up."[24] Unfortunately, Preston was diagnosed with active tuberculosis. She was granted permission to depart on furlough as soon as she could make the necessary arrangements. The idea was that she would go as far as India and, if no steamer were available, she would enter a hospital or sanatorium there. "The doctors feel that it would be better for her to get away from China as you know [Sichuan] climate is not the best for folk with TB. We are indeed sorry that this had developed," Adelaide Harrison wrote, "as we will miss her from the work here as she has proved a very valuable worker."[25] The departure of Clara Preston from Chongqing on 27 January 1943 meant ramping up the pursuit of Cora Kilborn.[26] Although Kilborn did eventually return to China, she did not arrive until November 1944 at which time she was appointed to the General Hospital.[27]

Before Kilborn could return, the WCM lost yet another nurse: Dorothy Fox tendered her resignation on 23 May 1943. She was leaving "because of ill[ness and the] difficult conditions under which she has been working."[28] Her decision was a "real grief" to the WMS, since she was so capable. In a letter now only partially intact, Adelaide Harrison of the WMS noted,

> Because of [illegible] and financial conditions our hospital find[s] it impossible to get even [a minimum] of what our missionaries consider necessary in the way of [equipment]. Consequently, we are sorry to say, the quality of work being done is [less] than when it used to be. Also, the action of the Chinese government in [conscripting] 50% of all the graduates in medicine and nursing, whether of Mission [or] government institutions has made it exceedingly difficulty to staff our hospitals. Especially is this true in the nursing departments.[29]

The wartime conditions, Harrison acknowledged, were wearing: "having had so many years of nursing at [illegible] more or less ideal conditions [Fox] has found it particularly hard to [adjust] herself to the makeshift conditions under which medical work out here [is being] carried on at present."[30] Fox had found it somewhat easier when the General hospital was temporarily housed in the junior middle school. There, she had been superintendent of nurses and, after the departure of Caroline Wellwood, superintendent of the hospital. With so much authority, Fox was able to keep the standard of that particular hospital as high as was possible under the existing conditions. However, when the School of Nursing expanded to include the new University Hospital on the WCUU campus, Fox was no longer superintendent of nurses; this was the responsibility of Canadian missionary Dr. Allan E. Best, superintendent of the United Hospitals of the WCUU – that is, the University Hospital and the General Hospital. And Allan Best was "not an easy person to work with."[31]

According to Harrison, "Miss Fox found it next to [impossible] to get [Best's] cooperation in those things which she felt were essential to giving the student nurses the proper practical training – cleanliness and sanitation of the building, rules governing the patients, supplies etc."[32] Dr. Leslie Kilborn had a different view on the matter, and was more sympathetic to Best. A month before Fox resigned, Kilborn wrote,

> Best has been unit superintendent of the new hospital ... and has done a good job, but wishes to give up and spend more time on his

clinical work. Dorothy Fox is not turning out too well. She is an extreme pessimist and can find absolutely nothing good in her surroundings or in her colleagues, either Chinese or foreign. I'm afraid the new hospital job is really too big for her. I wish Cora were back here running it. Margaret Lee is better than Dorothy, but also inexperienced.[33]

The conflict between Fox and Best would foreshadow a similar conflict between Best and dean of nursing Vera Nieh once the PUMC School of Nursing opened on the WCUU campus later in 1943, just a few months after Dorothy Fox's resignation. In the meantime, Fox was experiencing ill health, possibly sprue. "The task of moving the hospital out to the Campus was not only a heavy one," wrote Harrison, "but nervewracking as well." This combination of events simply became too much for Fox, "so she decided the only way out was for her to resign."[34] After Fox's departure, her housemate Margaret Lee would move into the University Hospital with the Chinese nursing students and staff. This not only would lessen her expenses, it also would help bridge the gap between the Chinese and the remaining Canadian nurses.[35]

In June 1943, Dorothy Fox was selling all her personal belongings, and "with the prices now prevailing is realizing a tidy little sum, so will be able to not only pay her passage home, but have a considerable sum besides."[36] This was helpful since, as Fox had not completed the four years of her term, she had to return one-half of her travelling and outfit money.

VYING FOR THE REFUGEE PUMC

The reopening of the PUMC School of Nursing in Free China in July 1943, eighteen months after the Japanese closed the PUMC in Beijing, is one of the most remarkable stories of nursing in wartime China. During the three-year period that the refugee PUMC operated in Chengdu, it admitted four classes of undergraduates and one class of postgraduate students. The PUMC did not take any students with it to West China. The "School of Nursing" was, in fact, Vera Nieh and nine refugee nursing faculty. They welcomed their first cohort of new first-year students in Chengdu in September 1943, just two months after they arrived on the WCUU campus. Dr. Allen Best was delighted, and knew the public relations value of their arrival. In an annual letter to supporters he gushed, "perhaps the most significant from points financial, teaching and prestige has been the coming to our midst of the Peking Union Medical College and its attendant high grade school of nursing."[37]

There had been no concerted plan to move the School of Nursing to West China in the same way that other refugee institutions migrated. Nieh and PUMC faculty made independent decisions to migrate to Free China, thus joining the millions of other refugees from the Japanese-occupied regions seeking stability or an opportunity to help with the war effort. Some came almost a year before Vera Nieh. For example, in a telegram sent on 9 September 1942 to Edwin Lobenstine of the RF China Medical Board (CMB) board member Wong Wen-hao commented that he was in Chongqing with PUMC professor I.C. Yuan, two nursing instructors, seven medical students, and three nursing students.[38] Wang Hsui-ying, a PUMC nursing faculty member, noted that, between 31 January 1942 (when the PUMC closed) and June 1943, "practically all our nursing faculty came to Free China" in small groups, over a period of about five months.[39]

Although there were rumours in early 1943 that the CMB was considering reopening the PUMC in Chongqing, nothing was set by the time Vera Nieh and other PUMC faculty and staff started arriving in that city in mid-1943. Given that the PUMC name was synonymous with the Rockefeller Foundation, hosting the former would inevitably mean financial support from the latter. Perhaps this explains why a number of institutions in West China, upon learning of potential plans to reopen the PUMC School of Nursing, started vying for the privilege.

One of the earliest conversations about relocating the PUMC School of Nursing to West China was in December 1942, when Dr. Marshall C. Balfour, director of the RF's International Health Division (IHD), made a trip to West China to assess the situation there. On 22 December, he discussed the possibility of reopening or re-establishing the school, and a "project began to take form,"[40] with the approval of the CMB.[41] To

Edwin Lobenstine, this seemed the "most feasible way of maintaining a PUMC project, worthy of the parent institution."[42] The idea seemed feasible for a number of reasons: nursing staff from the PUMC Hospital were already in West China; there was a greater need for a "good Nursing School in Free China" than for a medical college; re-establishment of the PUMC School of Nursing could be accomplished in association with an existing medical college and hospital; and the Ministry of Education would presumably be okay with establishing the school in Sichuan since the PUMC was already registered with the government.[43] Marshall Balfour met with Hsu Ai-Chu, a PUMC nursing alumnus who was also president of the Nurses Association of China (NAC) and chief of public health nursing for the National Institute of Health.[44] In January 1943, at the request of the CMB Advisory Committee, Hsu Ai-Chu and other nurses prepared a proposal for the new school. At a meeting of the Advisory Committee on 19 January 1943, a "war-time" School of Nursing was approved. The next day, a Preparatory Committee was established that included Dr. M.C. Balfour, Dr. Wong Wen-hao, Dr. C.K. Chu or Dr. W.W. Yung, and Dr. Gordon King, as well as PUMC nursing alumnae Hsu Ai-Chu and Bernice Chu Chen.[45]

To Marshall Balfour, there were two overriding reasons to reopen the PUMC School of Nursing. First, there was a need to continue the supply of nurses "with higher educational background and good professional quality, able to meet the opportunities and needs in the rapidly developing fields of preventive and curative medicine." There had been constant demand for PUMC nursing graduates for "responsible positions in nursing education and administration," and now, with wartime conditions, the need for nurses with thorough professional education and a "spirit for service" was more acute. Second, PUMC nursing students required continuation of their education and, Balfour noted, "it is impossible to arrange studies for them in existing schools, such schemes are not conducive to the welfare of the students and in fact would be [a] regressive step derogatory to their academic standing as well as the development of their professional quality." In other words, with the closure of the PUMC, only lower-grade nursing schools were left in China. In comparison, PUMC graduates "have been drawn from college students or graduates and have received instruction and training for careers in nursing education and administration."[46] Thus, although PUMC nursing students could continue the clinical portion of their studies after the PUMC closed, there was a real need in China for a university-level school of nursing with the lofty ideals and high standards of the PUMC.

To the Preparatory Committee, it would be "comparatively simple" to reopen the school. "Quite a number" of the nursing faculty had already made their way into Free China. Furthermore, "those who are still in the occupied area, as most of them are single women, will be able to leave for the cause if the School is ready to reassemble," given that they did not have family responsibilities to keep them in Beijing.[47] Also, nursing students could be recruited from Ginling College, Yenching University, and other universities of the same standing, now in Free China as refugee institutions. In the proposed plan, administration of the school would be independent, under the direction of a board of directors whose membership would include members of the Preparatory Committee, plus PUMC alumnae Chou Meiyu and Eva Liu. The committee also made recommendations as to who could take leadership roles in the school. Interestingly, it recommended Sia Yun-hua, rather than Vera Nieh, as dean. It recommended that Vera Nieh (or Edith Hseih) be the principal of the school and superintendent of the hospital. Of the fifteen names listed to be possibly hired as regular staff for the school, eight were already in Free China, and four (including Vera Nieh) had expressed the desire to come to Free China.

On 22 February 1943, the Preparatory Committee, now renamed the Subcommittee on the School of Nursing, agreed unanimously that the school be located in Koloshan, about twenty-two kilometres outside of Chongqing, where the Central Hospital and Shanghai National Medical College were situated.[48] The authorities of these institutions had already signified their goodwill and willingness to cooperate. They also agreed that Vera Nieh should serve as principal of the school.[49] However, within weeks, the committee changed its mind on Koloshan, a decision that would spark controversy, and even death threats.

It was shortly after this, on 19 April 1943, that Dr. Claude Forkner, who had previously taught at the PUMC Medical School, headed to

China as the new director of the CMB.[50] He arrived in Chongqing on 5 May 1943 to the realities of a community that had been at war for six years. He found "great difficulties in transportation and communication," with letters slow, telephone service unsatisfactory, and telegrams delayed or not reaching their destination.[51] Rickshaws were not of much use on the hills, chairs (used for carrying clients up the steep steps) were infrequent and expensive, buses were dirty and "jammed," and "of course no taxis are available."[52] It was an inauspicious start to his tenure.

Claude Forkner met with Bernice Chu Chen on 18 May 1943. A member of the Subcommittee on the School of Nursing, Bernice was the principal of the School of Nursing in Koloshan. She believed that the PUMC School of Nursing should not be in Koloshan but, rather, at a national college in Chengdu. She listed four reasons. First, there was already a nursing school at Koloshan that was using the Central Hospital in that city for its teaching and practice. That school had 94 students and had plans to increase the number to 200 within the next two years to help support Chiang Kai-shek's call for 232,000 physicians and 600,000 nurses within ten years.[53] To Chu Chen, there was simply not room in Koloshan for another school of nursing. Second, she believed that PUMC nursing students should be in the same city as a group of PUMC medical students who had evacuated from Beijing – that is, in Chengdu. This would centralize teaching, strengthen and improve the local hospital for both PUMC nursing and medical students simultaneously, promote more unity within the PUMC group, and simplify their wartime administration. Third, in Chengdu there were quarters that could be rented instead of built, and this might result in better quarters at less cost. Finally, Chiang Kai-shek had made a ruling that no new schools were to be started within 200 li (6 miles) of Chongqing. These were all compelling arguments.

Claude Forkner also conferred with five other PUMC nursing alumnae. Four were at Koloshan: Sia Yun-hua was superintendent of nurses, Chen Liang-yu was supervisor of nurses, and Hilda Wang (Wang Ia fang) was assistant supervisor of nurses, all in the city of Koloshan. Hsu Ai-Chu was head of the Nursing Department of the National Institute of Health in Koloshan. Liu Ching-ho was the temporary secretary to the Wartime Advisory Committee on the PUMC School of Nursing.[54] These nurses disagreed with Chu Chen, preferring the PUMC School of Nursing to open at the Central Hospital in Koloshan. They liked the atmosphere at the Central Hospital and thought the PUMC school would add to its efficiency. In their view, the alternate site being considered – the National Central Nursing School in Chengdu and its affiliate hospital, the National Hospital – were unsuitable. They had heard that nurses did not like working with the superintendent, Dr. S.N. Cheer. Furthermore, the "academic morale" there was low; medical faculty were all secretly working in private practice, dividing their loyalties at the expense of teaching. They had also heard rumours of inadequate living facilities, that students had difficulty studying because of the overcrowding.

Forkner visited the Central Hospital in Koloshan to see the conditions there for himself. He found a number of significant defects.[55] The first had to do with sanitation. There was no running water or well, the water supply source being a ditch that could not be kept clean. The lack of water meant that admission baths could not be given, and bedpans and sputum cups were not properly sterilized. Cleaning was inadequate, and all the rooms had bugs. Second, although there were electrical lights, they could not be used because of the expense of coal and lack of water to run the steam engine that powered the generator. In essence, there was no electricity. Third, the hospital was a temporary building and in a constant state of disrepair. There were no window or door screens, and no facilities for keeping the building warm: inside and outside temperatures were the same. The space, he concluded, was simply not suitable for the PUMC.

While sorting out the best location for the refugee PUMC, Claude Forkner and Dr. Stephen Chang, now also in West China, started to recruit PUMC nursing alumnae to come to Sichuan. On 26 June 1943, they sent a letter on behalf of the CMB to "all the teaching staff and graduates of the PUMC," notifying them that they anticipated the reopening of the PUMC School of Nursing in the fall at either Chongqing or Chengdu.[56] "We know that all of you would like to join us," they wrote, noting that they realized there was uncertainty as to jobs and salaries, and difficulties and dangers in travelling to Free China. However, they opined, "there may be greater danger in remaining in Occupied Areas than in traveling west."[57] Forkner and Chang assured recipients that the CMB would do everything to take care of any teaching staff who came to Free China, whether from occupied regions or abroad. "Your crossing through No-mans land will be as safe as we can make it," they promised. However, "we do not propose to offer beds of roses," they continued. "This is war time and we expect all of us to sacrifice something."[58] At that point, about thirty-five PUMC medical and nursing alumnae were already in Sichuan, along with about thirty-five medical students.

Claude Forkner knew well how tough it was to live in Free China. A couple of weeks prior to writing the recruitment letter, he had climbed aboard a Friends Ambulance Unit (FAU) truck heading to Chengdu from Koloshan. About two hours after departing, the FAU truck had a head-on collision with a Chinese Air Force truck "which was coming fast down a hill around a corner on the wrong side of the road."[59] No one was injured, but both trucks were out of commission. "After thirty hours of work in the boiling sun and in great filth in the midst of a tiny Chinese village street," Forkner wrote, "the chauffeur and I succeeded [in] repairing the vehicle."[60] During the two nights on the road, they slept on boxes on top of the truck.

A turning point in Forkner's decision regarding a location for the PUMC came when he was in Chengdu, at the home of Canadian missionary Dr. Ernest Struthers. A long-serving United Church of Canada North China missionary, Struthers had evacuated from Qilu Medical School at the Shandong Christian University. "Before my trip to Chengdu," Forkner reported, "I had learned that the [PUMC] students [in Sichuan] were extremely unhappy and that they were praying for someone to come and help them with their difficulties." Consistent with the message he had heard from the nursing alumnae in Koloshan, the professors at the National Central College in the city "seemed to have lost their interest in teaching and are for the most part engaged in private practice or business, hence they neglect their university duties."[61] Dr. S.N. Cheer, for example, was "heavily engaged" in private practice. The medical students felt that they were not learning anything and wanted to transfer to the WCUU. Forkner also found the National Central staff to be unhappy, "displeased with the deterioration of medical education." Furthermore, "not a single PUMC graduate nurse wants to work in Dr. Cheer's institution. They feel that he regards nurses as inferior and that he is not in sympathy with their point of view."[62]

Having visited both institutions recommended by the Subcommittee on the School of Nursing – the Central Hospital and Nursing School at Koloshan and the National Central Hospital and College at Chengdu – Forkner was of the view that neither would be suitable. However, now that he was in the home of Ernest Struthers on the WCUU campus, and having just heard from PUMC students of their desire to transfer to the WCUU, a new idea quickly formed. He now thought it wise to explore the possibility of "properly accommodating" the medical students at the WCUU while "simultaneously opening the nursing school in that institution."[63] This new development would change the trajectory for nursing education at both the PUMC and the WCUU.

Forkner stayed seventeen days in Chengdu. On 2 July 1943, the CMB Wartime Committee met, including Drs. Wong Wen-hao, Y.T. Tsur, P.Z. King, Gordon King, and Forkner himself, to discuss the location of the nursing school. P.Z. King preferred the site in the city of Koloshan; Gordon King also preferred Koloshan but saw advantages in the WCUU. The others preferred the WCUU. Edwin Lobenstine, in New York, was to make the final decision.[64]

On 3 July 1943, Claude Forkner and Dr. Leslie Kilborn, dean of medicine at the WCUU, signed a letter outlining a tentative general agreement between the CMB and the WCUU that was then approved by the Wartime Committee. The letter noted that the CMB was considering reopening the PUMC School of Nursing to "function temporarily at the United Hospital until the PUMC can become reestablished in a permanent home."[65] The School of Nursing would require between fifteen and twenty-five staff, with about twenty-five "college-grade" students admitted to each class. The nursing program would consist of three years of training after completion of pre-nursing (university) requirements. The refugee PUMC School of Nursing would take "complete charge" of the nursing services (i.e., patient care) at the University Hospital and would work "in affiliation with the existing Ren Chi [Renji] nursing school associated with the United Hospital."[66]

This was exceptionally good news for the WCM and the WCUU. Not only would they now have enough personnel and students to run the new University Hospital, they would also have the opportunity to learn how to upgrade their own School of Nursing to offer a baccalaureate degree. "It is hoped," Claude Forkner noted, "that this PUMC school may provide a basis for a university-grade [school of nursing] which you have planned to continue here after the PUMC returns to its new quarters which we trust will be in the PUMC buildings in [Beijing]" after the war.[67]

In addition to what it meant for the PUMC, the CMB "nursing project" also encouraged the missionary community. For the Associated Boards of Christian Colleges in China, for example, the opportunity to host the PUMC would help missionaries to further the Christian mission. They wanted to take full advantage of this windfall:

> The question arises, how can this contribution in money and well-trained student body, with background of high educational standards, be so used as to make the largest contribution to medical and nursing education during the war period and to leave the medical and nursing education of WCUU in a stronger position when the visiting institutions and students leave for their own campuses?[68]

The "contribution in money" referred to here was the means to complete two unfinished buildings on the WCUU campus. The CMB offered to supply the WCUU with the necessary funds to complete buildings that would be used by the PUMC School of Nursing and for PUMC medical students completing their studies at the WCUU.[69] It was further agreed that, if the CMB made certain expenditures, it would "be entitled to the occupancy of the quarters as listed free of charge and for the purposes stated for a period of two years or for the duration of the war whichever of the two is longer."[70] The "duration of the war" was understood to mean not only the end of the war, but also the time needed for the PUMC School of Nursing to settle back into its own quarters in Beijing, or to be re-established elsewhere if the Beijing quarters were destroyed.[71]

The advantages to the WCUU were precisely some of what other institutions had hoped to gain by hosting the PUMC. In a confidential letter dated 11 July 1943, Claude Forkner outlined to Edwin Lobenstine and Agnes Pearce some of the context for what was quickly becoming a controversial decision regarding the location of the nursing school. "Everything here seems to be dominated by political maneuvering," he wrote, adding:

> Everyone is scheming to get everyone else's job. Everyone wants to be a "general" and if he is not made one he feels mistreated ... I fully appreciate that this country has gone through 6 years of desperate struggle, that security is threatened, that they have been for years abandoned by other nations. It has frayed their nerves, made them to an extent bitter, has promoted nationalism and intensified anti-foreignism. All of the criticism which one might level against what is happening is quite easily explained. They have fought a good war and have held on when almost anyone else would have capitulated ... I have faith in their future.[72]

On 15 July 1943, Edwin Lobenstine sent a telegram to Forkner saying that, "assuming full cooperation [of the] PUMC nursing staff," the Executive Committee of the trustees of the CMB approved the reopening of the PUMC School of Nursing at the WCUU.[73] The next day, Vera Nieh sent a confidential telegram to Edwin Lobenstine, stating that the "nursing faculty favors West China."[74] The decision was made.

Claude Forkner outlined eleven reasons for choosing the WCUU as the refugee PUMC site. First, the difficulties with medical education at Koloshan were "apparent to everyone" and "no one knows how to remedy them."[75] Second, the PUMC medical students were already at the WCUU; thus, CMB grants could serve the double purpose of benefiting both PUMC medical and nursing students. Third, the WCUU had two unfinished buildings for which they required funds to complete. It would cost the CMB less money to complete these buildings than to build new temporary quarters. Moreover, the buildings were "almost ideal" for the

PUMC medical students and the nursing school.[76] Fourth, Koloshan would cost US$50,000 more than Chengdu. Fifth, the CMB had contributed to the WCUU in the past; supporting the university through funding permanent buildings would be consistent with existing policies of the board. Sixth, the WCUU needed and would welcome additional staff from the United States or occupied regions of China. Hence, some of the PUMC staff currently in those areas might be attracted to come to the WCUU. Seventh, the facilities at the WCUU were far better for the care of patients and for teaching than were those at the other sites. "Water is plentiful," Forkner wrote, "whereas in Koloshan it is almost absent at certain critical periods of the year."[77] Furthermore, electricity was available at the WCUU. Eighth, there was a good academic atmosphere at the WCUU. There were five universities on the WCUU campus (and three thousand students),[78] which could provide a good pool from which to recruit medical and nursing students. Ninth, the WCUU was "relatively free from the political maneuvering which is present in government universities" and especially in the wartime capital of Chongqing. Tenth, Vera Nieh and her assistants who knew both places preferred the WCUU. Finally, Forkner could see "no advantages" for the PUMC in being associated with a national university. "It is like comparing Harvard with the University of Vermont," he wrote.[79]

Once word got out about the CMB decision, the controversies began almost immediately. First was Dr. C.K. Chu's "surprise" that PUMC medical students were departing National Central University at Koloshan for the WCUU.[80] This was followed by the minister of education's choice to delay the registration of the nursing school. Most distressing, however, was a threatening letter sent to PUMC nursing alumnae, warning them not to go to the WCUU. The letter was delivered by mail to the secretary of the Preparatory Committee for the Re-opening of the PUMC School of Nursing. The letter, written to "Lady Members" (i.e., Bernice Chu Chen and Hsu Ai-Chu) derided the decision to go to Chengdu, calling it a demonstration of a complete lack of patriotism. The letter was filled with insults, calling the recipients "girls of loving comfort and merriment" who, by living in foreign buildings, associating with foreigners, and enjoying a Westernized way of life, were being distracted from the need to focus all their energies on resisting the Japanese and "saving the nation."[81] The letter suggested that Chu Chen and Ai-Chu were "obey[ing] the words of foreign masters because they give you money." By receiving this kind of money, the letter stated, they were committing a "very big crime" because it meant they were obeying foreigners rather than the Chinese government. By "flattering foreigners," the women were giving them an opening to take over China. The letter called the women naïve and recommended they go to the Central Training Corps to receive training to understand the Chiang Kai-shek's writing entitled "China's Fate." The letter ended with a threat: "We have sent persons to watch you. Afraid that you will not be easy to reach [in Chengdu]. Do not think that foreigners are almighty. Can they protect your body?"[82]

Although Claude Forkner considered the letter a "pernicious piece of nonsense," it was not the only surprising response.[83] His predecessor, Marshall Balfour, was also critical of the WCUU decision. Balfour believed that the minister of education preferred that the PUMC associate with a national medical college rather than a missionary one. "To call a spade a spade," he wrote to Forkner, "the fundamental question is a choice between what is national policy of China, and what are primarily missionary interests."[84] In Balfour's opinion, the PUMC should go along with the "national movement and spirit," even though "there may be disadvantages and slow progress at times."[85] Although the WCUU had the best physical layout and the least cost, Balfour was concerned that once the PUMC was involved with the WCUU, "it will become very difficult to become dissociated from the interests and financial responsibilities assumed."[86] If the PUMC *were* to move to the WCUU, Balfour preferred that everything associated with the PUMC – the hospital, medical college, nursing school, and nursing services – be placed under the direction of the PUMC trustees rather than the missionaries. He also realized that was unlikely to happen.

Balfour was puzzled that Forkner had chosen to go against the wishes of the PUMC alumnae who had clearly favoured Koloshan. He also thought that the criticism directed at S.N. Cheer was an insufficient reason not to use the National Hospital in Chengdu. To Balfour, this school and faculty was "still the best" in terms of "quality medical education in Free China today."[87] Mostly, though, he was concerned that going to the WCUU would damage the CMB's good relationship with the Chinese government. "Whatever the developments may be [in terms of the PUMC's postwar future], I believe personally that the future relationship with government should be in such fashion that it meets with the sympathetic interest and support of government representatives, or difficulties and misunderstandings will be greater than in the past."[88]

Likely at the behest of Balfour, Edwin Lobenstine contacted Vera Nieh directly, asking whether the decision in favour of the WCUU was "fully supported by yourself and other members of the nursing faculty."[89] Reading Nieh's positive response was all Lobenstine needed to throw his support behind the decision. Having heard from Nieh, he expressed delight "that the way is open of the carrying on of the fine work which the Peiping Union Medical College nursing school has done in past years." He also expressed hope that the nursing school would find its new location satisfactory. "That you will be crowded," he presumed, "must be taken for granted since there are so many students brought together on the university campus." However, he anticipated that Vera Nieh would find the atmosphere congenial and predicted that her "presence will be inspiring to those who have the service of their fellow countrymen and women and children at heart."[90]

THE REFUGEE PUMC ARRIVES AT THE WCUU

Vera Nieh arrived in Sichuan in May or June 1943. She, like many individuals, decided to migrate to "the interior" once there was no more work for her in "this invaded area [Beijing] under the Japanese control."[91] After making arrangements for the well-being of her family, including her mother, Nieh and her brother set off for Sichuan. She hoped to find work there, possibly to "start the nursing education." Other nursing faculty had similar, albeit indefinite, plans.

Vera Nieh's recollection of her migration from Beijing to Chongqing was that it was "a very difficult and dangerous trip."[92] It took her, her brother, and the small group they travelled with, two months by various modes of transportation to get there. They were inspected by Japanese soldiers "every day and night" along the way, as they crossed from occupied regions to "the free area." There were bandits and others that would "take advantage of you, the chance to get money and what not." The travel itself was difficult and "sometimes in the middle of the night, the inspectors would come in and [ask] you, where are you going ... and why and so forth; inspect your things."[93]

One of the most significant parts of Vera Nieh's journey is almost completely absent from the archival records: the death of her brother. In the thousands of documents I reviewed, this tragic event is mentioned only once, by Claude Forkner, director of the CMB, in a note to Edward Lobenstine on 21 October 1943, where he wrote, "Also, as I believe you may know, [Vera Nieh] had quite a shock on her way from [Beijing]. Her brother who was in the party was killed."[94] Forty years later, in an unpublished interview with Anne Davis at the University of California at San Francisco's, Nieh brought up this subject herself:

> VERA NIEH: Unfortunately, to my own personal great loss was the death of my brother. 'Cause my younger brother went with me and died in the middle of the way. And I don't want to say too much about it.
>
> ANNE DAVIS: He died on the way to Chengdu?
>
> VERA NIEH: On my way to the interior my brother died. Killed.
>
> ANNE DAVIS: By the Japanese?
>
> VERA NIEH: No, by the Guomindang [Chinese] soldiers. Well, anyway, I don't want to say too much about that.[95]

After her brother died, Nieh received help from some friends to carry on to Chongqing, "At just that time," she recalled, "the CMB was also planning to help get this nursing education started in Chengdu."[96] After she arrived in Chongqing, where a number of CMB trustees and PUMC alumnae had found work, she became involved in discussions about reopening the PUMC. Once it was decided that the school would reopen in Chengdu, most of the PUMC nursing faculty that were in Chongqing travelled almost immediately to Chengdu, moving into the WCUU nurses' dormitory on 13 August 1943.[97] They "got busy right away," immediately starting negotiations with the WCUU and the other evacuated universities to find students who had already completed appropriate pre-nursing courses.[98]

In August 1943, Nieh was appointed the general superintendent of nurses at the University Hospital, with charge of the outpatient department and sanatorium. "She is an excellent person to deal with," wrote Dr. Ed Cunningham, the acting dean of medicine at the WCUU. "She is busy installing her nurses and getting things whipped into shape. The CMB are supplying cash to finish two top floors of service unit, not enough money to finish tower. The PUMC nurses [are] to use these two top floors."[99]

The first official meeting of the PUMC Preliminary Committee on the School of Nursing was held on 5 August 1943 in Chengdu, with five in attendance: Vera Nieh, Eva Liu, Wang Hsui Ying, Sia Ming Be, and Liu Ching Ho.[100] All were graduates of the PUMC – three from the Class of 1936 – and had been on faculty at the college since the late 1930s.

By 1 October 1943, there were nine nursing faculty members at the refugee PUMC (see Table 5.2). Three others were listed as head nurses, who would have provided leadership on the hospital wards. Only three PUMC nursing faculty were *not* in Chengdu by this time, and one of these arrived the following month. The commitment of these women to the PUMC and to each other was remarkable, and perhaps best explained by the fact that all were PUMC School of Nursing alumnae. This fits with John Z. Bowers's assertion that "the mutual admiration and respect generated between teachers and students, the excellence of the educational program, as well as the stimulating ambience of PUMC, made the nursing alumnae as devoted to the college as were the graduates in medicine."[101]

While the arrival of the refugee PUMC gave a boost in morale to the WCUU, the WCM's staffing difficulties got even worse. On 13 April 1944, the WMS put out an appeal for five missionary nurses: "during the past two years, by retirement and resignation the nursing forces of the Mission have been further depleted by three and ... of those on the field four are likely in their fourth term, and three of whom are unlikely to

TABLE 5.2 PUMC nursing faculty at the WCUU as of 1 October 1943

Name	Alternative name	Likely starting date	PUMC graduation year
Faculty/teaching staff			
Nieh, Vera	Nieh Yuchan	July 1943	1927
Kwan, Chung-hua	Mrs. Pai; Kuan Chung Hwa	August 1943	1930
Wang, Hsui-ying		July 1943	1931
Sia, Ming-be		July 1943	1936
Tso, Han-yen		August 1943	1936
Lui, Ching-ho		July 1943	1936
Lu, Hui-ching		September 1943	1938
Ho, Pei-fen		September 1943	1937
Lee, Margaret		September 1943	n/a
Liu, Chih-chen	Eva Liu	July 1943	1936
Head nurses			
Li Han-chiang			1940
Hsu Sze-mei			1940
Jen Chih-chih			1939
Faculty not yet in Free China by October 1943			
Chen Chi			1931
Wang Loh Loh	Wang Yi	November 1943	1932
Li Shun-sheng			1936

return to the field after their furlough."[102] By 1944, the WCM was down to four nurses (from ten in 1940; see Tables 3.1 and 5.1). In January 1945, the United Church of Canada WCM Seventh Joint Council made notice of the attrition of missionary nurses. The "loss of missionary nursing personnel becomes increasingly serious, so much so that [of] all of the nurses who have come to the field during the past fourteen years, not one remains," the council noted.[103] It resolved that the WMS Medical Committee "be requested to make careful investigation of the causes leading to this inordinate depletion of the missionary nursing personnel, and if necessary make such changes as will give full opportunity and expression of initiative for missionary nurses thereby ensuring their continued interest and devotion to their share of the missionary task."[104]

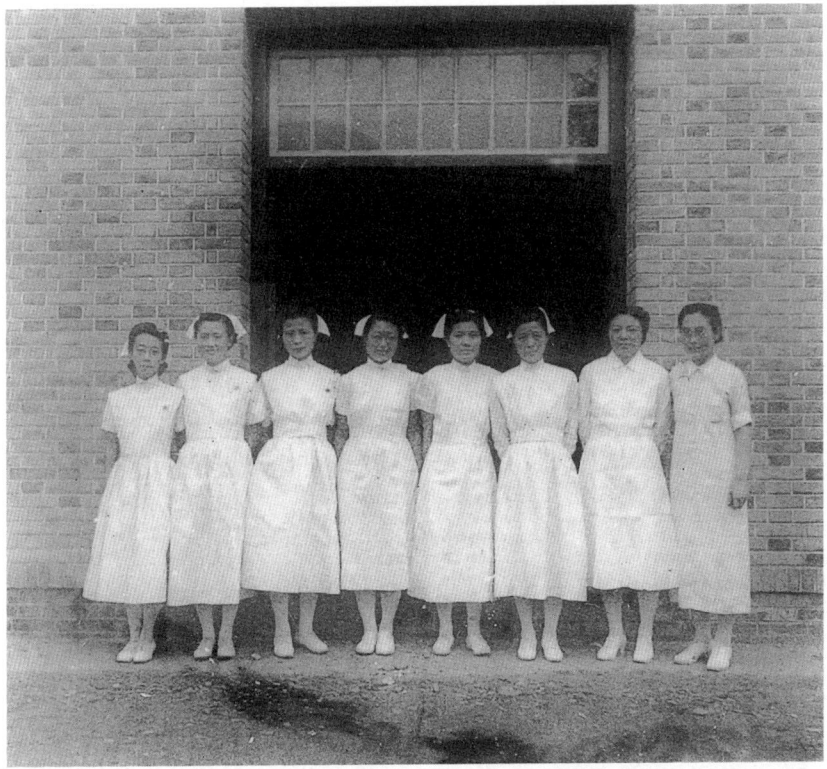

FIGURE 5.2 PUMC nursing faculty in West China, ca. 1943. Vera Nieh is third from right. | Courtesy Rockefeller Archive Center, RAC-CMB_FA065_B1144_F1042_002.

The investigation, if it indeed occurred, did not help the nursing situation. In 1945 and 1946, the WCM was down to two missionary nurses: Cora Kilborn and Irene Harris.

There was very little turnover in the PUMC faculty as well during this period. Vera Nieh later commented that the main reasons for departure of nursing faculty were marriage and "political changes" – similar reasons to those for the departure of Canadian missionaries.[105] However, there was an additional reason for attrition of the Chinese nurses: the "tremendous demand for teaching and administrative personnel by other medical institutions."[106] Between 1943 and 1946, thirty-three nurses worked at various points for the PUMC. Of these, twenty-two (67 percent) were PUMC alumnae, and thirteen (39 percent) had been PUMC faculty before the Japanese takeover in 1941. In other words, during and immediately after the difficult refugee years in Chengdu, the PUMC School of Nursing was able to rely on alumnae and former faculty to help with the wartime and rebuilding effort.

Perhaps one of the most interesting names associated with the PUMC was WCUU nurse Margaret Lee, whose name is also listed alongside PUMC faculty in the PUMC School of Nursing Faculty Meeting minutes starting with the first faculty meeting on 24 September 1943.[107] As discussed in Chapter 3, Lee was a Canadian missionary nurse of Chinese descent. In 1943, she moved into the Chinese nurses' dormitories then located in the University Hospital. She was, it seems, a bridge between the WCM and the PUMC, helping each better understand the other. For example, she was well aware of the conflicts that her colleague Dorothy Fox had had with Dr. Allan Best before she resigned in 1943. When Vera Nieh also had conflicts with Best, Lee was able to provide support. "Margaret Lee was in the other day," wrote WMS secretary Adelaide Harrison in November 1943, "and was telling me that Miss Nieh, principal of PUMC Nurse Training School and Supt. of the Nurses at the University Hospital is finding things just as difficult as Dorothy [Fox] and Margaret [Lee] did, and complains of lack of co-operation on the part of the hospital supt [Best]."[108] Lee was a supportive figure during the first year of the refugee PUMC, until her marriage and subsequent retirement in July 1944.[109]

The opening of the PUMC School of Nursing in Chengdu was newsworthy enough to be announced in the *American Journal of Nursing* (*AJN*) in January 1944. The journal noted that Vera Nieh was dean, that a number of former faculty members were now on the new faculty, and that twenty-nine students were enrolled.[110] By May 1944, the *AJN* reported that the faculty had grown to thirteen nurses, all graduates of the PUMC School of Nursing. "For the time being," the journal reported, "this school is conducted jointly with the already established school of West China Union University Hospital."[111] The *AJN* also noted that four nurses who were formerly on staff of the PUMC "returned safely to the United States on December 1, 1943 on the *Gripsholm* after months of internment in China and the Philippines."[112] These were Elizabeth Hirst, Ethel Robinson, Faye Whiteside, and Margaret Wyne.[113]

SETTING UP SHOP IN CHENGDU

Vera Nieh and the small group of PUMC nursing faculty wasted no time in getting the program set up in Chengdu. They had charge of the nursing service at the University Hospital and intended to introduce "PUMC systems" into it.[114] They divided up the first tasks: Vera Nieh and Liu Ching-ho would organize nursing uniforms (as nursing schools provided these for their students), Sia Ming-Be would arrange for the forms used on the hospital wards, Wang Hsui-ying would take care of "letters" (likely ordering letterhead and stationary), and Liu Ching Ho would look for "places where to get instruments and supplies."[115] By the end of August 1943, their attention was turned to admitting students. Enrolment of new, first-year nursing students started on 15 September. "To our great surprise," Wang Hsui-ying wrote, "there were forty-two applicants from different universities on the campus."[116] Over the course of the next three years, the refugee PUMC School of Nursing would take in three classes of "our own" students, who had taken pre-nursing at various universities on the WCUU campus; it also offered one two-year program for postgraduate students. In total, the PUMC ran four classes.[117]

Within its first seven months of operation, the nursing faculty opened two new wards (medical and surgical) at the University Hospital for teaching first-year students (Figure 5.3). It also improved the obstetrical, gynecological, and outpatient services, which had been fully moved to the University Hospital from the former Women's Hospital in February 1943 and were being used by the Renji School of Nursing students (see Figure 5.4).[118]

One of the earliest decisions – "moved, duly seconded and unanimously agreed to" – was to continue using English as the language of instruction. Although English had always been used for instruction at the PUMC, the faculty raised the question of whether this practice should continue in Free China. Not only were there no foreign nurses on the

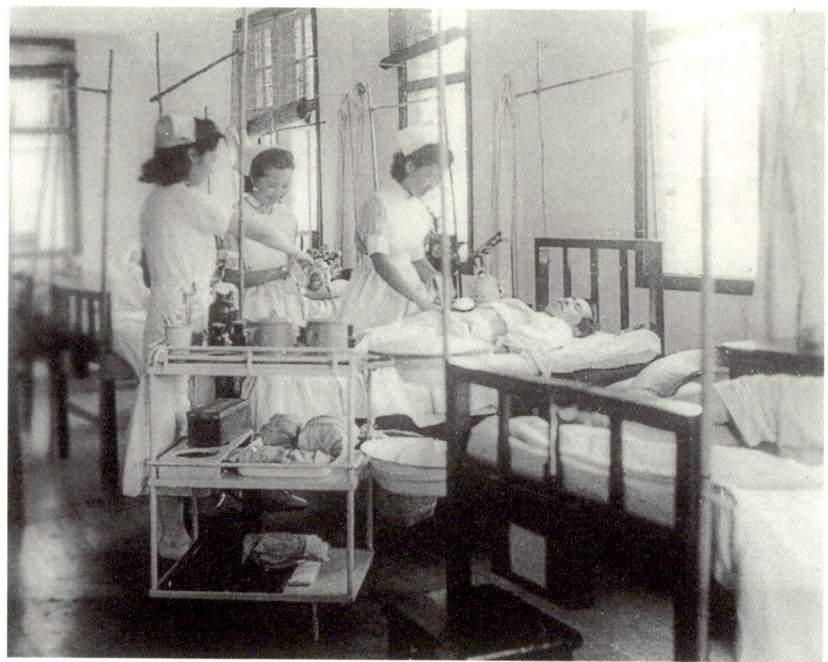

FIGURE 5.3 Surgical ward in the WCUU University Hospital, ca. 1943. | Courtesy Rockefeller Archive Center, RAC-CMB_FA065_B1144_F1042_006.

PUMC staff, it is unlikely they would find as many English-speaking students in remote Sichuan as they had in cosmopolitan Beijing. At the same time, most reference books were in English, "and medical terms used on the wards are in English too."[119]

The question of whether to teach in English is an interesting one, and came up at various times in nursing history in China. Canadian nursing programs at the WCM, the NCM, and Qilu were taught in Chinese. Indeed, missionary nurses – including Margaret Lee, who spoke Cantonese, not Mandarin – were required to take two years of language study when they first arrived in China. Nor was the PUMC absolutely required to teach in English. In 1936, the PUMC board of trustees had granted the dean of nursing discretion as to whether subjects would be taught in English or Chinese.[120] In some circumstances, it made more sense to teach in Chinese – such as in the postgraduate courses in public health, where students might not know English.[121]

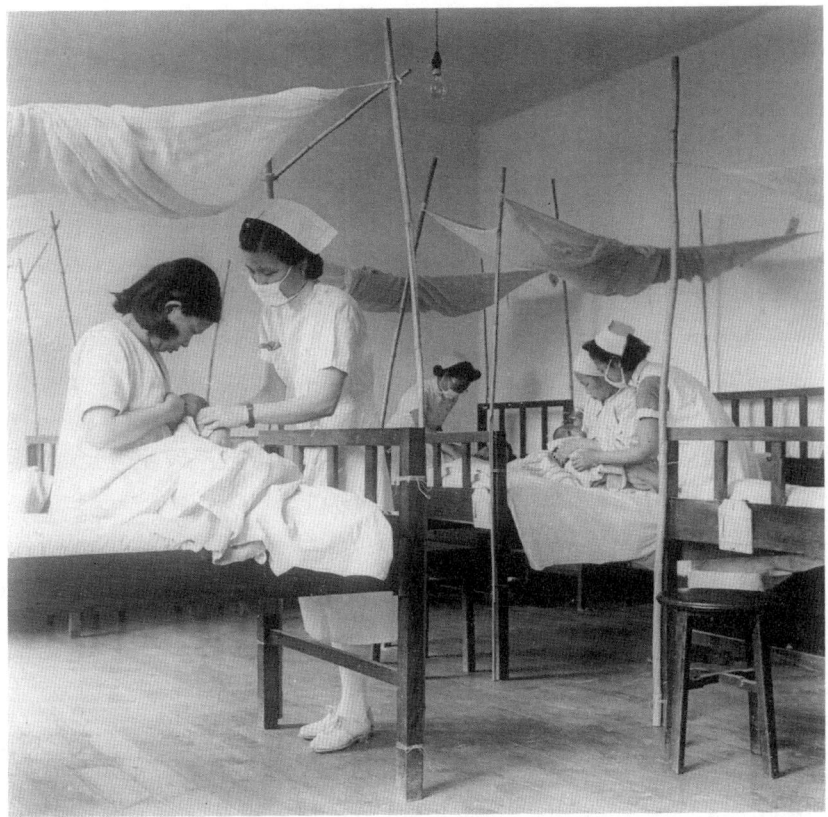

FIGURE 5.4 Renji nursing students in the WCUU University Hospital, ca. 1943. | Courtesy Rockefeller Archive Center, RAC-CMB_FA065_B1144_F1042_008.

That the now all-Chinese PUMC Faculty Committee unanimously voted to keep teaching in English is quite remarkable; there must have been more to the decision than the practicality of English textbooks. The most likely reason was that it set the PUMC School of Nursing apart as an elite institution. Refugee PUMC nursing faculty member Liu Ching-ho described it this way:

> We nurses are looked up to because we can speak English, and not many people can do that. We have attended college, and not many people have had the opportunity of attending college. We are immaculate. We have starched uniforms pressed by American laundry

machines, which people admire. But it is not because of the nursing profession. We see that. We can see it in the fact that in the recruitment of students in [Chengdu], when the School of Nursing of the PUMC was re-established there. I met on the campus the applicants coming to the nursing profession. They were all from [Beijing], not one from [Chengdu]. Not one of the applicants came from [Chengdu], the local place.[122]

With forty-two applicants on their doorstep as soon as they opened, the PUMC nursing faculty recognized that part of the attraction was not that they were bringing nursing education to Sichuan, but that they were bringing China's most exclusive nursing school within reach. By 1945, however, the PUMC had to look pragmatically at the realities associated with continuing to teach exclusively in English. On 27 September 1945, Vera Nieh announced that "all classes may be conducted either in English or Chinese, in any way which can express one's ideas most clearly. But the technical terms should be taught in English with Chinese translations if possible."[123]

China scholar Mary Brown Bullock noted that the PUMC had difficulty adapting to wartime conditions in Sichuan and that "wartime experiences were a rude shock for some of the former ivory tower graduates."[124] Mary Ferguson, who was sent back to China by the CMB after the war, similarly noted that it had become apparent during wartime that the PUMC had kept itself too isolated from other medical schools. "Formerly," Ferguson noted, "there was a tendency toward keeping too closely within our walls, described by some as 'monastic' isolation."[125] Such a tendency also explains, in part, why the PUMC School of Nursing worked parallel to, rather than in collaboration with, the Renji School of Nursing. The priority, then, when the refugee PUMC started setting up in Chengdu, was for faculty to do what they could to demonstrate all that made the PUMC unique, and superior. And it worked. Their impact was already felt on the wards of the University Hospital less than a month after their arrival, where the PUMC faculty arranged a well-organized set up (see Figure 5.5). In August 1943, Canadian missionary nurse Margaret Lee, who also worked at

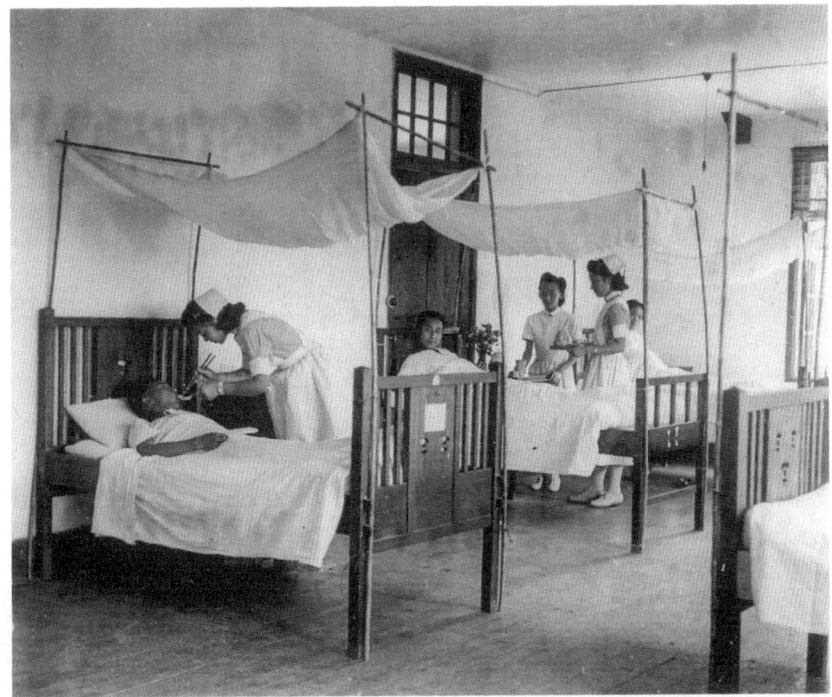

FIGURE 5.5 Nursing students in medical ward of the WCUU University Hospital, ca. 1944. | Courtesy Rockefeller Archive Center, CMB_FA065_B1144_F1042_007.

the University Hospital, was excited about some of the changes already underway:

> Both [Vera Nieh] and her staff have helped us to make some im-
> provements. We have improved methods and techniques, have
> been able to change or develop and maintain certain policies, meth-
> ods which we had partially succeeded because we could not get the
> co-operation of the other departments, and because our numbers
> (of senior staff) were too small to give constant supervision to the
> various phases of the work. Miss Nieh has brought with her a well-
> qualified staff whose ideals and ideas of nursing are similar to mine;
> I hope that we shall be able to work hand in hand toward one goal,
> namely the betterment of nursing education in [Chengdu] and in
> [Sichuan].[126]

The Renji School of Nursing, in the meantime, was reportedly "flourishing," with over ninety students in August 1943.[127] Renji students received the major portion of their training at the United Hospital (Si Shen Tsi) and then came to the University Hospital for four months to obtain their required obstetrical and gynecological experience. In 1943, the Renji school also started taking in two cohorts of students per year, in the spring and fall. This was a way to ensure that "we would have enough nurses to care for the patients when we expand our work out here on campus."[128] The original plan was for the Renji and PUMC nursing programs to work together. Indeed, on 8 December 1943, Vera Nieh proposed at the regular PUMC faculty meeting that they "start a teaching program for the Jen Chi [Renji] students who are here [at the University Hospital] and for the staff nurses."[129] The connection between the two nursing programs was instead limited to support for the Renji students during their third-year practicums at the University Hospital. However, although the Renji school was not directly associated with the PUMC, it did benefit from the association. PUMC alumnus Eva Liu became principal of the Renji School of Nursing and superintendent of nurses at the General Hospital and Eye, Ear, Nose, and Throat hospital units.[130] When Liu resigned, on 1 December 1944, she was replaced by PUMC alumna Bernice Chu Chen.[131] In this way, the PUMC's influence extended across both nursing programs associated with the WCUU.

Faculty meeting minutes give a sense of the lengths to which the Faculty Committee went to ensure that the PUMC school was properly set up. For example, on 24 September 1943 they made the following decisions: nursing services should have a separate kitchen from the one for patients; nurses should not take responsibility for collecting money from patients; new patients should wait downstairs until the ward was ready for them; ward visiting hours should be limited to 3:00–5:00 p.m. daily for "second and third class patients"; and tips from patients to the ward should be handed to the nurse in charge, who would divide them among all the ward servants. Wang Hsui-ying noted that the nurses had to do "all kinds of work; from coolies' up to accountants and secretarial work besides routine nursing, as nurses are hard to get."[132]

The faculty also set regulations related to working conditions for both students and graduate nurses. It is helpful to remember that nursing in China, as elsewhere, was provided by women who lived on site, either at or near the hospital. School of nursing offices and classrooms were normally in the hospital itself. Schools of nursing and associated hospitals worked closely together, the dean of nursing typically also being the superintendent of nurses at the hospital. Nursing schools oversaw the "nursing service" at the hospital, meaning that, in addition to running the education program, the dean was responsible for ensuring that hospital wards were adequately staffed. Hospital rules and regulations were, therefore, ultimately determined by the dean of nursing. In October 1943, the PUMC Faculty Committee set out rules regarding time off. Graduate nurses were allowed one day off each week, whereas "dressers and attendants" were allowed one afternoon off each week, and one day off each month. Dressers and attendants worked nine-hour days; "coolies" worked ten.[133] Everyone worked two hours less on holidays.[134] Nurses would be on night duty for eight weeks at a time. Before going on night duty, they would be granted a whole day off, which was counted as their day off for that week.[135] Such rules allowed for the smooth running of the nursing service and ensured that the hospital was adequately staffed twenty-four hours a day. As new structures were put in place, the WCUU Hospital started to resemble the PUMC Hospital in Bejing (see Figure 5.6).

While ward servants helped to ensure the smooth running of the work site, dormitory servants helped support nurses at home. Hospitals were typically responsible for providing nursing staff (including students) with lodging, food, and uniforms. Nurses were responsible for purchasing their own shoes and stockings. At the refugee PUMC, dormitory servants ran "errands for everyone on Tuesday and Friday afternoons." Servants also provided laundry service for uniforms and personal items, personal laundry being "returned on Wednesday and Saturday evenings."[136] By April 1944, the refugee PUMC had established "all necessary routines and regulations both in the hospital and in the school."[137] To Wang Hsui-ying, "things generally are put into shape,

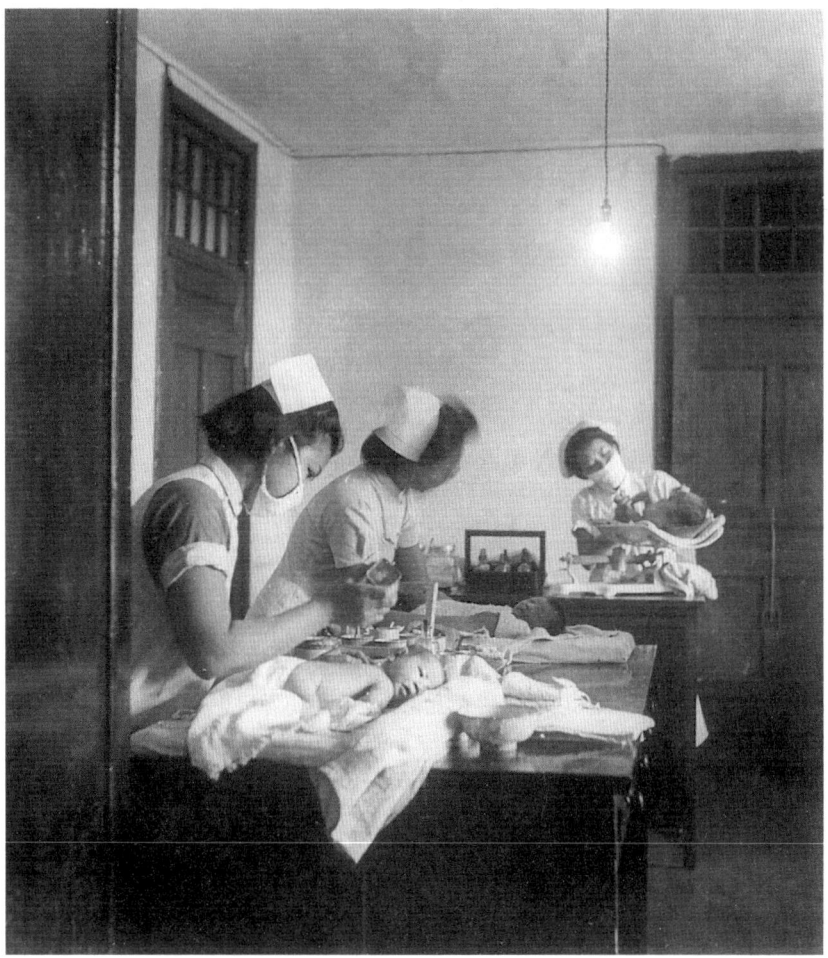

FIGURE 5.6 Nursing students in the WCUU University Hospital nursery, ca. 1944. | Courtesy Rockefeller Archive Center, RAC-CMB_FA065_B1144_F1042_009.

and we feel with comfort that we have really started something worthy of our effort."[138]

As much as Vera Nieh was intent on having expectations and provisions in Sichuan that were similar to those in Beijing, this proved difficult. Wartime conditions complicated matters; both the hospital and the nurses' resources were stretched so thin, the regulations had to be constantly adjusted to ensure that nurses' physical needs were met. Nurses who did not live in the hospital (and therefore did not have access to hospital food) were soon provided with a food allowance.[139] To balance the cost, time off became more restricted, as did the provision of uniforms:[140] by 1944, nurses could no longer keep their uniforms if they left before one year of service. By May 1945, they were still required to provide their own shoes and stockings, but it was no longer required that these be white.[141] In winter time, the students added socks to their uniforms to keep warm; their colour had to match the shoes and stockings.[142]

On first glance, the change in uniform, stocking, and shoe expectations might seem minor. In fact, this was an important indicator of how difficult things had become. For most nurses in China and elsewhere, for most of the twentieth century, the uniform was critical to their identity. Belts, colours, pins, and caps all had particular meanings, setting probationers apart from student nurses, first-year students from third-year students, students from graduate nurses, and staff nurses from head nurses. For example, even in the 1960s, at the Vancouver General Hospital, when a new rule called for *all* students to wear white stockings, effectively eliminating the rite of passage from black to white stockings previously preserved for upper-level students, senior students revolted.[143] The PUMC uniform was a blue dress with a starched white apron, cuffs, and distinctive cap – and students were expected to care for (and wear) their uniforms with a military precision. In short, the PUMC uniform was both a source of pride and a marker of prestige. It is also why arranging for uniforms was the first order of the day when the Faculty Committee met for the first time in Chengdu in July 1943, and the first order of business for the dean. The significance of the PUMC uniform is exemplified by a concern raised by the PUMC in 1945, when someone pointed out that "it was said that Jen Chi [Renji] student nurses' uniforms are like ours. Miss Wang HY [Wang Hsui-ying?] was elected as a representative to inquire about it."[144] For the PUMC, the distinctive uniform was central to its identity. For the CMB, however, the cost of the uniforms was prohibitively high; Claude Forkner could simply not understand why specific uniforms were so critical. The uniform budget would be just one source of consternation for Forkner, and just one cause for conflict between him and Vera Nieh.

* * *

While Vera Nieh's role in the establishment of the PUMC School of Nursing in West China is well recognized, in reality many people were involved. Indeed, the actual decisions regarding the opening of the school did not involve Nieh at all. Instead, led by Dr. Marshall Balfour, Dr. Claude Forkner, and Dr. Edwin Lobenstine, it was other PUMC nursing alumnae who were intimately involved with the decision-making process before Nieh arrived in West China, most notably Bernice Chu Chen and Hsu Ai-Chu. PUMC alumnae were deeply involved in the planning, founding, and operation of the refugee PUMC, as well as in the support of nursing education at the Canadian West China Mission. The first nine faculty to work at the refugee PUMC were all PUMC alumnae, and almost the entire PUMC faculty eventually migrated to Chengdu to work there. The nursing leaders in Koloshan who contributed to Claude Forkner's decision regarding the location of the school were also PUMC alumnae. And, even though they did not work at the refugee PUMC, alumnae Bernice Chu Chen and Eva Liu provided leadership at the WCM United Hospital. Thus, the refugee PUMC story is really one of a remarkably committed and engaged group of PUMC alumnae – approximately twelve in all – who firmly believed that the PUMC had something critical to offer the war effort in China.

Although the PUMC tended, as Mary Brown Bullock and Mary Ferguson noted, to work in isolation from other schools and with ivory tower ideals, the PUMC nursing alumnae who took up leadership positions in West China adjusted remarkably quickly to the wartime conditions. This is exemplified, in part, by the contrast between the attrition of missionary nurses in West China and the relative stability of the PUMC workforce. It is also evidenced by the swift impact the PUMC had on the organization of the new University Hospital, evidenced by the descriptions provided by Margaret Lee. In 1942, Lee had decried the "comparatively low" standards in Chengdu, which she blamed on the wartime conditions. Ten months later, she praised the PUMC for helping the

WCM improve methods, techniques, and policies at the hospital. While she credited some of this improvement to the increase in the number of nursing staff, she attributed most to the excellence of the PUMC leaders. While dire wartime conditions and shortages were in part to blame for lower quality nursing care, it was the quality of the nursing faculty and staff that really mattered – a belief that was central to the PUMC philosophy, but not fully tested until its refugee years.

CHAPTER SIX

Fighting the Foundation's "Darling Child" (1943–46)

Conflicts with the PUMC

It is an open secret that that [the PUMC School of Nursing] was the darling child of the Rockefeller Foundation, and regarded by that body as the most satisfying of its large family of projects through the world.

– *Dr. Allen Best, University Hospital Superintendent, WCUU, 1943*

Vera Nieh was a fighter. Although she had not been the first choice of the Peking Union Medical College (PUMC) as dean of the School of Nursing, she proved herself capable of adhering to and fighting for her own deeply held principles – and supporting women's leadership at the same time. Her first priority was the well-being of her nursing faculty, and then of her nursing students. And, underpinning her priorities, was a patriotism that kept her focused on the future: China needed nurses. More to the point, China needed nurse leaders. The PUMC had prepared Nieh to be a leader, and she took the role seriously, planting her feet firmly as she went toe to toe, time and again, with various men who were in authority over her – breaking Chinese, gender, and nursing social norms everywhere she went. When she believed something was right (or wrong), she would not back down. As a result, clarion calls for her resignation came regularly, and from different corners. However, she knew how to position herself, how to nurture and then draw upon allies. At just over five feet tall and one hundred pounds, she was a formidable force. In this chapter, we zero in on the contentious relationships between Nieh and her contemporaries, suggesting that, in order to be seen, heard, and taken seriously, she had to assert herself and her principles into every decision made by others regarding the PUMC School of Nursing. She was a jealous defender of PUMC ideals.

BESTING BEST

From the very beginning, Claude Forkner, director of the Rockefeller Foundation's China Medical Board (CMB), and Vera Nieh had an uneasy relationship. In a letter to his colleague Edwin Lobenstine on 21 October 1943, Forkner expressed frustration with Nieh, blaming her for "difficulties in getting the nursing school properly adjusted." He did concede, however, that Nieh was not the only "difficult personality." Indeed, "there are lots of them here," he wrote, "among both foreign and Chinese staff." Forkner appreciated that Vera Nieh was a "very efficient and straightforward person," and graciously, if insincerely, stated, "I think she is going to run an excellent school."[1] These were, after all, wartime conditions, and difficulties and discouragement were inevitable. Still, he considered Nieh to be a "nervous person" who had "some difficulties in getting along with the hospital business and superintendent's offices." In addition, "she gets excited and in her manner incites considerable antagonism. We have had many talks together and she realizes some of those facts and is keeping herself more under control. She has a hard task and I sympathize with her."[2] As their relationship grew increasingly strained over the next number of months, Forkner settled on a view of Nieh as mentally unstable and unfit for her role.

The "difficulties in getting along" that Forkner was referring to were Nieh's difficulties with Dr. Allen Best, the West China missionary who was the superintendent of the United Hospitals in Chengdu. For his part, Best had been overjoyed at the news that the PUMC was coming to the West China Union University (WCUU) campus; it would give him the opportunity to leave the administrative position he really did not like, as the PUMC would provide a hospital administrator of its own: "Getting this 'little institution' [a reference to the relative newness of the University Hospital] out of its swaddling clothes and well through the toddling stage," he wrote, "has been a star example of muddling along. Now there is real promise of getting back at last to my main interest in life, working with patients and students." Pleased that the PUMC was planning to provide the new University Hospital with an "experienced hospital superintendent," Best was "preparing joyfully to unload that irksome, time-consuming and patience-absorbing job onto the strong shoulders of one of our Chinese, foreign-trained friends."[3] Little did he realize that some of the strongest shoulders would belong to the diminutive Vera Nieh.

On 26 December 1943, Best wrote a gleeful circular letter to "Friends of Centennial" that outlined the arrival of the PUMC, and his view of it. "Perhaps the most significant [thing that has happened here] from points financial, teaching and prestige has been the coming to our midst of the Peking Union Medical College and its attendant high grade school of nursing."[4] He continued, "we have been over the years rather proud (perhaps a little too proud) of our own college and school of nursing but I think that in all fairness we should have to admit that from the standpoint of uniformly high-grade efficiency their set up is all-in-all the best in China." Best informed his readers of the events that led to the PUMC's presence on the WCUU campus, writing that, two years earlier, the Japanese had "made it impossible" for the PUMC to continue in Beijing, so "gradually the twos and threes of both staff and students (mostly students) began their long trek up here into Free China." As Best told it, they were "months on the road and for months they kept straggling in." Word of their desire to see the PUMC reopened in Sichuan "trickled through to New York and apparently after much deliberation Dr. Claude Forkner (of 'iron lung' fame) was appointed as the Director and sent out here to see what could be done." Best had great respect for Claude Forkner. He commented that Forkner, having studied the situation, came to the conclusion that building a new campus was out of the question, and thus the wisest plan would be for the PUMC to "cast in their lot with one of the existing medical colleges here." Once people began to hear of the possibility of hosting the famous and well-resourced PUMC, "there was immediately as you might guess something of a scramble." That the PUMC "chose to smile" on the WCUU meant the latter institution "had much reason to congratulate itself."[5]

For Allen Best, having the PUMC gladly join up with the WCUU was "one of the most heartening things that has happened to us for many years."[6] He would not be of the same opinion three months later.

The conflict between Vera Nieh and Allen Best started shortly after the refugee PUMC arrived at the WCUU. In part it was a personality conflict. Other nurses – most notably Dorothy Fox, who resigned from the West China Mission as a result – had difficulties working with Best. While the details of the conflict are not clear, it was significant enough for the CMB to send former PUMC dean of nursing Ruth Ingram to Chengdu to investigate. She concluded that the issue was not, as she had been told, the local nurses' distrust of Vera Nieh. Rather, the issue was Best's "peculiar temperament and strange administrative policies."[7]

In March 1944, Best turned over the superintendency of the University Hospital to Dr. Li Ting-an, formerly of Central University Medical College.[8] "The situation [at the University Hospital] has not been satisfactory," Canadian missionary Dr. Gerald Bell wrote to the Canadian Mission headquarters in Toronto,

> especially since the PUMC Nursing School came in. The Director, Miss Nieh, was too much for Best and most of the others on his staff. Li [Ting-an] happens to be a sort of Executive Secretary of the PUMC Nursing School Board of Directors with a great deal of authority given to him since the members are widely scattered. This solution seems to be working out very well and he has already laid down the law to Miss Nieh and conditions are much improved, so far as the general running is concerned.[9]

That Nieh was willing to clash with superiors – typically male physicians in administrative authority over her – seems clear. There are records of significant personality clashes with Dr. John B. Grant (Health Station, 1932, 1933), Dr. Claude Forkner (1944), Dr. Stephen Chang (1944), Dr. Allen Best (1943, 1945), and Dr. C.C. Chen (1944). We learn a bit of how she was perceived from an undated diary entry of Marshall Balfour, who noted that, on 23 May 1947, Vera Nieh, who was in New

York after the war, came in to talk with him.[10] He reviewed with her discussions he had had with PUMC trustees and others related to a proposal to continue the Rockefeller Foundation grant to the PUMC School of Nursing for the same amount as in 1945–46. At first, Nieh seemed satisfied. "All went well," he wrote, "until she finally lets go and makes serious accusations about the character and integrity of certain Trustees, particularly C.C. Chen." Balfour declared himself "rather appalled," as he had complete faith in Chen. He let Nieh know "fully of his dismay, disgust and discouragement."[11] Balfour considered this his final interview with Nieh, and he subsequently conveyed the substance of it to Drs. C.C. Chen, Li Ting-an, and Y.T. Tsur.[12] For Balfour, being witness to Vera Nieh's fury only served to confirm the prevailing view among the men in the various CMB-related offices that Nieh was unfit for a leadership position.

A THORN IN OUR FLESH

From the outset, Vera Nieh was committed to ensuring that the refugee PUMC School of Nursing – and herself as dean – had similar prestige and privileges in Chengdu as it had had in Beijing. Of particular concern to her was the organizational structure set up by the PUMC board of trustees, whereby the School of Nursing was (incorrectly) considered a Department of Nursing, and the dean of nursing (incorrectly) considered a principal of nursing. In the Beijing structure, the School of Nursing had existed under that name since 1924, the same time that the baccalaureate program had started, and its first head, Anna Wolf, was designated dean.[13] At that time, structural changes were meant to indicate that the PUMC was not a run-of-the-mill, hospital-based nurses' training program. Rather, nursing was a full partner in the overall university enterprise. The dean of nursing held much of the decision-making authority (including related to the budget) for the School of Nursing as well as for the nursing service at the associated hospital. At the refugee PUMC, however, the principal of the Nursing School reported to the CMB director (a position held by Claude Forkner) and to the hospital superintendent (a position held by Allen Best). Thus, when, in early 1944, the PUMC nursing faculty and alumnae recommended to the board that the name of the school be changed (back) to the PUMC School of Nursing, it was in recognition of the political disadvantages of the new structure.[14]

Although the refugee PUMC opened in September 1943, it was not until December of that year that the CMB board of trustees was able to meet to discuss its vision and priorities. This delay was, in part, because of the disruption caused by the internment of enemy aliens in China. On 16 December, the trustees met at the CMB headquarters in New York, two weeks after the arrival of the MS *Gripsholm* in New York brought ten PUMC faculty and staff among its 1,500 passengers. Seven of the trustees were now in the United States: three had returned on the *Gripsholm*, four were already there. Three trustees (Dr. Li Ting-an, Dr. Y.T. Tsur, and Dr. Wong Wen-hao) were in West China, and eight others were in occupied China – presumably interned. At the New York meeting ("informal" because of the lack of quorum), among the items discussed were the many problems of personnel, policy, and finance related to the reestablishment of the School of Nursing in Chengdu. They also discussed how to reconstitute the CMB trustees, given the number of board members who were caught in occupied China. They worked this out by appointing three new trustees while removing the eight in occupied China. One of the new trustees was C.C. Chen, a physician. Chen's father was the first Chinese to be ordained as a Methodist minister, in Beijing. Dr. Y.T. Tsur was selected as chairman of the trustees in Free China. The refugee PUMC now had someone to whom they could direct their concerns.

The first meeting of the PUMC trustees in Free China, on 17 January 1944, was held in Chongqing with Wong Wen-hao, Y.T. Tsur, and Li Ting-an. Claude Forkner and Vera Nieh were guests.[15] The purpose of the meeting was to discuss the administrative management of the PUMC School of Nursing, which, since its reopening, had been under the administrative charge of the CMB Wartime Committee and of Claude Forkner.[16] One item was about the budget: Nieh had added almost 800,000 CN Chinese "dollars")[17] to the budget originally submitted just three months previous – from 1,042,680 CN to 1,800,000 CN; she said it was due to inflation. A six-month budget for 827,250 CN was approved. The group also discussed concerns related to Dr. Allen Best: "Many difficulties have arisen between Miss Nieh and her staff in relation to the Hospital Superintendent and Business Manager. It was pointed out that the present Superintendent is not trained for his post and is anxious to be relieved of it."[18] The board recognized Best's desire to depart, and decided that Li Ting-an be asked to take up Best's duties. Li accepted, provided arrangements could be made with the National Centre Medical School to release him of his duties there, and with hospital authorities "to relieve the present incumbent of the office, the latter being left to Dr. C.H. Forkner to negotiate."[19]

Five weeks later, upon receiving the minutes of the meeting, Vera Nieh immediately wrote to Claude Forkner to ask for corrections. She asked him to change "many difficulties have arisen between Miss Nieh and her staff in relation to the Hospital Superintendent and Business Manager" to "many difficulties have arisen between the nursing faculties and the Hospital Superintendent and Business Manager" to clarify that the problem was not between Nieh and her staff, as, she noted, "we are working in the best of harmony."[20] She also noted that one of the items in the minutes had not actually been discussed in the meeting – that is, that decisions of the board of trustees in Free China would require approval from the trustees in New York. "If decisions of trustees in Free China have to be approved in New York the school administration will be greatly handicapped," she noted.[21] The depth of Nieh's frustration with Claude Forkner is glossed over in her letter to him but unmistakable in a cablegram she sent the same day, 23 February 1944, to Edwin Lobenstine: "Forkner is great hindrance to nursing school," Nieh complained, "not desirable in China. School must have budget. Letter follows."[22] A flurry of cablegrams followed. On 26 February 1944, Lobenstine sent a cablegram to Y.T. Tsur, chairman of the PUMC board of trustees: "cable received from Vera Nieh concerning Forkner's relations nursing school stop am replying such problems should be handled through PUMC committee."[23] On 3 March 1944, Forkner responded with a cablegram of his own:

VERA NIEH EMOTIONALLY UNSTABLE FIGHTING EVERY-
ONE INSUBORDINATE NO SENSE ABOUT ADIMINISTRA-
TION UNAWARE WARTIME CONDITIONS REFUESES TAKE
DIRECTION FROM ADMINISTRATIVE COMMITEEE RE-
FUSES INFORM LI TING AN CONCERNING HER CABLE
TO LIU STOP DEMANDS PERSONAL UNSUPERVISED CON-
TROL ALL MONEY ALLOCATED BY CMB FOR NURSING
SCHOOL HAVE PREVIOUSLY RECOMMENDED TO TSUR
HER REPLACEMENT STOP[24]

He finished the cablegram with the enigmatic statement – "Suspect other
influences." That same day, 3 March 1944, Li Ting-an also sent a cablegram to the CMB in New York:

NURSING SCHOOL HAS MANY FRICTIONS STOP VERA
NIEH AND MOST NURSING SCHOOL FACUTLY CONSIDER
FUNCITON OF ADMINISTRATIVE COMMITTEE ADVISORY
ONLY THEY WANT COMPLETE CONTROLE SCHOOL AD-
MINISTRATION INCLUDING FINANCE AND THREATEN
TROUBLE OR MASSIVE RESIGNATION IF I AS EXECUTIVE
OFFICER INTERFERE STOP CONDITION SERIOUS HAVE
WIRED Y T TSUR STOP WELCOME INSTRUCTIONS[25]

Three days later, Earle Ballou,[26] Executive Secretary for the United
Board for Christian Colleges in China, responded to Li:

GREATLY DISTRESSED NURSING SCHOOL DIFFICULTIES
STOPLACK TOO MANY DETAILS TO SUGGEST SOLU-
TION BUT CONSIDER IMPORTANT THAT RELATIONSHIP
SCHOOL TO TRUSTEES COMMITTEE BE CLEARLY DE-
FINED PERHAPS ALLOWING SCHOOL ADMINISTRATIVE
AUTONOMY WITHIN BUDGET APPROVED BY TRUSTEES
SUBJECT TO PROPER ACCOUNTING CONTROLS BY UNI-
VERSITY OF COMMITTEE APPOINTEE STOP PLEASE

CONVEY FOREGOING TO MEMBERS ADMINISTRATIVE
COMMITTEE AND NIEH.[27]

The situation was rapidly escalating; Claude Forkner considered it to
be acute. He wrote to Dr. Y.T. Tsur of his concerns about Nieh, using
increasingly strong language.[28] He noted that both he and Dr. Li were
"distressed" at the nursing school's "lack of cooperation" and "lack of
appreciation" that he and Li were attempting in every way to help them.[29]
To Forkner, the nursing faculty interpreted any help as interference, and
rejected any proposals he and Li made. His proposed solution was for
full authority of the school to be delegated to the CMB Administrative
Committee in China, rather than having the trustees in New York "continue to interfere with the nursing school about which they have no concrete information."[30] By this time, Forkner had become incensed with
Nieh: "My experience with Miss Nieh has been sufficient to arrive at the
very definite conclusion that she is not the person to head the school and
that the school will fail under her administration."[31]

WEIGHING IN: STEPHEN CHANG'S PERSPECTIVE

Dr. Stephen Chang also weighed in on the PUMC trustee criticism of
Vera Nieh. In a confidential eight-page, single-spaced letter to Edwin
Lobenstine on 18 March 1944, he outlined his work in West China over
the previous ten months.[32] The first two pages of his letter praised the
work and character of Dr. Forkner. "He was my favorite teacher," Chang
noted, and students and alumni alike were "thrilled" with him. The focus
for Forkner was the opening of the Nursing School and the placement of
PUMC medical students. Although the decision to use the WCUU as the
site of the School of Nursing was a good one, it "gave us a few choice ene-
mies." "As much as I regret to say so," continued Chang, "our capital is
soaked through with intrigues and politics and to have come out with
only so few scratches is a real credit to anybody." Chang exclaimed that
he himself was not afraid to sacrifice anything, "even imprisonment would
not deter me"– something he had already proven during his work at the
PUMC under Japanese occupation. "I can only say," he emphasized,

"that I have never been under anybody who is more fair and straight-forward and sincere than Dr. Forkner." Furthermore, he had "done much better than many of the foreign missionaries here." Chang claimed that he himself had never worked so hard in his life, "but when a fellow who is not Chinese works so hard for China, what can a Chinese do but be inspired?"[33]

After two full pages of praise ("This letter sounds like a high-pressure eulogy," he admitted), Chang suggested that all was going as well as could be expected within the refugee PUMC, except at the Nursing School, "which I must say has disappointed us a great deal." He viewed it as ironic that the Nursing School, which had been the PUMC's "greatest purpose and pride from the beginning," was now the source of such strife. "We have tried to nurture it from its rebirth with care and zeal and we have left no stone unturned to make it a success," he noted. The whole campus and medical community "held their breath" he suggested, to see what would come of this "wonderful" school. According to Chang, the WCUU had for years wanted to create a college-grade nursing school, but did not do so because it feared that young Sichuanese women would not "condescend" to become nurses. Both Claude Forkner and Stephen Chang believed that, with such a "fine bunch" of nursing faculty, and "an able woman like Miss Nieh as the dean," a "wonderful mine where raw materials could be drawn," and such interest on all sides, "the School could not help be a success." "Who would imagine," he wrote, "that it has turned out to be a thorn in our flesh?"[34]

Stephen Chang described Vera Nieh as "a dynamic go-getter" who "has no fear for anybody." These were necessary qualities for her role, he conceded. "The only trouble," he noted, "is she also has several rather damaging shortcomings." In Chang's view, Nieh acted as if there was no war going on. Instead of focusing on the fundamentals of nursing, she was spending energy on outside appearances. Furniture and living quarters had to be just so. The school printed stationary on (more expensive) foreign paper "and they must give teas to every new and departing faculty member." Of particular concern to Chang were the uniforms" she expected nursing students to wear the same style uniform, stockings, and shoes as they did in Beijing. "You can imagine the effect,"

Chang wrote, "when these [PUMC] students made their debut with dazzling uniforms when the local Jen Chi [Renji] Nursing School also work in the hospital [and] are wearing the simplest of uniforms." In the winter, most of the PUMC nurses got chilblains because their stockings were too thin. "When the Superintendent out of kindness suggested warm Chinese cotton-padded shoes and warmer stockings, he was told by Miss Nieh that the nurses must keep up their traditions chilblains or no chilblains."[35]

In Chang's view, the PUMC nurses did not want to work with medical doctors. He suggested that the animus might have originated because Nieh herself did not complete medical school: "I have only recently learned that Miss Nieh tried the medical course and failed and so has got a complex there." This statement offered an inaccurate account of Nieh's experience (she did not fail; she withdrew) but a convenient analysis. Chang also complained about Nieh's insubordination. "She argues with every Tom, Dick and Harry," he complained. "She must get everything by quarrelling." She "bangs on the table" and she "shouts," and yet, the nursing students, he noted, were very proud of her. At one point, Chang noted, the whole nursing school threatened to go on strike if Dr. Li interfered with the nursing school. To Chang, the threat to strike could have only come from Vera Nieh: "They do not really mean it for [if] they had, I would say that anybody who strikes during wartime should be shot as saboteurs."[36]

Still, despite his criticism of the nurses (and perhaps because he started to think his letter was becoming a bit harsh), Chang also admitted that they were doing good work. They have "absolutely cleaned up the wards in this University Hospital," he noted. The staff had done a "wonderful piece of work" and "it is a joy to see a ward well run." The nurses knew their job and did it well. "If only they would not quarrel and display themselves, all would have been well." Chang believed that Nieh did not accept him in his position. She looked down on him, he believed. Yet, "even so, I have no grudge against her," he wrote – never mind that he had just spent two pages praising Forkner and the next six criticizing Nieh. "She did graduate many years before I did from the PUMC and seniority in China counts a lot." He said that he realized early on that he was not welcome in the Nursing School and therefore, with Dr. Forkner's permission, had as little to do with the School as possible. "You cannot blame us," he wrote, "for [sometimes] wishing we had never started the School."[37]

In Stephen Chang's view, Vera Nieh had been an excellent dean at the PUMC in Beijing. However, "if you put such people in a totally new place and virgin field they go hayway and lose control of their own power and ability." And there was the rub. In Beijing, he noted, Nieh was content to be under the authority of Harry Houghton and Trevor Bowen. But, "as soon as you put her in a new place and call her a principal according [sic] to the government custom then she goes out of her boundary and thinks she is responsible to nobody except herself." This, after all, was Nieh's complaint – that she was called and considered someone less in Chengdu than she had been in Beijing. Stephen Chang, like Claude Forkner, thought that Nieh should be replaced. "She is a bad example to her students and she is the most outstanding example of the criticism [illegible] at PUMC." Although Chang claimed that he held no grudge against her, he also suggested to Lobenstine that, "if I may be allowed to say so I am afraid she really needs some psychiatric attention." He also believed that, if Nieh did not have the support from "unhealthy influential people," she would "not have dared to be so bold to everybody." According to Chang, Li Ting-an "will not hesitate to ask her to resign if she keeps up with her attitude."[38]

NUDGING NIEH TOWARD RESIGNATION

Li Ting-an, who replaced Allen Best at the University Hospital, was well known to Vera Nieh; they had worked together at the Health Station in Beijing a decade earlier. At that time, Nieh had complained that Li Ting-an and John B. Gant were making important decisions without consulting her, and that the organizational structure at the Health Station left her with little to no authority. She was not going to let this happen again. Thus, when Li, now the executive officer of the Administrative Committee for the Nursing School, and newly appointed as the superintendent of the University Hospital, wrote to Vera Nieh requiring her to follow the regulations outlined by Y.T. Tsur, she and the nursing faculty revolted.[39] At issue was the "Outline of Regulations Governing the Administration of the PUMC School of Nursing," as approved by Tsur on 1 March 1944.[40] In this two-page document, Tsur had outlined five principles and twenty-five rules governing appointments, salary payment or remuneration, the handling of funds, and custody of school property.[41] Faculty appointments, for example, could be suggested by the dean, but were to be made by the chairman of the Administrative Committee. Increases to salaries proposed by the dean would need to be approved by the Administrative Committee. The faculty disagreed.

On 20 March 1944, the nursing faculty wrote a detailed letter to Tsur, outlining a number of their concerns since the school was reopened in Chengdu.[42] One concern was the title of the head of the school – specifically, the assumption by those in Chengdu that a "dean" did not have the same authority as a "director." In Beijing, they noted, the title of the head of the nursing school in Chinese was "director" while in English it was "dean" – the point being that the dean "in reality had the same authority and responsibilities as those of a Director."[43] This mattered because, in Chengdu, Vera Nieh did not have the same authority, responsibilities, duties, and rights as those in charge of a nursing school normally would have. She should serve as an ex-officio member in board meetings, they suggested, or at any meetings where school affairs were discussed and planned. The organizational structure in Chengdu, they believed, gave too much authority to the executive officer, who, essentially, had been "given the rights as a Director of a nursing school," which made the administrative structure unnecessarily complicated. The faculty also requested that the dean be given the right to appoint school staff. Not only was this right "stated in the constitution of the Ministry of Education," but also, since the dean was a nurse, she would know more about nursing than someone who was not a nurse. Finally, they noted that the dean should have a "free hand" to use the approved budget – presumably as compared to having to get permission from Li Ting-an regarding budget items. In other words, the faculty was asking that the dean have the full right to use the budget within limits approved by the board.[44]

During this time, Li Ting-an was also becoming fed up with Vera Nieh. He sent a confidential letter to Y.T. Tsur on 19 March 1944 noting that he had been calling upon PUMC alumni to try to "smooth out matters," but that, "due to Miss Nieh's stubborn attitude," he had not had much success.[45] He had told Claude Forkner (himself agitating for Vera Nieh's resignation) that he did not wish to "sacrifice the services of Miss Nieh and some of her capable staff members unless I am one hundred percent convinced that all efforts have been exhausted." However, if Vera Nieh *were* to be replaced, Li thought that Chou Meiyu would be a suitable substitute. He also noted that "Miss Eva Liu is available [but she and Vera Nieh] cannot get along and work together, and she does not like Miss Nieh." Liu would be glad to take up the post, but Li thought Chou would be a better fit. Thus, if Vera Nieh did resign, Li wrote, "I will send you an express telegram asking you to approach [Chou] and I will wait for your final instructions." He further remarked,

> I have asked Dr. Forkner as to who suggested Miss Nieh's name and invited her to head up the school of nursing. Dr. Forkner said that before the Administrative Committee was organized, the PUMC nurses and some PUMC graduates and possibly others (I myself not included) took it for granted that since she was dean of the school she should be requested to come in to Free China to serve as dean. Officially we are not obliged for such an appointment and Dr. Forkner said to me: "No official appointment has been sent her yet."[46]

All of this intrigue was starting to wear on Edwin Lobenstine, who was usually the recipient of the missives sent by various players in the unfolding PUMC drama. On 21 March 1944, Lobenstine wrote to PUMC board trustee Dr. Wong Wen-hao that "a new misunderstanding seems to have arisen."[47] There were "certain difficulties" between Claude Forkner and Vera Nieh in connection with the administration of the nursing school. He noted that Nieh had sent a cablegram to Dr. J. Heng Liu and, ten days later, to Lobenstine. Both "attacked Dr. Forkner in strong terms." Lobenstine had turned them over to Ballou. A few days later, Ballou was provided additional cablegrams from Li Ting-an and Forkner on the same subject. "These were of sufficient importance to make it seem desirable to Mr. Ballou and Miss Ferguson to call together the Trustees of [the PUMC] now in this area." He further noted that, on 17 March, a trustee meeting had been held in New York. It was reported at that meeting that "this was by no means the first time there had been friction between the nurses and the authorities of the PUMC." As Lobenstine understood it, "the nurses had always been jealous of their authority and desired to run the school without interference from the Medical School authorities."[48] In this, Lobenstine was correct. PUMC nurses had been taught to be leaders, after all; that was part of the distinctive approach of the PUMC School of Nursing. It is ironic, then, that the CMB and PUMC members themselves seemed surprised to find that one of their strongest alumnae, Vera Nieh, was exercising the authority the PUMC itself had helped to instill in her.

Bringing in Allies: Hodgman and Tennant

With the PUMC men finding ways to disparage her, Vera Nieh turned to her group of allies – the CMB women. Or, more to the point, Nieh's faculty members turned to Gertrude Hodgman and Elizabeth Tennant for support on her behalf. In a letter marked "Personal" and sent from Chengdu on 5 April 1944, Wang Hsui-ying, who had been on the PUMC nursing staff since 1937, wrote that she wished to "unburden my mind" with something she thought both women would be interested to know.[49] She wrote that, when the Japanese had closed the PUMC School of Nursing on 31 January 1942, "practically all" the nursing faculty migrated to Free China over a five-month period. Most were in Chongqing when the decision was made to reopen the school in Chengdu. According to Wang Hsui-ying, Vera Nieh was appointed as the "General Superintendent of Nurses" in the WCUU University Hospital. "The whole nursing service," she noted, "was transferred to us." After outlining everything the small group of faculty members had accomplished in Chengdu over the previous seven months, Wang noted that, before the school was closed in Beijing, the dean of nursing had had the "same position, authority and responsibility which are comparable to that of the director of any progressive nursing school." Since, at the present time, the whole PUMC was no longer in existence, the Nursing School, she posited, should be an independent administrative unit. Understandably, then, the dean had continued to carry out her duties with the presumption that she had the same rights as in Beijing.[50]

Wang Hsui-ying informed Hodgman and Tennant that, at the first PUMC board meeting, held on 17 January 1944, a budget was passed. However, "after the meeting, the budget has never been given to our dean." A month later, a set of regulations governing the School of Nursing was "drawn by some one and sent to the chairman for his signature." A signed copy was delivered to the dean on 10 March 1944. By that time, "the school budget has been given to the executive officer whose function, according to the regulations, is comparable to that of the director of the school." To Wang, these new regulations "put our school in a very weak position," and, furthermore, "put the dean into difficulty and embarrassment after all the hard work she has done to start the school." Nursing faculty members, Wang wrote, could not understand why the position and administration of the nursing school would be "so unnecessarily weakened – particularly as it is the only leading nursing school in China." She noted that the faculty had also written to the chair of the PUMC board for his help.[51]

Wang Hsui-ying appealed to Hodgman and Tennant's deep knowledge of nursing education and administration. "Among the four executives," she noted,

> Drs. Y.T. Tsur and W.H. Weng are so busy and know little about nursing education in general. On the other hand, both Drs. T.A. Li and C.E. Forkner have given us the impression that they do not seem to know well enough about the nursing education and administration. Hence such regulations are written. We have no support and we do not know to whom we should appeal ... Therefore we decided to write personal letters to our nursing leaders in America for guidance.[52]

To Wang, it seemed necessary for the CMB to have some "American nursing leaders who have profound interest in nursing education in China as members, or to form a separate board so we could have some backing and our school would be in a sound position." The faculty was, then, aware of the value of American nursing support, and was requesting to leverage the same. Wang ended on an ominous note: "Should anything happen to our school after July, 1944, you understand why."[53]

On 30 June 1944, Gertrude Hodgman wrote to Vera Nieh, Wang Hsui-ying, Mary Sia "and others of the Faculty and Alumnae" of the PUMC[54] in response to the letter addressed to Hodgman and Tennant, and forwarded to Hodgman, who was in Rio de Janeiro. She first noted that "nothing must keep [the PUMC School of Nursing] from going and going well." The next part, which she later deleted, read: "You will know that only the PUMC School can produce the kind of nurse which China needs for the present war effort, and also, and especially, for the great needs of China when this horrible fighting is over, victoriously for the Allies, even though the days now must look pretty dark to you." She gave some advice about how often Nieh should attend which committees, and argued that the "function of the Dean or Director is then as executive officer of the School to carry it on according to its aims and within the limits of budget and personnel approved by the Committee, to be responsible for school property, personnel, students, curriculum, etc."[55] Mary Tennant added her belief that, "the School of Nursing means more to the PUMC nurses and they should spend every effort to make this venture in S.W. China successful, give thoughtful and wise decision on controversial questions, not fly off the handle; otherwise, people become intolerant with nurses who do."[56]

A FINAL (UNSUCCESSFUL) PUSH

Initially, Vera Nieh's agitating seemed to pay off. Within three weeks, she learned that the regulations for the school would be changed, and that Claude Forkner had resigned from all PUMC responsibilities. Dr. C.C. Chen was added to the PUMC board of trustees in Free China. Furthermore the PUMC trustees confirmed Nieh's appointment as dean of the PUMC School of Nursing in Chengdu.[57] On the surface, the relationship between the PUMC board and Nieh seemed markedly improved. However, it appears that the trustees had simply changed their tactics. The PUMC board now approached the problem by offering Nieh a two-month study leave – to Ceylon and India.

The idea of sending the dean of nursing away for two months in the middle of the war must have seemed preposterous. Although Nieh had been the happy recipient of study leaves abroad in the past, they had centred on gaining university credentials. In this case, the aim was to dampen her expectations of what the PUMC could and should achieve in West China. The trustees claimed that it was a disadvantage that Nieh's experience in administration of a nursing school "is limited to her American contacts."[58] Given the similarities in the socioeconomic makeup of Ceylon, India, and China, the trustees expressed interest in learning reasons why "nursing education in India is backward and that in Ceylon somewhat better."[59]

> After an extended discussion on the personslity [sic] problem of the School of Nursing, it is agreed that Miss Nieh ... needs more knowledge of the evolution in nursing education of the world and more contacts with British experiments under complicated conditions. The present difficulty of transportation does not allow extensive travel and Miss Nieh's responsibility in Chengdu also speaks against a prolonged period of leave of absence. A short study on this specific subject may improve her physical and mental status and better equip her to deal with the most difficult time.[60]

A letter from Dr. C.C. Chen gives perhaps the clearest reason for Vera Nieh's study leave: it was a last-ditch effort to try to ensure that the PUMC board had given her "every opportunity to improve her knowledge and experience" before concluding that she was "inadequate for her present position" as dean of the School of Nursing. Having listened to her verbal report at the recent trustee meeting, Chen noted that, while Nieh "undoubtedly tried to do her best," there was evidence of her lack of experience."[61] The trustees felt that most of the problems she was facing had to do with the independence of the School of Nursing – and that issues she had to deal with in Chengdu had, in Beijing, been taken care of by the PUMC administrators. They hoped that a study tour of nursing education in a relatively poor nation would "constitute a source of inspiration and may help develop practical intelligence in a person like Miss Nieh."[62]

For his part, Claude Forkner, while no longer directly involved in the PUMC, still held out hope that the trustees would be eventually able to take over the "real responsibility" of running the Nursing School.[63] In terms of Vera Nieh's study tour, Forkner wrote, "I must be frank in my admission to you that I do not think this will result in improvement of the fundamental defects in the administration of the School."[64] In the end, it was a moot point. When Nieh heard about the proposed study tour, she took it as an insult. Marshall Balfour conceded that it was an "ill-conceived notion."[65] To him, there was "little reason for sending her to India and Ceylon unless it be for a rest or with the Chinese technique of retirement."[66] The offer was thus rescinded.[67] Like her mentor the indomitable Gertrude Hodgman, Vera Nieh proved herself a force to be reckoned with. Considering how many of her male superiors expressed exasperation with her – John B. Grant, Allen Best, Claude Forkner, Stephen Chang, and C.C. Chen – it is a testament to her tenacity that she survived and succeeded in her role as dean of nursing of the refugee PUMC.

NIEH ABSOLVED

Throughout the war years, Vera Nieh was perceived and portrayed by her (male) superiors as a difficult personality – with descriptors ranging from the bland "inexperienced" to a loaded "psychiatric instability." However, for the most part, those who criticized her during the war came around to admire her afterwards. For example, on 25 August 1945, ten days after the surrender of Japan following the bombing of Hiroshima and Nagasaki, Dr. Y.T. Tsur wrote a letter to one of the PUMC trustees, Dr. Sao-Ke (Alfred) Sze, expressing his analysis of Vera Nieh.[68] To Tsur, she was "sensitive, earnest, and serious about her duties." She would become "irritated" with "any criticism of the Nursing School which to her is unjustified." However, she also admitted her faults sincerely and frankly. Indeed, most people who had had associations with her in recent months told Dr. Tsur that "she is much changed." To Tsur, most of the difficulties that had arisen in the past were due to "an insufficient knowledge of her personality." Tsur admitted that he himself had misunderstood her – in part because of her strained relationship with Claude Forkner, whom Tsur described as "also" strict, earnest, and inexperienced. When the two clashed, Tsur took the side of Forkner, whom Tsur felt he had to back since Forkner was the "higher authority." Tsur, it must be noted, lived in Guiling. It was not until he spent two months in Chengdu (to have his teeth fixed) that he was able to study the situation closely – and conclude that "the atmosphere had radically changed." Vera Nieh, Tsur determined, "is a very dynamic character" who "runs the Nursing School like a watchful mother over her child." He believed that she would be less excitable once the situation returned to relative normalcy in Beijing.[69] In a similar way, Marshall Balfour, who had sworn off of Vera Nieh, later wrote that he heard that she was "transformed and is quite a different person with whom to deal."[70] By the time Nieh returned to Beijing, she was welcomed warmly, any negative personality traits now glossed over.

Between 1943 and 1946, Vera Nieh approached her work at the WCUU with the same determination and adaptability that had characterized her work in Beijing. Much of her administrative time was spent recruiting students, supporting faculty, and adapting the PUMC curriculum to local realities. Her fierce advocacy for faculty members brought as much admiration from them as it brought ire from her superiors. In August 1945, for example, she sought (and received) a salary increase for the nursing faculty, which lifted them to "approximately ... the same level as those of the faculty of the five universities" operating on the WCUU campus.[71] Furthermore, "whenever there are special subsidies given to faculty members of the five universities, our faculty members will enjoy the same privilege even though the fund will be drawn from our school budget."[72] It is little wonder her faculty and staff stayed strongly committed to her, even when others attempted to discredit her or devalue her work. Ultimately, for Nieh, quality is what distinguished the PUMC from other nursing schools: "Let PUMC Nursing School take care of quality," she wrote, "and the Chinese government nursing schools take care of quantity."[73]

After the war, Mary Elizabeth Tennant went out of her way to support Nieh, introducing her to the directors of various schools of nursing in the United States as the first Chinese dean of the PUMC School of Nursing and as someone who, "due to her courage and interest, kept the School of Nursing functioning during the war years in [Chengdu]."[74] Emphsizing that this work was done under great difficulty, Tennant then concluded, "anything that you are able to do to assist Miss Nieh I would deeply appreciate."[75] If Vera Nieh was admired among her nursing colleagues before the war, the admiration only increased afterwards, and likely laid the foundation for her subsequent election as president of the Nurses Association of China in 1947.

MAKING THE (UNIVERSITY) GRADE: GROUNDWORK FOR BACCALAUREATE EDUCATION AT THE WCUU

For all the conflicts involving Vera Nieh, the fact remained that she did an exemplary job as dean of nursing at the refugee PUMC. She also is credited with the initiation and early development of a baccalaureate degree in nursing at the WCUU. On this front, Nieh was, as always, forceful in her views – and yet, in the context of assisting the WCUU to emulate the PUMC, she proved herself a strategic thinker rather than a reactionary.

On 27 January 1944, the WCUU College of Medicine and Dentistry appointed an Executive Committee of the University Hospital, with Eva Liu and M.E. Streeter co-opted to consider the organization of a school of nursing of college grade.[76] Starting in the 1920s, the PUMC was the only school of nursing in China offering "college grade" (university-level) nursing. Part of the WCUU's attraction to having the PUMC as part of its campus community was the opportunity it gave for the WCUU to start a college-grade nursing program of its own. Given the wartime conditions, ongoing conflicts, and lack of missionary personnel, it is surprising that the WCUU and PUMC were able to keep this opportunity on their radar, never mind find a way to realize it.

Based on the report of the Executive Committee, on 16 March 1944 the WCUU College of Medicine and Dentistry, resolved that:

> (1) the College approach Board of Trustees of the PUMC with a request that students from the Women's College of WCUU may be trained in the PUMC nursing school, leading to a degree, (2) that the College approach the Women's College, College of Science, and Committee of studies WCUU [sic] for permission to accept in 1944–45 ten students in nursing, working towards a degree in arts of science: the nursing course to be in association with the PUMC Nursing, (3) that the following constitute a standing committee of College on preparatory plans for University Nursing School: T.A. Li, E.R. Cunningham [acting dean of medicine] with Miss Streeter [dean of women, WCUU], Miss Nieh, Miss E. Liu, co-opted.[77]

At around this same time a "Tentative Plan" for a college-grade nursing school was presented to the WCUU.[78] The proposed aim of the school was "to provide health workers of the highest type in the nursing profession who will be able to meet the opportunities and the needs in the rapidly developing fields of preventative and curative medicine."[79] The plan noted that demand for nurses with a background in medical and social sciences and a "thorough education for their profession" was high.[80] The proposal recommended that Canadian missionary nurse Cora Kilborn be appointed to the staff of the Women's College so that she could "arouse the interest of the students in the work of the nursing profession."[81] There would be two program options: one for students wishing to acquire a diploma in nursing (four years, including a nine month "pre-clinical" course) and one for students desiring both a diploma in nursing and a bachelor of science degree (two years study in the College of Science, followed by the three-year nursing curriculum).[82]

On 18 March 1944, Dr. E.R. Cunningham wrote M.E. Streeter outlining the plan.[83] The hope, expressed further in a 21 March 1944 letter to H.S. Chang, dean of the College of Science, would be that "the PUMC might during the war period undertake the actual nursing training of these nursing students. After the war our University would organize a University Nursing School of our own."[84] Cunningham also wrote Dr. Li Ting-an to permit the admission to the WCUU of ten female students trained in the PUMC School of Nursing. The rationale for admission was "with a view of starting a nucleus of a student body for a future Nursing School for our University Hospital."[85] Finally, he wrote S.H. Fong, dean of studies at WCUU, asking that a similar arrangement be made between the WCUU and its associated School of Nursing as between Yenching and Ginling Universities and the PUMC School of Nursing – that is, that the WCUU grant degrees to nurses who took two years of pre-nursing at the university and then went on to finish their training in the nursing school.[86]

The Women's College board agreed to the co-institutional degree on 10 April 1944.[87] Li Ting-an and Claude Forkner agreed on behalf of the PUMC board later in the month.[88] Everything seemed to be falling into place. However, Vera Nieh, true to form, was not going to hand over expertise without some clear benefit to the PUMC.

In 1945, Nieh took stock on just how much the PUMC was benefiting the University Hospital. She noted that the University Hospital benefited financially from having PUMC nursing students, staff, and faculty helping to maintain its nursing service.[89] She was responding to a study completed by Dr. Allen Best that, in her view, underestimated the number of nurses needed to staff the hospital in the following year. She was "in full sympathy with [Dr. T.A. Li] and other authorities in the financial status of this hospital."[90] She also sincerely hoped that "the PUMC Nursing School can be of even more service to this hospital and that the China Medical Board or any other organizations will give to this hospital a generous donation so that we can give the best medical and nursing care to our patients and ... carry on our teaching properly."[91]

In Nieh's estimation, the University Hospital would normally require eighty-eight nursing personnel. Of this, the PUMC was providing forty-two staff nurses, twenty-nine second- and third-year students, and eleven nursing faculty – a total of eighty-two personnel.[92] The total cost to

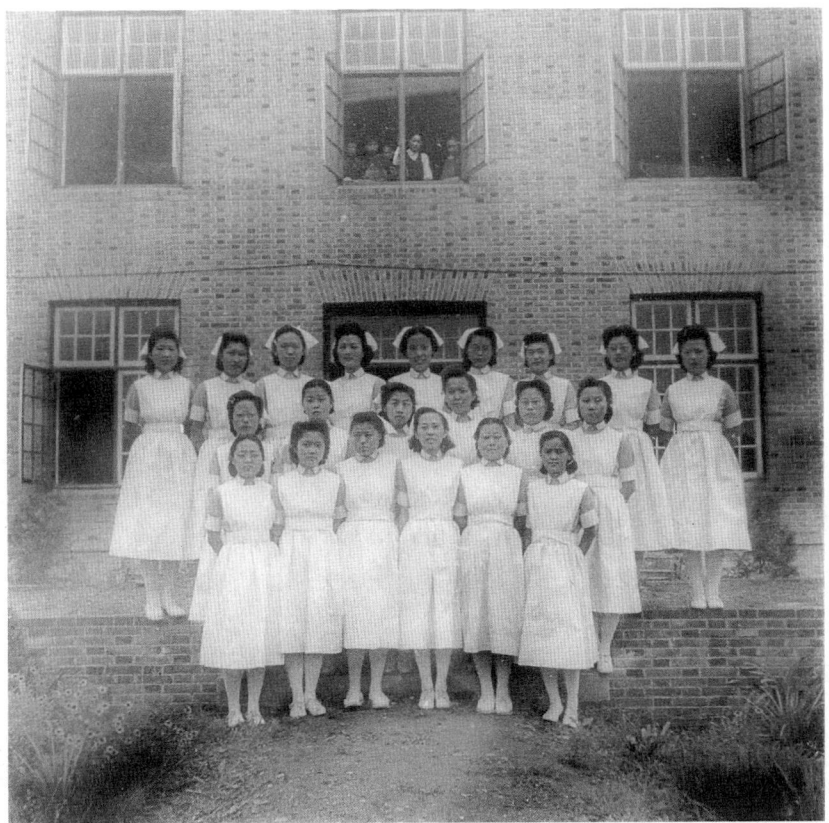

FIGURE 6.1 PUMC nursing students at the WCUU, 1946. | Courtesy Rockefeller Archive Center, RAC-CMB_FA065_B1144_F1042_003.

maintain nursing service at the University Hospital was over 68 million CN; the total cost of PUMC personnel was just under 45 million CN. In other words, having the PUMC School of Nursing providing nursing service in the University Hospital was saving the WCUU around 23 million CN each year. Furthermore, Nieh observed, the cost for maintaining nursing students (room, board, tuition) was normally provided entirely by the hospital where students did their practical work. In the case of the PUMC, the University Hospital was sharing no responsibility for the expenses of the school. The PUMC School of Nursing was a valuable commodity, and Vera Nieh wanted to ensure that its value was recognized.

In addition, Nieh outlined the following contributions to the University Hospital in connection with the PUMC School of Nursing:

- Buildings were completed by the CMB for the medical college and hospital of the WCUU because of the co-operative enterprise between the WCUU and the PUMC School of Nursing.
- The entire PUMC faculty and student body were rendering free service to the University Hospital, which in turn "only provided" maintenance for faculty who were doing hospital work and for second-year students. The first-year students paid the hospital one dou of rice per student per month (rice being a commodity used in lieu of cash).
- All clerical work of the nursing service was done by the PUMC School of Nursing.
- Nearly all stationary goods were supplied by PUMC nursing.
- PUMC nursing bore half of the bus fare for hospital staff coming from distant places.
- PUMC nursing shared fuel for ward patients in the winter months, and hot water all year round to the nurses dormitory.
- PUMC nursing lent equipment and supplies used by the University Hospital.
- The PUMC School of Nursing employed two servants at full wages and provided maintenance for the living quarters of nursing supervisors and head nurses.

All things considered, Nieh argued that that "quality of service is too important to be neglected both from the stand point of financial income of patients and of teaching value since this is a teaching hospital."[93] In other words, if the WCUU wanted to provide the same level of service after the war as the PUMC was providing now, it would have to start some serious planning.

* * *

If anyone doubted it before the refugee PUMC opened in 1943, there was no doubting it afterward: Vera Nieh was an indomitable force. Disliked by her male superiors, revered by her nursing faculty, and supported by

American nursing leaders, she had a vision of how the PUMC School of Nursing should be run, and she persisted with it. It is noteworthy how differently the male administrators, mostly physicians, and her female faculty and mentors, all nurses, viewed Nieh and her priorities. For example, Allen Best's and Li Ting-an's insistence that Vera Nieh was causing trouble and ruining things stands in sharp contrast to Wang Hsui-ying's and Margaret Lee's descriptions of how much she had improved services at the University Hospital. Perhaps most striking is Nieh's disposition, as a woman who absolutely refused to back down from something she believed was right. While she had always had an independent streak, in Chengdu she was particularly obstinate, in ways that irritated her superiors but endeared her to the nurses. In the end, it was Claude Forkner, not Vera Nieh, who resigned. Furthermore, even those who criticized her during the war eventually came to appreciate all that she ahd managed to accomplish. While Forkner believed that PUMC graduates had been too "Americanized, over-isolated from social conditions, and unable to adapt to problem situations,"[94] the PUMC nursing alumnae proved themselves up for the task.

CHAPTER SEVEN

"Our Triumphant Return" (1946–49)

Postwar Dreams and Dashed Hopes

Then we came on to the hospital and found the whole hospital force at the gate to greet us with firecrackers. It was a thrilling contrast to the way I left [with the Japanese taking me out].

— *Susie Kelsey, Canadian missionary nurse,*
28 January 1946

China's War of Resistance against Japan ended with the surrender of Japan after the United States dropped atomic bombs on Hiroshima and Nagasaki on 6 and 9 August 1945. The seventy-nine nurses who were still interned – primarily British, American, and Canadian – were released by the end of the month. The data are not complete, but it is likely that the internees returned to the West as soon as they were able to after their release, to restore their health and decide on their next steps. Canadian nurse Betty Gale and her husband Dr. Godfrey Gale, for example, left their internment camp on 1 September 1945, although but they not depart Shanghai until 2 November 1945, almost three months after Japan's surrender. Initially Dr. Godfrey had hoped to return to his work at the Shandong Christian University (Qilu). Conditions there, however, were uncertain; it was impossible to consider that possibility yet.[1]

The immediate postwar climate in West China was tumultuous. After the surrender, Canadian missionary nurses Irene Harris and Alma Tallman departed Chengdu, leaving only Cora Kilborn. In 1946, Kilborn was joined by Bessie Julien and, the following year, by three more Canadian nurses: Marjorie Alexander, Lillian Taylor, and Helen Turner. Turner, who had transferred from the North China Mission, which had since closed, transferred again a year later to Qilu, where she married

Peter Nelson of the English Baptist Missionary Society. They were among the last missionaries to leave Jinan, in June 1951.[2] During this unsettled postwar and civil-war period, the PUMC managed to continue its aim of educating baccalaureate nurses in Beijing until 1951, when the new Communist government closed the Peking Union Medical College (PUMC) in favour of a three-year Soviet apprenticeship model for nursing education. The West China Union University (WCUU) also closed in 1951, after graduating two classes of baccalaureate students. This chapter traces the final years of both the WCUU and the PUMC, examining how modern nursing and modern nurses – both Chinese and Western – continued to adapt to the changing socio-political context, staking a claim in China's health care system until their stake was unceremoniously pulled, in 1951.

CANADIAN MISSIONARIES RETURN TO CHINA

Months before the end of the war, Canadian missionary nurses Susie Kelsey and Clara Preston made plans to return to China. Susie Kelsey, a missionary nurse with the Anglican Church of Canada in Henan, had been repatriated to Canada in September 1943 after being arrested and interned under the Japanese. In February 1945, she requested, and was granted, permission from the Anglican mission to be seconded for work as a nurse with the United Church of Canada in Sichuan, since Henan was still under Japanese occupation. The plan was for Kelsey to work at the University Hospital in Chengdu.[3] In February 1945, the Woman's Missionary Society (WMS) of the United Church of Canada began to make arrangements for Kelsey's travel and inoculations.[4] She sailed from New York in June, arriving in Chongqing via India on 6 October. Japan's surrender occurred during her four-month voyage, and she came to view her time in West China as a stopover en route to her ultimate destination of Sanqui, Henan. While she waited in Chongqing to sort out travel plans, she stayed at the home of West China Mission (WCM) nurse Irene Harris. Like Kelsey, Harris was a graduate of the Winnipeg General Hospital (she had graduated in 1919; Kelsey in 1923).[5] Both were long-serving missionaries. Harris had served at WCM hospitals in Sichuan since 1921. Kelsey had served at the Anglican Mission's St. Paul's Hospital in Henan since 1924.[6] It was a natural choice, then, for Kelsey to stay with Harris while awaiting further passage. It was also a natural choice for Kelsey to help out Harris in the hospital while she waited. Although the Canadian mission hospitals in Chengdu had the extra help provided by PUMC nurses, the Canadian mission hospital in Chongqing did not. "I gather [Irene Harris] needs my help as much as anyone in the [Chengdu] hospitals," Susie wrote in a letter from Chongqing on 28 October 1945, "as they have a big work and nursing school, and [yet] she is the only foreign nurse [in Chongqing]."[7]

As China's wartime capital, Chongqing was the natural place to try to find a route to other parts of postwar China. It was therefore also a place where many were scrambling for transportation. Susie Kelsey's first attempt was to catch a ride on a Friends Ambulance Unit (FAU) truck with Dr. Bob McClure, which was heading to Henan for postwar rehabilitation work. "Mission heads," she wrote, "especially are anxious to get back to their places in liberated areas, to take back property while they can and resume work."[8] She reported that there were tensions between "those Chinese who remained in occupied areas and those who came out" – for example, the refugees in Free China.[9] "Only an experienced foreign missionary," she surmised, "can take the lead and steer through the troubled waters during early days of reconstruction."[10] Unfortunately, Kelsey's hope for a ride with the FAU fell through. So did her next option, where she was "promised a place on the next boat" to Hankou, but heard nothing further.[11]

Having had no luck securing transportation by truck or boat, Kelsey booked a plane to Nanjing, with the idea of taking a train from there to Henan. Altogether, it took her eight months to get to her mission in Sanqui, including three months spent at the WCM in Sichuan. "I cannot tell you how warmly I have been welcomed everywhere," she wrote Bishop Tsen, "a pleasant contrast to the way the Japanese took me out."[12] Bishop Tsen sent an immediate cablegram to Canada to let the Anglican mission know of her safe arrival, to which the mission responded "Laus deo" – praise be to God.[13]

Initially, Kelsey found the buildings were in better condition than she expected, with a few bullet holes from machine gun fire.[14] However, within a few weeks she realized that much repair was necessary. There was no electricity or running water, and many items were in limited supply: "It is discouraging to have the nurses coming to me for this and that and to have to keep saying we have none, but we are all counting on both funds and supplies being forthcoming in due time."[15] At least there were medications. Despite shortages, she was "pleasantly surprised at the amount of stuff left here, for I had heard that the houses had been cleaned out."[16] Currency, however, was a "nightmare" because of soaring inflation. "A million dollars would only buy enough cotton for 120 sheets and we need 300 and all that goes with them."[17] The hospital staff, she noted, was paid fairly well, but the other workers did not earn a living wage.

In March 1948, Kelsey reported that the previous year had been one of uncertainty in Henan, with "increasing deterioration in the political and economic situation in China."[18] Sanqui was regularly "threatened by Communist forces and each time at their approach the government troops fortified our hospital compound." The nursing school continued, however, under the supervision of Kelsey and another Canadian missionary nurse, Mary Peters, and nine students had graduated. For Kelsey, "the main purpose of our medical work, like all missionary work, is to bring men to Christ, but by direct teaching and preaching and by the example of Christianity in action in our service and love." She reported that all of the graduates and most of the students "are now Christians," a number of them "having been baptized or confirmed in our own hospital Chapel of Holy Love." Having provided much detail about the successful work in Sanqui, Kelsey ended her report with a sad realization that her years in China were likely coming to a permanent end: she wrote that she and Mary Peters had left the hospital and were, in fact, presently taking refuge in Shanghai:

> This was not only for our own safety in the event of a Communist attack but also because it is felt that it will be easier for the Chinese

Christians when the turnover [of government] comes if they have no contact with foreign missionaries. So the majority of missionaries in North China have had to leave their posts ... But the future of both the hospital and staff and of us missionaries lies in God's hands and we can trust His loving guidance who has so wonderfully led and protected us in the past."[19]

Although Kelsey left out details about the circumstances of her departure from Sanqui, Henan, Clara Preston filled these in somewhat with her description of her last days at the Canadian United Church North China Mission (NCM) in Weihui, Henan. Having been seconded to the WCM from the NCM in 1941, Preston had returned to Canada in January 1943 to recover from tuberculosis. Like Kelsey, Preston returned to Henan in October 1946, during the time that Bob McClure and the FAU were re-establishing the mission work there. Two new nurses were hired for three-year terms with the NCM: Margaret Hossie and Helen Turner.[20] Unlike at Sanqui, where little damage had been done to the buildings, many of the NCM buildings in Anyang and Weihui had been destroyed. The FAU successfully helped hospital work resume in both Anyang and Weihui, completing its mandate by early 1947. When Clara Preston arrived in Weihui, there were eight graduate nurses, including two Chinese nursing leaders (likely Li Shu-yang and Liu Qing-yin), ready to continue with nurses' training. During the war, NCM nurses had worked with the Red Cross hospitals, public health centres, and the military.[21] Now, Preston, like Kelsey, was eager to resume her missionary work. However, within months of her arrival, fighting broke out nearby between Communist and Nationalist troops. Missionary work was about to be interrupted again, and this time the Canadian mission would close permanently.

On 26 March 1947, "the enemy came upon us like a thief in the night," Preston wrote in a letter home. Some of the nursing staff left the mission compound to go to the walled city proper, "where they felt it was safer."[22] On 30 March, Preston heard bombs and shooting all night long. Remaining staff evacuated the mission compound, leaving Preston, Margaret Hossie, and Dr. Greta Singer in charge of seventy patients.

They prepared patients for evacuation and awaited ten trucks supplied by the Nationalists. But gunfire prevented the trucks from reaching the mission compound, leaving the nurses with little option but to escort by foot patients who could walk and leave the most critical patients behind with servants and volunteers. The normally thirty-minute walk took seven hours. As they evacuated out of the north gate of the mission compound, Communist forces were positioned at the east gate and entering through the south gate.

The experience was traumatizing. It also highlighted a new threat to China – civil war – and a new threat to Christian missions: Communist rule. Two months after Preston's departure, the sixty-year-old Canadian North China Mission evacuated all of its missionaries and permanently closed. Its closure foreshadowed the shuttering of the WCM four years later.

POSTWAR TRANSITION PLANNING

After Japan's surrender in August 1945, planning for a baccalaureate program at the WCUU began in earnest. Between October and November, a group of Chinese and Canadian nurses started meeting regularly as the Planning Committee on Nursing Education.[23] Comprising Cora Kilborn, Wang Hsui-ying, Miss R. Westra, Bernice Chu Chen, and Vera Nieh, the Planning Committee would make transition plans for nursing in Chengdu, as the PUMC would be heading back to Beijing as soon as conditions permitted and transportation was available. It was apparent to those assembled that, if ever there was a "time to open a Nursing School of College Grade in West China," this was it.[24]

The makeup of this committee was fascinating: it represented the two nursing programs operating, in one way or another, under the aegis of the WCUU, and was planning for a preferred future for Canadian mission-sponsored nursing education, yet it included only one Canadian nurse, Cora Kilborn.[25] PUMC alumna Bernice Chu Chen worked with Kilborn at the Renji School of Nursing; Chu Chen was principal of the school, and Kilborn superintendent of nursing at the United Hospital. Vera Nieh was dean of the PUMC School of Nursing, and Wang Hsui-ying superintendent of nurses at the University Hospital. Despite the over-representation of PUMC staff and alunmae, the new baccalaureate program was clearly a Canadian missionary endeavour: the meetings were held at missionary houses, and opened with prayer.

The Planning Committee members had a vague notion that some "negotiations" had been underway between the WCUU and "university authorities" regarding opening a college-grade nursing school, but they were not sure where these stood. Indeed, a Committee on Nursing School of College Grade had met in 1944, but it involved all different players, except for Vera Nieh. The Planning Committee on Nursing Education recommended that a new Preparatory Committee should be struck that would include the dean of women, the dean of medicine, the dean of science, a doctor from the WCUU, and four nurses. Cora Kilborn, the Planning Committee suggested, should be immediately appointed director or acting director of the new baccalaureate program with an able assistant, with the aim of taking in a class of students during the spring 1946 semester.[26] On the recommendation of the Planning Committee, Cora Kilborn followed up with H.D. Robertson (likely a WCUU administrator) to see the state of plans regarding the new school. On 17 October 1945, she reported to the Planning Committee that the request to open a School of Nursing had already been approved, so it was up to the Planning Committee to plan for it.[27]

Subsequent meetings were spent on details related to items such as the curriculum, fees, uniforms, entrance requirements, physical examinations, vacations, and grades. Committee members decided on the minimum nursing faculty required (eight, plus a director/dean and assistant director/dean).[28] Perhaps wishing to avoid the pitfalls experienced at the PUMC and at the Health Stations at Beijing and in Chengdu, they also determined that the director of nursing also be the director of nursing services in the hospital. To aid in the transition when the PUMC withdrew, Vera Nieh offered to hire Sichuanese nurses onto her staff so that there would be experienced nurses on the University Hospital staff – an important offer that, while sincere, drew criticism later on when it turned out that no PUMC nurses desired to stay.[29]

On 20 December 1945, after the last meeting of the Planning Committee, H.D. Robertson noted that the President's Council had approved the establishment of a Preparatory Committee on Nursing Education, as suggested. The committee members were Cora Kilborn, Dr. Fornot, Dr. Hsieh (until the return of Leslie Kilborn), Dr. Helen Yoh, Dean H.L. Chang, Vera Nieh, Bernice Chu Chen, and Evelyn Lin. The committee would consider the plan proposed by the Planning Committee on Nursing Education and report to the president of the WCUU.[30] The new committee met into 1946. One interesting additional member was Ruth Ingram, former PUMC dean of nursing, who was in China volunteering with the United Nations Relief and Rehabilitation Administration (UNRRA).

In February 1946, plans were underway to prepare a proposal for the Ministry of Education to establish a university-degree course in nursing, under the WCUU College of Medicine.[31] The program, which was drawn up in close cooperation with Vera Nieh and Ruth Ingram, followed "very closely" the PUMC School of Nursing curriculum.[32] In April, the WCUU College of Medicine resolved that, in view of the proposed incorporation of nursing as a faculty of the college, it would extend to Cora Kilborn "a hearty welcome to become a member of this College Faculty."[33] At the same meeting, members recorded the "thanks of this College to the [PUMC] Board of Trustees, Principal Vera Nieh and her staff, and to the students of the PUMC School of Nursing for the high grade of service rendered from their arrival in September 1943, to their going off duty preparatory to leaving, March 1946, and that best wishes be extended to them for a peaceful journey to [Beijing]."[34]

On 4 May 1946, it became official: the WCUU general faculty recommended to the board of directors that "the University be permitted to establish a four years' course in Nursing Education leading to the degree of BNS and that the Nursing [program] be a Division of the College of Medicine and Dentistry."[35] The idea was met with such enthusiasm by the WCUU Associate Board of Directors that it was recommended as a new model for missions beyond the WCUU. In 1945, the WCUU Associated Board of Director's Planning Committee recommended that,

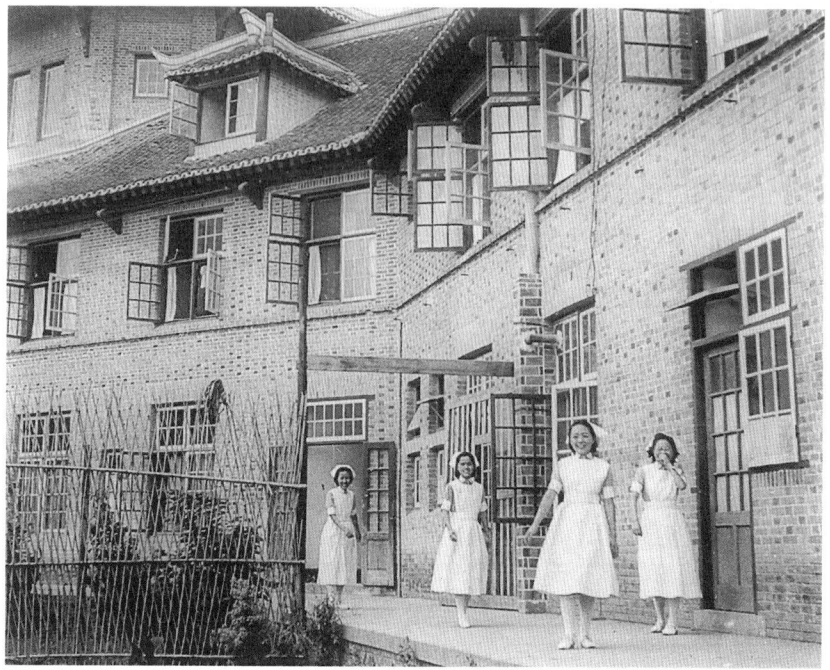

FIGURE 7.1 The WCUU nurses' dormitory, ca. 1946. | Courtesy Rockefeller Archive Center, RAC- CMB_FA065_B1144_F1042_011.

in association with each of the colleges of medicine connected with the Christian universities, that there should be a school of nursing for which graduation from a senior middle school would be an admission requirement.[36] Furthermore, in view of the Chinese government's request for assistance from the missions in the training of many more nurses during the next ten years, schools of nursing of similar grade should be established at other university centres that lacked medical colleges but had large, well-run mission hospitals (e.g., in Nanjing, Suzhou, and Fuzhou). Finally, it was recommended that the five mission medical colleges in China develop high-level health centres for teaching purposes to provide student nurses with a basic program of nursing and advanced preparation in public health.[37] There seemed to be no end of possibilities: it was as if the PUMC had provided the war-weary missionaries with a new lease on life. The proposal would now go to the Ministry of Education for final approval.

The reply from the ministry, dated 10 May 1946 and received by the WCUU a week later, was short: "We in the Ministry of Education are not yet in a position to consider this matter."[38] An excerpt from the note as filed states, "your letter, together with the programme proposed for Nursing Education has been put on one side."[39] The person who had typed up the excerpt summarized their suspicions about what "being put to one side" actually meant, adding the query "(? destroyed)" at the end of the note.[40] Now that the war was over, the Chinese ministry had little appetite to support any extension of the reach of Western missionaries. As the PUMC School of Nursing made plans to return to Beijing, it looked like the WCUU would lose not only its invaluable guests but also the opportunity to offer a baccalaureate program in Chengdu.

THE PUMC'S DEPARTURE FROM THE WCUU

Regarding Japan's surrender, Vera Nieh would later write, "Out of the dreary clouds, V-J Day brought us sunshine and hope."[41] V-J Day (Victory over Japan Day) was the day on which the Empire of Japan surrendered, ending the Second World War, but also effectively ending the War of Resistance in China. The PUMC School of Nursing almost immediately began to make plans to return to Beijing. The nurses were anxious to move as soon as possible, "being afraid of the extreme localism which prevails in this part of the country."[42] In a letter to fellow PUMC trustee Dr. Sao-ke Sze, Dr. Y.T. Tsur noted that he sympathized with the nurses' apprehension, but did not give further insight, commenting only that the "reason was very delicate to mention."[43]

It was difficult to know exactly what would be awaiting the PUMC nurses when they returned to Beijing. Anticipating that the PUMC Hospital might require repairs (as had the Canadian mission hospitals in Henan), Y.T. Tsur suggested that the returning nursing school might initially be housed in one or two large missionary hospitals in Beijing. Tsur also emphasized his stance that the PUMC in Chengdu was to be considered a "contribution of the College towards the national war effort" and not a continuation of the PUMC School of Nursing per se, which Tsur considered to have officially closed on 1 February 1942.[44] He made this point because the salaries in Chengdu had been adapted to the wartime conditions and were different than they had been in Beijing, and he was not keen to continue on Chengdu terms once the school returned to Beijing. In response, the nursing faculty members had sent a letter of complaint to the dean regarding their low salaries.[45] The postwar struggle over control and directin of the PUMC had begun.

Despite the desire of the nursing faculty to return to Beijing as soon as possible, they were forced to wait until transportation could be arranged and conditions were settled enough to travel safely. This did not happen until April 1946, as it turned out. In the meantime, not knowing the precise departure dates (and expecting them at any time) brought new sources of friction. For example, on 5 February 1946, Dr. Leslie Kilborn wrote to Dr. Marshall Balfour that the China Medical Board (CMB) offices, which had been housed on the WCUU campus, were closed a month previous but were still being used by the PUMC and therefore were not available to the WCUU.[46] Kilborn was frustrated that the offices had been turned over to the PUMC School of Nursing as bedrooms for their married students, without Kilborn's consent. At the same time, he did not wish to give the impression that he wanted to push out the PUMC. On the contrary, he noted that "we are not anxious to see the PUMC School of Nursing move away from [Chengdu] this year and would very much welcome a more prolonged stay with us."[47] Although the Ministry of Education had not come around to the WCUU request to open a baccalaureate school of nursing, the missionaries were pushing ahead. Leslie Kilborn wrote: "As we are now in the process of organizing our own school, [the PUMC] can continue to give us very valuable help, as they already have been doing."[48] Like his sister Cora Kilborn, Leslie Kilborn was aware of what nursing at the West China Mission would lose when the PUMC departed.

Inevitably, the time came. On 26 February 1946, the PUMC trustees approved the return of the School of Nursing to Beijing sometime between 15 April and 1 June 1946 or at such time that transportation could be arranged for staff and students.[49] The trustees also resolved that, on arrival in Beijing, the staff of the School of Nursing would be granted such vacation as was due them.[50] The idea was that staff would take vacation in the time between their arrival in Beijing and the time that the school reopened.[51] The trustees noted that "the authorities of West China Union University are aware of the plans of the School of Nursing for returning to [Beijing] before the summer ... [and that] it seems desirable to inform the West China Union University officially of the plans."[52] The trustees, on this point, had resolved that "the Dean of the School of Nursing be requested to inform the appropriate authorities" of the WCUU of the plans to return to Beijing "and to negotiate details of withdrawal of PUMC personnel from the Nursing Service of the Hospital in such a way as to minimize the inevitable problems consequent on their withdrawal."[53] A note about the trustees' resolutions went to Vera Nieh on 27 February.[54]

Vera Nieh was frustrated with the wait. On 12 April, she was informed that the PUMC would not, after all, be ready to reopen in Beijing in the fall.[55] Thus, even though the PUMC nursing faculty could return to Beijing, their work would not be able to continue right away, a state of affairs that left Nieh "very much disappointed."[56] Not only would this delay be a great disadvantage for current PUMC nursing students, it would also be "a great deal of trouble" for PUMC nursing faculty to prepare the nursing school.[57] It also left her in limbo, as, under the conditions noted by Tsur, her current headship of the School of Nursing would not be automatically transferred to Beijing. Likely desiring some stability (and authority), Nieh requested that the dean of nursing for Beijing be appointed immediately, citing the need to hire faculty for the next year and to start making clinical practice arrangements for the senior students. "The senior students have to step into public health right away" in Beijing, she wrote in a letter to Mary Ferguson, "and the few teachers who are to teach them must have appointments for next year before they can carry on their duty."[58] The current faculty contracts, Nieh noted, were expiring at the end of June 1946.[59]

After months of waiting, the end came suddenly, and the PUMC nursing faculty and students were simply told to pack up. On 20 April, Bernice Chu Chen reported that her husband, Dr. Henry Chen, had started the journey back to Beijing via a bus from Chengdu to Nanjing a couple of weeks prior. In a letter to Marshall Balfour, Chu Chen also noted that Vera Nieh and "the whole school" of nursing would start "their long and hard journey by busses" back to Beijing the following day.[60] The sixty-two PUMC students and staff planned to leave together. Three FAU trucks had been secured to transport them from Chengdu. These (and possibly more) trucks would take the group to Xian and then on to Nanjing either via Shaanxi or Shanghai, and then to Beijing. While they departed a few days later than planned, they were still unclear as to whether there were definite positions for the faculty at the PUMC. Nor was it clear what the "fate of the students" would be.[61] Dr. C.C. Chen had "painted a picture in the most gloomy fashion stating it was very clear that the PUMC would not open for a long time."[62] However, according to Elsie Priest (possibly a CMB secretary, in Chengdu), Dr. Chen was known to be "not very helpful at times."[63]

The departure of the PUMC faculty and students, while long awaited, weighed heavily on the Canadian (and other) missionaries remaining in Chengdu. The refugee PUMC had been in Chengdu just shy of three years.

A Residual Controversy

The PUMC faculty and student body departed Chengdu on 24 April, arriving in Beijing two months later. Their loss was immediately felt at the WCUU. Not only was it going to be difficult to start the new baccalaureate nursing program at the WCUU, but the departure of so many PUMC staff nurses meant that the University Hospital was experiencing a severe nursing shortage. Although Vera Nieh had expressed her intention to hire Sichuanese nurses so that there would be experienced staff members staying on at the University Hospital once the PUMC left, no hiring had occured and none of the PUMC staff was willing to stay.

Leslie Kilborn was frustrated. He shot off a letter to Marshall Balfour on the day the PUMC departed. In it, he mentioned the earlier resolution by the Executive Committee of the trustees that the "Dean of the School of Nursing be requested to inform the appropriate authorities" of the WCUU of plans for their return to Beijing. "We were informed of this action in early March," Leslie Kilborn noted, "and at the same time Miss Nieh informed us that she had decided to give her nurses two weeks of holiday, beginning April 1st."[64] This meant that the PUMC staff would no longer provide nursing care of patients at the University Hospital. Kilborn was annoyed at the "early withdrawal" noting that this, combined with the short notice, created many difficulties for the WCUU.

Because of the departure of the PUMC nurses, Leslie Kilborn wrote,

> we have had to very materially reduce the number of inpatients, so that the hospital is now running at about half capacity. We have moved nurses from the [United] hospital on [Si Shen Tsi] Street [to the University Hospital], but since the nursing staff is insufficient to staff both hospitals, we are having to close out most of our work in that [United] hospital, and within a short time will move the entire [Renji] School of Nursing to the University Hospital, thus making it impossible to carry on the [United] hospital in [Chengdu city proper].[65]

He added that, when the PUMC started its work at the WCUU in 1943, "one of our hopes was that they would be able to leave at least a few of their staff members here to help us get our new college grade school started. But all have left ... We are planning to open this School this year. We are grateful for the assistance that Miss Nieh and others gave in this direction, but are disappointed that none are willing to remain with us."[66]

Marshall Balfour refused to get involved. "I was also a bit disturbed by your cable and letters," he responded to Leslie Kilborn, but, "since my appointment with the Board was terminated I intended to forward them to New York."[67] Balfour made a private note on the bottom of a copy that "I am sending herewith only one of Dr. Kilborn's letters. There were two others with more wailing, but in the meantime matters seem to have settled."[68] Mary Ferguson, too, had a strong reaction to Kilborn's letter, writing in a "personal" letter to "Bal" about the letter in which, as she described it, Kilborn "bewails" the shortage of notice he had received regarding the PUMC departure.[69] Although, by that time (24 May 1946), it was all "water under the bridge," Mary Ferguson still wanted Balfour to be aware of her perspective regarding what had happened. "Beginning last August after the end of the hostilities," Ferguson noted, Vera Nieh began asking the WCUU administration what their plans were for taking over the nursing service whenever it became possible for the PUMC nurses to return to Beijing. The WCUU "consistently ignored the problem," Ferguson wrote, and Nieh "as consistently kept reminding them of it."[70] Ferguson suggested that it was only after much prodding that the WCUU finally took action by putting Cora Kilborn in charge of the new set-up – "an arrangement," she noted, "promptly vetoed by Dr. Best who then put Miss Kilborn over the [United] hospital in the city" rather than the University Hospital.[71]

When Ferguson, returning to China after war's end, reached Chengdu in the middle of February 1946, "*nothing* had been done by the WCUU people." Furthermore, she noted, "Vera was worried at the prospect of just the sort of criticism expressed by Dr. Kilborn in his letter to you." Whenever Nieh raised the question of the WCUU's plans, the response was that they hoped the PUMC nurses would not be leaving. Leslie Kilborn told Mary Ferguson that he hoped that some of the nurses would stay, to which Ferguson responded that, while the PUMC would do nothing to prevent them from staying, the WCUU "couldn't expect us to *order* any of the girls to stay."[72] At the next meeting of the Executive Committee of the PUMC trustees in Chongqing, the trustees had taken action, informing the WCUU of the plans to depart between 15 April and 1 June. This, according to Ferguson, was "in order to strengthen Vera [Nieh's] hands and to force the West China people into action." The last lines of Ferguson's letter exemplify some of the underlying animosity between the missionaries and the PUMC personnel. "Personally I can't help feeling," she wrote, "that it isn't a bad thing to have something force [the WCUU] to concentrated [sic] all their work in the hospital on the campus instead of spreading themselves thinly all over [Chengdu]!"[73]

The first leg of the journey of the PUMC nursing faculty and students back to Beijing was to end in Baoji, a city in southwest Shaanxi that was an important railroad junction for the line from Chengdu. However, the group got only as far as Xian before it decided to go on to Nanjing and reach Beijing via Shanghai (not Shaanxi), as the railroad was still disrupted in the north.[74] They were not the only PUMC refugees trying to return home. On 19 May 1946, Elsie M. Priest noted in a letter to Mary Ferguson that "our 20th truck of staff and students just left for [Baoji] –

we have six more and then there will be left only a few people who for one reason or another are waiting or will seek their own means of transport."[75] Of the families still in Chendgu, five stayed because they were expecting babies that month. Many had lived in "temporary" dormitories through the war – something that, for some, ended in calamity in early May 1946. As Priest related to Ferguson, "after using thatched-roof cottages and dormitories for nearly eight years in Chengdu, the whole colony burned within twenty minutes two weeks ago."[76] Fortunately, all of the students and the single staff member had already moved out. However, of the fourteen families left in the houses, five "lost very heavily."[77]

For the PUMC nursing faculty and students, the trip back to Beijing was long and arduous, but it differed completely from the anxiety-filled flight from Beijing in 1943. For one thing, faculty and students travelled together this time, and as a large, single group. The war and Japanese threat being over, this return trip was "adventurous, interesting and educational."[78]

RECOGNIZING EMERGING PUMC NURSING LEADERS

Now that the hostilities were over – a happy lull before violence erupted again in the form of civil war – faculty and staff had the opportunity to reflect. After attending a party held in honour of Dr. Alan Gregg and his colleagues in late May, I.C. Yuan raised the question of whether PUMC nurses had been suitably recognized for their work during wartime. He noted that, of the twenty-seven PUMC alumnae gathered at the party, fifteen were nurses. It was an opportunity to hear their stories. He was surprised and delighted by what he heard. "Several of them have distinguished themselves in their profession," he noted, suggesting that "the Commission may like to know something of what they have been doing during the period of the national emergency."[79] His list of the successes provides insight into not only the nursing work accomplished during the war but also the characteristics widely associated with PUMC alumnae after the war.

First, Yuan made note of Ravenna Tien (Tien Tsai-lee, Class of 1926), who was the Nurses Association of China (NAC) general secretary for many years. According to Yuan, Tien had guarded the new NAC property in Nanjing for many years, while resisting repeated attempts of the "puppet government" to have the NAC headquarters register under it. "By force of character and courage," he asserted, "she succeeded in preserving the NAC headquarters during the darkest period of war when practically all other public buildings in [Nanjing] were occupied and mutilated by the enemy."[80]

Another nurse singled out by Yuan was Hsu Ai-Chu (Class of 1930), who had been president of the NAC since 1942. She was, Yuan noted, "my chief public health nurse" at the Beijing Health Station before she went to the interior in 1940. During that period, many of the nursing schools were closed down, and there was a nursing shortage everywhere. Largely due to her efforts, three new schools were opened under the auspices of the NAC, at Guiying, Lanzhou, and Chongqing, and in cooperation with the government hospitals. As chief of the Nursing Department of the National Institute of Health, Hsu Ai-Chu organized postgraduate courses for nurses. Her home in Chongqing was the meeting place for many nurses – "they went to her, seeking advice and assistance," Yuan noted. Furthermore, "her attractive personality and warm hospitality must have meant a great deal to many a nurse."[81]

Finally, Yuan outlined what he viewed as the major accomplishments of Vera Nieh. Based on conversations at the party, he observed that, even after the PUMC was occupied by the Japanese in December 1941, Nieh and her faculty continued to teach their senior students, ensuring that they would be able to complete their practical training.[82] In 1943, she "and almost the entire faculty" went to the interior "across enemy barriers and traveled overland for many weeks before they reached their final destination."[83] With the recognition extended by Yuan, then, the PUMC nurses were finally starting to get their due.

THE PUMC'S TRIUMPHANT RETURN TO BEIJING

The trip from the interior back to Beijing was difficult; China was still experiencing wartime conditions, and, as Vera Nieh later noted, there were many "fatal accidents" among refugees returning home. Fortunately, the sixty-two PUMC nursing staff and students, "thanks to God, came home safe and sound!"[84] In an unpublished 1948 report to PUMC alumnae entitled "A Brief Account of the PUMC School of Nursing during and after World War II," Nieh divided her account into four stages: the Japanese occupation of the PUMC; the closure of the PUMC; The reopening of the PUMC School of Nursing in Chengdu; and the "triumphant return" to Beijing. Describing the fourth stage, Nieh noted that, although the homecoming filled the faculty and students with "hope and inspiration," there were difficulties from the start. They "were immediately faced with the serious handicaps of not having our own medical faculty and hospital facilities for the teaching of our students."[85] In other words, neither the PUMC Hospital nor the Medical School had yet reopened.[86] However, after having lived through almost a decade of war and other threats, there was a lot of goodwill in Beijing to see the PUMC nursing and medical schools reopen. Former members of the PUMC medical faculty and alumnae helped in the teaching program. They were able to open some of the laboratories – although these were in rough shape following the Japanese occupation.[87]

Trevor Bowen, by now released from imprisonment, helped the Nursing School open enough rooms, including the laundry, dining room, and classrooms, to get things running.[88] Local hospitals such as Chung Ho, the Children's, Tung Jen, and Peiping allowed PUMC students to use their facilities for their practical experience. Just as they had done at the Douw Hospital in 1943, and at the WCUU University Hospital in Chengdu, the PUMC School of Nursing supplied faculty to supervise the students at these clinical sites. Although not without its problems, having this range of experience "gave our instructors as well as our students opportunity to have a deeper insight into and a more thorough understanding of" the many common problems of the "outside hospitals."[89] Since PUMC graduates were expected to work in various medical institutions, and not just the PUMC Hospital, Nieh considered this experience to be of real value.

One of the first things the PUMC School of Nursing did after its return from West China was to negotiate with all of its affiliating universities for their consent to reduce the length of the baccalaureate degree program from six to five years.[90] Because the School of Nursing had been in Chengdu for only three years – and although students came into the PUMC having already completed one pre-nursing year – none of the students had been able to complete their degree requirements before departing West China. Instead of a "sandwich" program, which involved one year of university and three years in a hospital, followed by two more years at university, Nieh proposed a program where two and a half years of university study was followed by the same amount of time in a hospital. It was a clever move. By requiring students to have all of their university requirements up front, the PUMC ensured highly qualified students and could get students through the PUMC portion of their education in short order. It would be an attractive choice for students too: degree-bound students could earn a nursing diploma with only one additional year of studies; diploma-bound students could earn a degree in only two additional years. In December 1946, the PUMC announced that Yenching University, Tung Wu University, and Gining College were again affiliated with the PUMC School of Nursing, the Catholic University (Fu Jen) joining in the summer of 1947.[91]

The PUMC was also keen to continue its offerings of postgraduate programs. In Chengdu, the refugee PUMC had been able to offer only a two-year program in institutional (i.e., hospital) nursing, and only to nine students. Three of these students were from the Canadian mission hospitals in Chongqing and Chengdu – another way in which the WCM benefited from the refugee PUMC.[92] In Beijing, by contrast, the Nursing School had insufficient teaching personnel and facilities for teaching institutional nursing, and so it reopened the postgraduate program in public health nursing.[93] Three classes – forty-six students – enrolled in the public health nursing program between 1946 and 1948.

In September 1947, the PUMC Medical School, which had been closed since early 1942, reopened, with a new first-year class.[94] This meant that departments with relevance to nursing, such as Anatomy, Physiology, Bacteriology, Parasitology, Pathology, and Biochemistry, were set up again. On 4 May 1948, the PUMC Hospital reopened, with two private wards for general medical and surgical cases. In July, an obstetric and gynecological ward was opened, as well as a public ward for

medical and surgical cases. The operating room and outpatient department were enlarged and other services gradually added. Each of these
additions enhanced the ability of PUMC nursing students to return to
the PUMC Hospital to continue their clinical training. By September
1948, the PUMC buildings had been repaired and repainted, the equipment renovated or replaced. "The 'Queen Mary,' as our Director once
called the PUMC," wrote Vera Nieh, "is now sailing on rough sea in bad
weather ... but so far she is sailing on beautifully!" [95]

Nieh's 1948 report to the PUMC nursing alumnae was, in addition to
being a letter to garner support, a recruitment strategy for new faculty
and staff. Nieh was concerned about the high turnover of personnel.
Some of the faculty left the PUMC because they "got discouraged" with
the conditions of having to teach students at affiliate hospitals because
the PUMC Hospital had not yet been restored. [96] Others resigned due to
marriage. However, there was a third, new reason for staff shortages: a
large number of the PUMC graduates had left China for advanced studies in the United States. Since the PUMC relied heavily on its alumnae
for its own staffing (in 1948, the PUMC faculty was made up entirely of
PUMC graduates), the departure of promising graduates to the United
States significantly shrank the pool of prospective PUMC employees. Of
the 203 PUMC graduates (as of 1948), 125 were in active service (5 working in the United States), 34 were studying in the United States or in other
countries, 21 were not in active service (9 reportedly "keeping house" in
the United States), 6 were sick, 6 were deceased, and the whereabouts of
11 were unknown. Thus, of the 180 known graduates who were not sick
or deceased, 48 were in the United States or other countries. This meant
that a full quarter (27 percent) of the PUMC graduates were unavailable
for hire by the PUMC itself. [97]

Recognizing the need for a supportive alumnae base as the PUMC
headed into a period of rehabilitation, Vera Nieh ensured that alumnae
were aware of the value of their PUMC diploma. "The popular demand
for our graduates to fill leadership posts," she wrote, "makes us feel even
keener about the need to further lift our standard of teaching in order to
better fulfill our mission." [98] Furthermore, PUMC graduates should not
feel that marriage should limit their career, as it had prior to the war.

During wartime, 90 percent of the PUMC graduates had been in constant active service, despite family responsibilities. Nor was nursing a limitation to marriage: the twenty-one graduates listed as not in active service "are actually rendering invaluable service in their homes," Nieh wrote, "and are credited with the success of their husbands." Perhaps as a way to cast as wide a net of support as possible, Nieh quoted one PUMC graduate as stating, "I will always strongly support the PUMC Nursing School, because it produces good housewives."[99]

Now that the Nursing School was once again firmly re-established in Beijing, Vera Nieh assured PUMC alumnae that "we are beginning to set our feet again on the road to normal development" and "anxious to further improve our teaching program and place our School in a normal state again." The experience of the past years had been "tough and trying," but "also infinitely valuable." "May we rely on the continuous interest and support of our Alumnae for the flourishing of their Alma Mater?" she asked. "Your ideas will be much valued and given serious consideration in the re-construction of our curriculum and in the re-shaping of our school as a whole."[100] Within three years, the PUMC School of Nursing would certainly be reshaped, but in ways that neither Vera Nieh nor the PUMC alumnae could have predicted.

TRANSITIONS: UNSETTLING NURSING AT THE WCUU

Throughout most of 1946, Cora Kilborn was the sole Canadian missionary nurse at the West China Mission. Irene Harris and Alma Tallman had departed in 1945. Caroline Wellwood had departed on furlough in 1943, and subsequently retired; she died in 1947. After the North China Mission was closed, in 1947, the West China Mission was finally able to attract some new recruits. Isabelle E. Millar joined Lillian Taylor, Helen Turner, and Marjorie (Marjory) Alexander in 1948.[101]

In January 1946, before the refugee PUMC left and while Cora Kilborn was still on her own at the WCM, Leslie Kilborn wrote to Canadian missionaries Ed and Gladys Cunningham about the United (General) Hospital in Chengdu, proudly noting that his sister, Cora, "has achieved so much in getting [Si Shen Tsi] cleaned up" since her return to

West China two years earlier.[102] He also noted, however, that Dr. Allen Best, who had caused problems for both Dorothy Fox and Vera Nieh, was still stirring controversy. "Best has evidently been a problem to many," Leslie Kilborn confided.[103] The following month, Leslie Kilborn wrote again to the Cunninghams, noting wryly that Best "as an administrator [has] not been an overwhelming success."[104] Leslie Kilborn was feeling the pressure. Contrary to his subsequent complaint to Marshall Balfour, he was keenly aware that the PUMC nurses would be leaving soon, and he was desperately trying to think of ways to continue the work they had started. His letter to the Cunninghams reveals his confidence in his sister Cora to take over the leadership during the next chapter of nursing at the WCM:

> The PUMC School of Nursing is undoubtedly leaving us this Spring, and that will make the nursing in the new hospital a bit difficult for awhile. But Cora may move out to the campus soon and take charge. We definitely hope to start a university grade school of nursing this year and that has already passed the faculty again, and received the approval of the Women's College board, etc. But there is still much work to be done. It goes to the Board of Directors next month."[105]

It is unclear whether this confident report about Cora Kilborn was a clear-eyed assessment by a well-experienced medical administrator of her ability, or whether he was trying to convince them (and himself) of her fitness for a potential leadership role in the new university-level program. Undoubtedly he was aware that the pool of suitable applicants to head up the new nursing program at the University Hospital was shallow. Although he knew that both the Nationalist government and changing social norms favoured the hiring of Chinese nurses into leadership roles, he also knew that it would be difficult to find someone suitable for a position in a Christian university – that is, a degree-prepared, Christian nurse. Cora Kilborn, who held a BA, met the requirements.

On 25 July 1947, Leslie Kilborn asked WCUU president S.H. Fong that Cora Kilborn be appointed head of the Department of Nursing, now part of the WCUU College of Medicine, of which Leslie Kilborn was dean. The baccalaureate program had been approved, with the first group of students entering in 1946. "You will remember," Leslie Kilborn wrote, "that last year this position was held by Miss Wang Hui-yin, but this Spring she resigned and left [Chengdu]. I have tried to secure a Chinese successor to her, but have not succeeded."[106] Fong agreed, and offered the position to Cora Kilborn the following day.[107]

The story of Wang Hui-yin's resignation from the WCUU Department of Nursing is instructive. It is an early, pivotal example of how the attitude toward foreign missionaries was changing at the WCUU in the postwar period, well before the Communist takeover. Animosity toward Cora Kilborn took hold in 1947, partly over the resignation of Wang, and kept growing until Kilborn's departure in 1950. According to WCUU nursing alumna Ho Jin-chin, the reason for Wang's departure was that there was conflict between her and Cora Kilborn.

The perspective of a nurse who studied at both the WCUU and PUMC provides some insight into the issues underpinning this conflict. Ho Jin-chin entered the WCUU nursing program in 1947 at age seventeen, graduating from the baccalaureate program in 1950.[108] She was motivated to apply to the WCUU Nursing School because her family was Christian, and poor: the school required tuition for only one year; after that, students had to only pay for their uniforms. Out of 300 applicants, only 12 were chosen. To Ho Jin-chin, the best thing about the WCUU program was the English-language training – all the courses were in English. This enabled her to go to the PUMC afterward to take postgraduate training in public health and to work at the PUMC as a staff nurse. The worst part about the program, in Ho's view, was that the degree students – who would have entered the program having completed a pre-nursing year of university courses – were treated the same as the diploma students at Renji, who entered nurses' training after graduating from junior middle school. What stood out in Ho's recollection fifty years later was that the courses at the WCUU were simply not at the college level, as promised. Her suspicions were confirmed after she spent time at the PUMC for postgraduate work: clearly the WCUU was at a lower level. To Ho, Cora Kilborn wanted the nursing courses to be like those of Renji, whereas Wang Hui-yin, who was a PUMC graduate, wanted them to be at a higher level. This difference resulted in conflict between the women, and, in the end, Wang resigned.[109]

In Ho's view, Cora Kilborn did not like baccalaureate students as much as the Renji students she was used to teaching because the former were not as compliant; the Renji students, with their lesser education, were "easier to use."[110] To WCUU alumna Chin Shu-wen, Cora Kilborn had a strong character and was strict. Other nurses, both Canadian and Chinese, were afraid of her.[111] Alumna Deng Shipu, who graduated in 1942 from the Renji diploma program, recalled Kilborn as having high professional standards, but as extending kindness to students, inviting nurses whom she considered to be dedicated to her home at Christmas.[112] Chen noted that she went to Kilborn's house for lunch every Thursday and that Kilborn wanted her to go to Canada to study, but this turned out not to be possible.[113] Like Chen, Deng believed that Canadian missionary nurses Marjory Alexander and Lillian Taylor were afraid of Kilborn.[114] Luo Don xiu, a 1951 graduate from the Renji diploma program, agreed that Kilborn was strict, with high standards.[115] Both Ho Jin-chin and Chin Shu-wen believed that Cora Kilborn received special treatment because of Leslie Kilborn's position: "Her power," recalled Ho, "came from her brother who was Dean of Medicine."[116] The students, as she recalled, decided to protest against the apparent nepotism.

In October 1947, three months after replacing Wang Hui-yin, Cora Kilborn resigned, recommending that Chang Fang-hsiu (Zhang Fang-xiu) be appointed in her place.[117] Chang was a PUMC graduate from 1932. The complaints continued, despite the new leadership. Within weeks, Leslie Kilborn was receiving various complaints about the Department of Nursing, mostly from the nursing students themselves. A second-year student (likely Liu Chwan-ih) drafted a note called "Ideas and Opinions and Petition from 2nd Year Students of the Department of Nursing."[118] Upset about the conflation of the Renji school and the university-level school, the petition outlined a list of complaints:

- Under this unreasonable and unlawful system [meaning unclear] we are not willing to continue our study

- The present program and status are entirely different from the former aim of establishing this department
- This method of teaching program cannot promote the standard of high nursing but sending the future of our young people to the grave
- The establishing of nursing department is for building up nursing personnel but not for creating special kind of work. This is not what education is!
- There is no special nursing personnel and also no funds for our department; there is no definite plan for doing things for this department. We are very disappointed.
- For the administration, it should not be mixed together with the Jen-Chi [Renji] nursing school, they should be separated completely
- The students in this department are not students of the Jen-Chi [Renji] Nursing School
- Because the education bases are different in two side of students, therefore the teachers should be different and the teaching method is not like those who teach the students of Jen-Chi [Renji] School
- Don't do things only for them (Jen-Chi [Renji]) and bury our own welfare
- There should be a definite sign for our department just as Chinese old saying "without definite position or name one cannot speak right word."
- We should be treated just as well as any University student and we should have the privilege they have now
- Five years program for our department is pushing us to a worthless path. And at last our hope is still that there will be new and reasonable and lawful method for this department but not restricted by the old and unimproved method.[119]

Leslie Kilborn responded on 1 December 1947, writing to second-year nursing student Liu Chwan-ih that he was "very much disappointed that you have so little interest in being a part of the pioneer course in college grade nursing."[120] He suggested that, "if any or all of you wish to transfer to some other department, I shall do my best to help you transfer next summer, at the proper time."[121] He ended his letter on a rather ominous note:

> Nursing is primarily a service profession, and although our aim has been to get nurses with a better educational background for their work, if you are unwilling to do the work along with the [Renji] students, then it will be impossible to continue this [baccalaureate program] and I shall have to report to the Board of Founders that the attempt has been a failure, and we are therefore withdrawing our application for registration of this [program] with the Ministry of Education.[122]

Leslie Kilborn was fuming. The same day he fired off a letter to President Fong, stating that he was so "'fed up' with the attitude of these students that I am quite willing to discontinue the [baccalaureate program], and admit it is a failure."[123] Kilborn was frustrated that these students did not have the traditional view of nursing as service. "Anyone who wants to insist on 'face' by refusing to do class work with the hospital nurses," he concluded, "is not worthy to be called a nurse." If university students adopt this position, he lamented, "then I fear that all we can say is that they themselves have demonstrated their unfitness to enter a great profession, and the sooner we get rid of them the better."[124]

Fong became involved in the conflict, at the request of the Nursing Department head, Chang Fang-hsiu. He met with the students, which diffused the matter somewhat. He reported to Leslie Kilborn that the students' primary request was that they not be taught exactly the same way as the lower-grade students from the Renji School. If they could live in separate dormitories and have some separate courses, they would probably be mollified.[125] Given that most Renji students entered nursing at age fifteen, and most baccalaureate students at age eighteen or older, this would have seemed an obvious decision. In Ho Jin-chin's recollection, "after the protest, things improved."[126]

On 5 June 1948, Chang Fang-hsiu tendered her resignation. Her rationale was that her mother was getting old and weak and needed her, that her own health was poor, and that it is "more convenient to travel with my family folks."[127] She agreed to stay on for a few months, however, to help with the transition – a delay that extended into 1949.

* * *

Postwar transitions were difficult for everyone, whether at the PUMC, WUCC, or the NCM. Canadian missionaries who returned to Henan after departing years earlier, whether through evacuation or internment, settled into rehabilitating the hospitals and nursing schools, only to be swept up in 1947 in a new wave of violence and menace related to the Communist-Nationalist civil war. The PUMC School of Nursing returned to Beijing only to find the PUMC Hospital temporarily closed and unavailable for clinical teaching. And the WCUU university-level nursing program opened under the leadership of Cora Kilborn, only to find itself in conflict with Chinese leaders (PUMC alumnae) and the first group of baccalaureate students, who disagreed with Cora Kilborn's approach to university-level education. Out of these three groups, it was the PUMC School of Nursing that found its feet most readily.

Of particular interest are the rather negative recollections of WCUU alumnae regarding Cora Kilborn. While the archival evidence verifies the student protest and Leslie Kilborn's attempts to quash it, it is important to acknowledge the subjectivity of subsequent remembrances, the memories being shaped, in part, by the interviewees living under Communist rule for the past fifty years: it is possible that the strong sentiments against Cora Kilborn grew deeper in an anti-Western environment. Still, there is no question that significant conflicts between the Kilborn siblings and their Chinese staff and students simmered – and then boiled over – and that such conflict was something that Cora Kilborn had not experienced in her upbringing in Chengdu, nor in her two decades of nursing there. But it would only get worse.

CHAPTER EIGHT

The Last Chapter (1949–51)

Missions, the PUMC, and the End of Modern Nursing in China

With you, I deeply regret that the Peking Union Medical College should have passed out of the hands of the China Medical Board and been taken over by the Peking government ... But who are we to say that this may not be the Lord's way of achieving the intent of the founders, although it be a way so wholly different from what has been in our minds.

–John D. Rockefeller Jr., writing to a friend, 4 April 1951

During the wartime years, new forms of nursing had come to the fore in China – all of them patriotic. First was Red Cross nursing. Established in China as the Shanghai International Red Cross Committee in 1904, the Red Cross Society of China was primarily a relief agency, which responded to natural disasters both in China and in other countries. It also opened Red Cross Hospitals in Shanghai and elsewhere.[1] During the War of Resistance against Japan, it was common for Chinese nurses to gravitate toward the Red Cross – both hospitals and medical relief corps – as the best place to invest their energies. For Peking Union Medical College (PUMC) alumna Chou Meiyu, working in the Red Cross Medical Relief Corps was foundational to her subsequent development of military nursing – a second form of patriotic nursing that emerged in China during the war.[2] Chou Meiyu founded the first National Army Nursing School in Guiyang. This program opened on 1 July 1943, at the same time the refugee PUMC opened in Chengdu.

A third form of patriotic nursing was volunteer nursing. As Nicole Elizabeth Barnes has argued, wartime opened up new avenues for women desiring to provide voluntary service as nurses, midwives, and physicians, including work with non-governmental organizations such as the

YMCA. Offering such services provided women with opportunities for practical expression of their nationalist ideals. Volunteer female medical workers performed both the medical labour that kept civilian and military medical institutions running, and the emotional labour that cemented bonds between civilians. Furthermore, Barnes convincingly credits the infrastructures (and relationships) formed by myriad volunteer organizations (and their members) as a key reason the Communist government was able to create a functional state so quickly in 1949 after decades of warfare and social upheaval.[3]

A fourth form of patriotic nursing that emerged during wartime was humanitarian nursing. Although Red Cross nursing was also a type of this nursing, the prolonged war in China sparked new manifestations of humanitarianism initiated by newly formed international organizations, offered in the shape of short-term medical relief projects. The Friends Ambulance Unit (FAU) and the United Nations Relief and Rehabilitation Administration (UNRRA) are two such examples. As Susan Armstrong-Reid has argued, new frontiers in humanitarian nursing were opened though the FAU China Convoy, which operated in China between 1941 and 1951.[4] In this venture, Chinese nurses joined teams of British, Canadian, American, and New Zealander Quakers – a Christian sect characterized by its commitment to peace – to provide practical assistance to victims of war. Their mantra was to "Go Anywhere, Do Anything" to relieve suffering, regardless of race, religion, or politics.[5] Humanitarianism was also the purpose of the UNRRA, which opened its China office in Chongqing in 1944. As Rana Mitter argues, the UNRRA (and its Chinese form, the Chinese National Relief and Rehabilitation Administration) provided a path for the international community to meet newly realized obligations to secure and support human rights. At the same time, the UNRRA relied upon, and reinforced the idea of, centralized health care; it depended on Nationalist government records and structures to determine needs and track aid.[6] In this way, the UNRAA helped reinforce a view of public health as a government responsibility in China.

Wartime, then, brought these four new forms of nursing to China, each highly valued and each attracting Chinese nurses wanting to express their patriotism. Two other existing forms of nursing also gained social currency during wartime, because of their demonstrated value to the war effort: public health nursing and its foundation, baccalaureate and postgraduate education – that is, university-level education for nurses. Public health nursing, while not new to China in the way military, FAU, and UNRRA nursing were, was newly invigorated during wartime. The Nationalist government viewed and promoted public health as a way to strengthen China's citizenry. Morbidity and mortality from injuries, illness, and infections exacerbated by wartime conditions could be prevented or reduced by attentiveness to (and education about) hygiene and communicable disease. Whereas Red Cross, military, volunteer, and humanitarian nursing were, along with traditional hospital-based nursing, *responsive* to illness and injury, public health *prevented* illness and injury. In other words, if the former contributed to nation *mending*, the latter was about nation *building*. Little wonder, then, that the Nationalist government supported public health.

There was just one problem. Public health nursing education – all university-level nursing education, in fact – was rooted in a Western worldview and firmly enmeshed with Western institutions and personnel. Indeed, neither the PUMC (the institution most readily associated with public health nursing education) nor the West China Union University (WCUU) (a newcomer to university-level education) were nationalized institutions. Regardless of the fact that, by this time, virtually all the nursing staff, students, administrators, and educators at both institutions were Chinese, the institutions themselves were foreign-owned, -funded, and -operated. Although the Nationalist government accepted foreign support as a necessary part of nation building, the Communists had a different view; after 1949, the prevailing government stance would be that reliance on foreign support was decidedly *un*patriotic.

A NEW CONCEPTION OF NURSING

The end of the War of Resistance against Japan triggered an identity crisis for nursing in China. For Canadian nurses at the WCUU, the long-awaited shift to baccalaureate nursing proved more complex than anticipated. Valuing and wanting to hold onto the time-honoured Western and

Christian view of nursing as a form of sacrificial service (serving others as a form of serving Christ), it was not quite clear to WCUU administrator Cora Kilborn or her brother, Leslie, how to retain traditional mission values while also supporting progressive educational ideals. Students in Chengdu were clearly eager for the latter; not only were there 300 applicants for the new baccalaureate program in 1946, but the students themselves were not afraid to be vocal about their elevated expectations. At the PUMC, a postwar shift in nursing ideals was also occurring, but in quite a different way than for the missionary nurses. Of course, their starting points were different too; in contrast to the Canadian WCM, the PUMC had never framed nursing in Christian terms nor was it new to baccalaureate nursing. Rather, for the Chinese nurses at the PUMC (and quite likely for the progressive Chinese nursing students enrolled in the baccalaureate program at the WCUU), what was being unsettled was the place of nursing as a patriotic profession in a postwar world. No longer part of the frontline of patriotic resistance, Chinese nurses (and their supporters) had to reimagine a role for nursing in China's future.

PUMC nurses had proven themselves during the war. It is instructive to consider what it meant that those who rose to the challenge by taking on significant formal leadership roles obtained their nursing education during a specific socio-political period in China: the Nanjing (or Nationalist) Decade (1927-37) (see Table 8.1). During this period of moderate peace, the fledgling Nationalist government ruled from Nanjing. John Watt describes this decade as "one of the more auspicious periods in the development of nursing in China."[7] He gives four reasons for this. First, nursing reduced its dependency on foreign missionary leadership – particularly in the Nurses Association of China (NAC). Second, the Nationalist government's Ministry of Health became interested in the promotion of public health and health education training for nurses. Third, the Ministry of Education established a subcommittee on nursing to register and supervise nursing education. Finally, during this decade, the profession became predominantly the domain of women.[8] For PUMC alumnae, the wartime period had solidified the value of a PUMC education. It had also reframed nursing as a primarily patriotic profession. In the postwar period, however, it was more difficult to identify Western

TABLE 8.1 PUMC alumnae leadership roles, prior to 1949

Name	Alternate name	PUMC graduation year	Key leadership role before 1949
Lin Sz-sing	Evelyn Lin	1926	NAC president
Tien Tsai-lee	Ravenna Tien	1926	NAC general secretary
Chu Pi-hui	Bernice Chu Chen	1926	Renji nursing head; United Hospital superintendent of nurses
Nieh Yuchan	Vera Nieh	1927	PUMC dean; NAC president
Chou Meiyu	–	1930	Army general
Hsu Ai-Chu	–	1930	National Institute of Health Nursing Department head; NAC president
Sia Yun-hua	–	1931	Koloshan superintendent of nurses
Wang Hsui-ying	–	1931	WCUU University Hospital superintendent of nurses
Wu Zheying	Lillian Wu	1932	NAC president
Chang Fang-hsiu	–	1932	WCUU Nursing Department head
Wang Loh Loh	Yi Wang	1932	Koloshan assistant supervisor of nurses
Chen Liang-yu	–	1936	Koloshan supervisor of nurses
Liu Chih-chen	Eva Liu	1936	Renji nursing head; United Hospital superintendent of nurses
Liu Ching-ho	–	1936	PUMC temporary secretary to Wartime Advisory Committee

institutions, including the PUMC, with patriotism. Where was the place for nursing – and, more specifically, the PUMC – in postwar China?

Mary Elizabeth Tennant, assistant director of the Rockefeller Foundation (RF) International Health Division and a nursing consultant, did her best to defend nursing's place in the new China. In 1947, she wrote a letter to Dr. Hu Shih, chair of the PUMC board of trustees, emphasizing the importance of nursing education, and urging him to view nursing as significant to China as medicine or public health.[9] Given the power dynamics typically at play between (mostly male) medicine and (mostly female) nursing during this period, it is not surprising that Tennant would be working to defend and secure a position for nursing within the newly reopened PUMC. What is surprising is how rarely the archival records show tensions between physicians and nursing, at least in their clinical work. Rather, the tensions appeared more often to be between administrators – that is, over who "owned" administrative control of nursing. Nurses typically fought for administrative control of nursing by nurses – and the RF China Medical Board generally backed this up. Therefore, in 1947, it seems that Mary Tennant found it necessary to educate Dr. Hu Shih as to the value of nursing as a full partner in the PUMC. She had noticed that the RF Commission report of 15 November 1946 on the PUMC postwar development of public health medicine had left out nursing. "The nurse," Tennant pointed out, "is an essential worker in the health team, whether it is in a hospital field or in the public health field." Furthermore, "if the nurse in a leadership position as instructor, supervisor or administrator is to function effectively, she will require an equally high standard of education as the doctor."[10]

To back up her claim, Tennant referred to bylaws of the PUMC that "established the School [of Nursing] on safe and satisfactory grounds." Commenting on the RF Commission report, she noted that training teachers of nursing was an important activity for the PUMC and that "the high principles necessary for medical education are also needed in nursing education." She concluded, pointedly, by highlighting the accomplishments of the PUMC School of Nursing during wartime – during which, of course, the PUMC College of Medicine was shuttered: "It is most gratifying to observe that the PUMC nurses have made such a distinguished record during the war years. I am sure that you and the Trustees will make it possible for the PUMC School of Nursing to continue to prepare nursing leaders for China."[11] If PUMC trustees (mostly physicians) did not recognize the value of nursing, Tennant would make sure they did.

Mary Tennant was not the only one to leverage the wartime success of the refugee PUMC. Vera Nieh also wrote a letter to Hu Shih in early 1947, informing him that, at the NAC conference held in Nanjing the previous October, she had been elected president.[12] In this role, Nieh would be expected to attend the International Council of Nurses conference in May 1947 in Washington DC. Nieh intended to make the most of her visit, asking for a six-month leave of absence to also visit various university nursing programs. Requesting that her trip be financed by the PUMC, she reminded Hu Shih of her extraordinary commitment to the PUMC. She informed him she had worked at the PUMC since August 1938, and that she had managed the challenges when the Japanese took over the institution in December 1941. She had reopened the PUMC School of Nursing at Chengdu "upon the request of the Trustees and with the support of friends and alumni of the PUMC." "During the past few years the work was carried on with much strain and difficulty,' she reminded Shih. "Under those circumstances, I found it too difficult and almost impossible to take any vacation for the past years."[13] The tone of the letter signalled confidence and a solid sense of self-worth. Her boldness paid off; Nieh was provided funding. Nieh was in Carmel, California, visiting former PUMC director Harry Houghton and his wife when she received from Dr. C.U. Lee a letter offering to reappoint her as dean of the School of Nursing and concurrently superintendent of nurses in the PUMC Hospital.[14] She accepted.

THE LAST DAYS OF MODERN NURSING AT THE PUMC

For foreigners in China during the postwar period, the country remained an unsettled, uncertain place. The eruption of civil war between Communist and Nationalist forces was felt most immediately in North China, where, in 1947, the violence was severe enough to force the (permanent) closure of Canada's earliest missionary venture, the North China Mission in Henan. It would be a few more years before the results of the civil war would be fully felt in Beijing and Chengdu.

According to Vera Nieh, once the PUMC School of Nursing was up and running, things progressed normally, even after Mao Zedong's victory in 1949.[15] In November 1950, she completed a report on the School of Nursing covering the period from 1 July 1948 to 31 October 1950. In it, she painted a picture of a dynamic, successful school, adjusting itself to the postwar milieu. To Nieh, there was "definite progress" in the work of the School of Nursing. There were 219 students registered at the time of the report, including ninety-five undergraduate, fifty-six postgraduate (a six-month course in public health nursing), three in departmental graduate work, twenty-five "observers," and forty "affiliating" – the latter categories suggesting that the PUMC was a go-to place for students from other institutions.[16] In comparison, the largest cohort before the war, in 1936, had only a third of the number of undergraduate students. The PUMC now had five affiliate universities, which offered pre-nursing courses and became the main pipeline for nursing students at the college. These included one new university – St. John's (Shanghai), which became affiliated with the PUMC in 1950.

In Nieh's view, interest in university-level nursing education in China was growing. "There has been evidence that more and more college students are becoming interested in choosing the type of nursing education offered by [the PUMC]," she wrote, and there were now more students applying than the college had room for.[17] Of particular interest was the postgraduate course in public health nursing, which had a hundred applicants for thirty-six seats. Most of the students were sent (and presumably funded by) government hospitals and health institutions, afterward returning to "definite posts in their own institutions." The PUMC accepted more public health nurses than it could reasonably accommodate, "in view of the great need for public health nurses by government as well as private health enterprises."[18] Clearly, nursing was being recognized as a resource for the people. Given that nursing was introduced to China sixty years earlier as valuable support for missionary physicians, the fact that it was now recognized as valuable support for the Chinese populace reflects the movement toward naturalization of nursing knowledge.

Beginning in 1950–51, the PUMC also provided opportunity for a limited number of "our older graduates" to return to the School of Nursing for either a refresher course or further study under local fellowships. Nieh believed that providing such opportunities for alumnae would be beneficial, since it was difficult for many to go abroad for such purposes. Alumnae who had "been left behind in their career mostly due to marriage" but who now desired to return to nursing were no longer restricted from nursing. They could come to the PUMC for a refresher course.[19]

The "observer" students were graduate nurses from various hospitals who came to the PUMC for observation and practice in different clinical services. There was a great demand for such experience. Finally, the "affiliating" students came for practical experience that was either unavailable or inadequate in their own schools. These students were typically in their senior year of an undergraduate program in the Beijing-Tianjin area. In this area as well, the demand was more than the PUMC could accommodate, but it took in forty students from five different local schools in any case. As these examples demonstrate, the PUMC School of Nursing was not only open for business, it was keen to reinforce its patriotic postwar self-identity and to live up to its reputation as a place that developed Chinese nursing leaders.

Vera Nieh was concerned about efficiency of services, but she also had a strong sense of when savings were not useful. In her 1950 report, she revealed her ongoing commitment to the ideal that PUMC students should not be responsible for carrying out the day-to-day tasks of staff nurses as a way to keep down personnel costs. This was a difficult position to maintain, particularly considering that the postwar shortage of staff nurses was compounded by a postwar surge in maternity leaves. However, Nieh was steadfast in her belief of "non-exploitation of student service" and ensured that this policy was kept in place.

A last part of her 1950 report is especially noteworthy. It outlines a change in the long-held PUMC policy regarding use of English. After having often raised the question of whether English should remain the language for teaching at the PUMC, Nieh noted that "the teaching work is being gradually converted into Chinese." This was a "heavy task" for the already overloaded staff, but was "meeting a need and trend" both within and outside the institution.[20] The change in language, that most critical marker of identity, is the clearest indicator that modern nursing in China was being "Sino-fied." The PUMC was completing some unfinished business.

Another piece of unfinished business was the formalization of the graduation of PUMC students whose education had been interrupted after the closure of the PUMC in January 1942. After the war, the PUMC had resolved that "the members of the Class of 1943 who completed their course in the School of Nursing at Douw Hospital [in Beijing] during the war years be considered as regular graduate nurses."[21] They were, however, still required to make up six months of additional practical work in order to "meet the standard" of the PUMC school. This condition could be met by taking a postgraduate course or staff nurse position abroad, or by working at the PUMC as a paid staff nurse. If nurses were unable to go abroad or return to the PUMC, they simply would not be granted a PUMC diploma. Students from the Class of 1943 were given three years, until 1 July 1951, to complete the requirements for the nursing diploma. In 1951, only one student fell into this category: at a faculty meeting on 18 January 1951, nursing faculty were given opportunity to vote on whether to grant Huang Che, of the Class of 1943, a diploma, by signing their names under columns headed with the words "approved" or "disapproved." The entire group of fifteen, including Vera Nieh and Dr. C.U. Lee, individually signed as "approved."[22]

This meeting would be the last of the PUMC School of Nursing.

In 1951, the new Communist government took over the PUMC. The Communists had decided to stop university-level education for nurses, and therefore the School of Nursing stopped taking pre-nursing students from other universities. Only senior and junior students were allowed to remain; they were able to complete the program and take examinations as graduates of the PUMC. The other students were distributed to various universities, to medical colleges to study medicine, or to pre-clinical programs such as biology, anatomy and physiology, pharmacology, or bacteriology.[23] The School of Nursing's involvement in nursing service at the PUMC Hospital ceased, and a member of the Communist Party replaced Vera Nieh as superintendent of nurses. According to Immanuel Hsu, "with Russian advice and all the zeal of revolutionaries, the Chinese Communists resolutely and rapidly carried out a gigantic and far-reaching educational reform which included the complete reorganization of all institutions of higher learning and their educational programmes and methods."[24]

Vera Nieh's recollections from this period were captured in a 1985 interview.[25] According to Nieh, "for quite a long time" there were "different movements" at the PUMC as the Communist Party worked to "make

THE LAST CHAPTER (1949–51)

people understand ... the Communists' goal," how Communists think, and "what was wrong with the past." Then, suddenly,

> the whole thing stopped. The organization was taken over entirely. No more nursing school ... The nursing personnel were distributed to different posts outside PUMC. [*Falls into silence.*] And then I was ... well, in 1953 that's the end of the PUMC Nursing School. [*pauses*] As far as the school is concerned, that's official. [And] also as far as I am concerned.[26]

THE END OF MISSIONARY NURSING

Although political unrest had been associated with China for as long as missionaries had been there, something seemed different in this postwar period. On 28 November 1948, Canadian West China Mission (WCM) missionary Dr. Ed Cunningham received a note from Nanjing, likely from the Canadian ambassador. The letter warned missionaries in West China of political stirrings in other regions of the country that would impact the WCUU. "I felt I should make known to the Canadian Community in [Chengdu and Chongqing] and elsewhere up in that section, the seriousness of the present situation in order that they might at least be giving thought to the question of whether they would remain where they are or attempt evacuation."[27] The letter noted that, while things seemed peaceful on the surface in Sichuan, and Canadians may feel far removed from any "Communist threat," the American Consulate had been instructed to warn Americans of the dangers, suggesting that Canadians should be warned too. As a result, the author noted, he had telegraphed Mr. Price, British consul at Chongqing, as well as a Mr. Veals, the following: "Will you please advise all Canadians in your section that in view of generally deteriorating situation and likelihood that a means of exit from China may later be unavailable that those who are not prepared to remain under hazardous conditions where they now reside should plan at once to move to places of safety."[28]

Three Canadian missionary nurses were living in Chengdu at that time. Marjory Alexander lived with Cora Kilborn, and Isabelle Miller had just arrived, in October 1948.[29] On 2 December, conditions were "quiet in West China," and "our missionaries are considering the best course of action should there be a turnover in the government."[30] Some suggested that all should leave at once rather than planning to remain through "the possibility of a Communist regime."[31] American missionaries with small children evacuated. By 7 December, the Canadian Woman's Missionary Society (WMS) was preparing for possible evacuation, working out who would be prioritized to depart first. "I presume those of our WMS missionaries on these lists [of medical priorities] will be among the first to leave in the event of an evacuation," wrote WMS secretary Winifred Harris.[32] Among the priorities were Misses Holt and Rouse, WMS missionaries in the WCM outpost at Rongxian. Shortly after, on 28 December, WMS missionary Violet Stewart wrote that she also wanted to be included on the priority list.[33] She was on the "B" list because she had been through an evacuation before. Stewart accompanied Holt and Rouse from Rongxian to Chengdu, from where they would take a plane to evacuate. The plan was for Stewart to evacuate in a second group "if a really serious situation developed."[34]

On 23 March 1949, the WMS home office noted that, "in view of the whole situation at present we [did] not send short-term nurses to China this year, even though [the] West China Mission Council has requested them."[35] The nursing situation, which was already tenuous, became worse when Marjory Alexander became ill in May 1949. "The climate does not suit her," was the reason given.[36] Alexander's illness compounded difficulties experienced by Cora Kilborn, who, in April, had met with a painful accident. She scalded her right leg from knee to toe when a pail of boiling water, which she was heating on the grate, tipped over."[37] The situation was growing increasingly tense as the Communists advanced in other areas.[38] Xian had fallen ("liberated," in the Communist lexicon) and Hangzhou was threatened. Missionaries with small children were given permission to evacuate.[39] Everyone was waiting for something to erupt. And it did.

On 22 August 1949, Cora Kilborn reported an astonishing incident to Dr. Clifford Tsao, WCUU dean of medicine and acting General Director of the University Hospital. A nursing supervisor had slapped Kilborn's face, "twice as hard as she could." Incensed and confused, Kilborn "did not say anything but merely asked her to go." The nurse left without saying much more. "Miss Lin had gone to bring her back and demand the meaning of it all for we are all in the dark," Kilborn wrote. Kilborn wanted Tsao to ask for the nurse's immediate resignation, writing, "I do not think that such a person is fit to hold the position she does, and the sooner she leaves the better."[40] The person in question was Chang Fang-hsiu, who had stayed on after previously resigning. After assaulting Kilborn, Chang resigned again, on 30 August 1949.

The incident was so unsettling that WCUU nursing alumna Ho Jin-chin recalled it fifty years later. Ho's recollection was that Chang hit Kilborn in the face during a head nurses' meeting. In Ho's view, the reason underpinning Chang's behaviour and her consequent departure was similar to that of as Wang Hui-yin's, as discussed in Chapter 7: Kilborn, who was the superintendent of nurses at the University Hospital, continued to push her ideas about nursing education onto Chang, who had replaced Wang as the head of the WCUU Nursing Department. "All the students wept when [Chang] left," recalled Ho Jin-chin, "because they could see that she wanted to remain."[41] Cora Kilborn's social capital, built up over a lifetime of living and working in Chengdu, was quickly disappearing.

Chang Fang-hsiu's departure triggered a rotating door of leaders in the Nursing Department. First, Dr. Greta Cunningham was appointed acting head of the Nursing Department. She was able to "resolve the problems" and stepped down on 11 February 1950.[42] A month later, Cora Kilborn took up the headship herself, now called the "chairmanship."[43] However, the students of the senior class objected to Kilborn being the head of the department. Thus, on 21 November 1950, Dr. Helen Yoh (Yoh Sh-chen) agreed to accept the headship.[44]

While the WCUU School of Nursing offered a degree program, the Renji school continued to offer its traditional diploma-level nurses' training. In 1950, Leslie Kilborn noted that, while Renji, "for the most part," took in junior middle school graduates, who then took a three-year nursing program, "one improvement was made": "a minimum age of 18 [at the time of entrance] is now enforced."[45] To Leslie Kilborn, some of the former difficulties associated with the Renji school arose because "many fifteen year old girls [who] got into the Hospital Nursing Course ... were too immature to accept the responsibility that is usually placed on a nursing student."[46] As of October 1950, the WCUU was providing a four-year nursing program, accepting only senior middle school graduates who had taken the same entrance exams as other university students. The nursing degree program was financed entirely by the University Hospital. Leslie Kilborn noted that, since the academic standing of Renji was "below that of the University students, it is not reported as a University School, but its relationship to the university is very intimate."[47]

In September 1949, shortly after Chang Fang-hsiu resigned, the WCM executive was asking new missionary appointees and applicants to "state definitely whether or not they are willing to work under a Communist Government."[48] The executive also requested that, "due to the instability of the times and potential difficult future facing those of us who remain, ... those who receive appointment be more than usually carefully chosen from the standpoint of health, nervous and psychological stability."[49]

On 1 October 1949, Mao Zedong declared victory. China was now under Communist rule. Within two weeks, the WCUU was the only one of thirteen colleges (likely colleges of medicine) that remained outside of the sphere of influence of the new government. Nonetheless, "reports continue to stress the peaceful condition of most areas":

> Private colleges and universities have been required to register with the Government Educational Commissions but as yet there is not evidence that this action in any way threatens their independence.
>
> The avowed policy of the new regime is religious freedom. They recognize protestant Christianity as a real social force, capable of cooperating in the new united front. On the other hand, Religion is generally regarded by the new regime as superstitious and reactionary, and from what is already known as to happenings in some areas, Christianity may be in for difficult times and probably for persecution.[50]

By early December, Communist troops had entered Chongqing and were on their way to Chengdu.[51] As Canadian missionary Lewis Walmsley later recalled, "when the National Government forces met defeat after defeat, an atmosphere of fatality descended on a large proportion of the WCUU community. However, many on campus still hoped they could continue the whole program without too great an adjustment."[52] He further recalled that "report and rumour spread throughout the campus community. Fabulous stories circulated in [Chengdu] about corruption at the University."[53] Prices skyrocketed as the currency became almost worthless. At first, the Communist regime imposed no serious restrictions on the WCUU. Gradually, however, as they consolidatd power, the freedom of the university decreased. With the outbreak of the Korean War in June 1950, conditions at the WCUU rapidly worsened. As Zhou Enlai reportedly stated, "While China is putting its house in order, it is undesirable for guests to be present."[54]

On 10 April 1950, Violet Stewart had written from West China that "everything is going well here and no interference with our work in any way. We are all being registered this ten days or two weeks by quite friendly and pleasant young people."[55] There were, however, no opportunities for missionaries to go, or return, to China; no entry permits were being allowed.[56] The university hospitals were starting to feel the pressure of working under the new Communist government. "In view of the very serious situation in the Hospitals of West China because of losses of income and heavy taxes," the WMS assistant treasurer wrote, the WMS Executive Committee was requesting funds from Canada to help with the costs.[57] Moreover, as Lewis Walmsley recalled, by fall 1950, anti-foreign feeling in general, and anti-American antagonism in particular, was evident. When the American government froze all Chinese assets in the United States, Chinese government retaliation was immediate. Banks stopped payment on accounts of all American citizens in Chengdu, and all other foreign citizens as well.[58] The attitude toward Christian institutions became openly antagonistic.

Canadian missionaries Cora Kilborn, her sister, Mary Kilborn, and Lillian Taylor decided to evacuate. By 27 October 1950, Cora and Mary

Kilborn were back in Canada.[59] By 5 January 1951, Lillian Taylor had also returned.[60] Marjorie Alexander departed sometime in 1950. Apparently Eleanor Burwell, a missionary nurse who was born in Zhengzhou, Henan, and who arrived in West China in 1944, also left in 1950.[61] Violet Stewart finally evacuated West China with a number of other Canadians in early 1951. Late February saw her in Hong Kong, waiting for Winifred Harris to arrive.

As WCUU nursing alumnae described it fifty years later, students had mixed emotions when missionaries started to leave. Many thought that the Communist government was treating the WCUU teachers unfairly, but "nobody dared to speak out."[62] After 1949, students felt that a time of great change was coming. Indeed, in terms of modern nursing, it already had.

Following an interview with WCUU nursing alumna Ho Jin-chin on 22 October 2000, Janet Beaton wrote: "Ho Jin-chin notes that the level of nursing education was lowered in 1951 because the government [said] that nurses did not need such a high level of education. When asked what she thought about this she stated emphatically, 'It was a mistake, a mistake that continued until 1981.' Having said this, she started to weep."[63]

POSTSCRIPT

There is a day coming ... when all this can be told, but most missionaries feel it is not at this time.

— *Violet Stewart, Canadian Missionary in West China, 1951*

The WCUU

On 4 January 1951, the Communists marched onto the WCUU campus and took control of the university.[64] Indoctrination by the new government began in earnest. A "University Protection Committee" comprising students and junior staff was organized, and it arranged a thorough search of the households of all foreign staff and about fifteen Chinese staff members and had lists made of all "suspicious objects."[65] Missionary meetings stopped. To many of the leading Chinese, at the WCUU "it seemed that the presence of the foreigners was an embarrassment and a cause of constant misunderstanding with Government authorities."[66] All missionaries gave up positions of authority in the university.[67] Winifred Harris, long-time WMS secretary at Chengdu, noted in a letter written from Hong Kong on 10 July 1951 that "when things began to tighten and investigations seemed to be the order of the day we felt we should destroy all our correspondence as we learned from bitter experience that things which to us seemed insignificant took on quite large proportions when viewed by the eagle eye of representatives of the People's Government."[68] WMS staff went carefully through all the books and files, destroying anything that might be incriminating, "comb[ing] the attics until we were just as sick of it as anyone could be. We spent nights burning anything that might have come from N. America."[69]

On 8 March 1951, the government passed "a new law imposing [a] death sentence on all who oppose the new regime. Number of the gentry class in West China have been killed."[70] On 28 June, a directive to the executive of the WMS Overseas Mission Committee noted that, "in view of the decision of the Church of Christ in China to accept no further subsidy from abroad and the inability of our missionaries who are still in China to carry on missionary work, our Society join the Board of Overseas Missions in closing our China Missions as from this date and recalling all the remaining personnel at once."[71] The formal takeover of the WCCU occurred on 5 October, 1951.

Although the attitudes of some Canadian missionaries toward the Communists in earlier days had been somewhat positive, this did not spare them from being targeted as the new regime came into power.[72] Dr. Stewart Allen, superintendent of the United Church of Canada hospital in Chongqing, had reported favourably on Communist hospitals in Sichuan following the war with Japan.[73] In October 1951 Allen and the nurse who worked with him, Constance Ward, were "invited" to attend a meeting that turned out to be a four-hour ordeal of accusations. They had to kneel on the stage, their backs to the audience, facing a portrait of Mao Zedong, while hospital employees screamed prepared stories.

While there was some accuracy to the charges, they were blown out of proportion – the most serious one being that, by not paying taxes amounting to one dollar on certain UNRRA drugs, Allen had denigrated the government.[74]

The treatment of Allen and Ward alarmed the Canadian missionaries. To Violet Stewart, writing from Hong Kong after her evacuation, the Communist "programme has been most intense in [Sichuan], and the foreign community has been living in a tense atmosphere in [Chengdu and Chongqing]. Ohu [?] Stockwell & Stewart Allen," she noted, were "still in prison."[75] The situation there was distressing: two Methodist missionaries in Chongqing, Jane Surdain and Luella Cater, were brought to their mission house under guard to get their clothes, and then were taken back to their station, "for trial no doubt."[76] They were forbidden to talk; five soldiers guarded them. Constance Ward had had to report every week for questioning since her release from hospital imprisonment, but now she was permitted to apply for an exit permit. Stewart also relayed the awful news that the sisters and husband of Doreen Wu, a supporter who lived in Toronto, had died in Rongxian:

> I heard it on the way down river the whole story, from a Chinese woman from [Rongxian]. However, before they suffered too much they managed to get hold of some poison. Since my arrival in Hong Kong a letter from [Winifred Harris] has confirmed their death. Others in the gentry in [Rongxian] whom I know have been killed. Our High School principal & her husband there are [illegible] afraid having their day for I hear that Pastor Chow has had to leave [Rongxian] ... Fortunately John Kitchen has been released to leave & is on his way now ... So far as we know the situation on the [WCUU] Campus is still the same. [We have] had some news notes from [Earl William?] in which he talks of leaving in the next 6 months. Says westerners not wanted.[77]

Violet later learned that, while Doreen Wu's sister (surname Chang) indeed died of self-administered poison, her husband was still alive.[78] He had contracted pneumonia but later recovered. He lost everything, however, and Wu was attempting to get him out of China to be with her in Canada.

In a letter to Violet Stewart in Hong Kong on 15 March 1951, Mrs. Hugh Taylor noted that the Department of External Affairs was aware of the arrest of Dr. Stewart Allen and Constance Ward but "warned us most particularly not to let any reference to it get into the press as that might have an adverse effect on the possibility of their being released."[79] Consequently, the United Church of Canada mission was being "very quiet about the whole thing" and were "dismayed" to find a press report from Hong Kong getting into the papers in Canada. "It is very hard to know just what to give publicity to and what to keep quiet about and still keep the Church informed, intelligent and sympathetic about the church in China."[80] According to Steward, censorship on the WCUU campus "had become very real and very serious after the University had been taken over." She commented that there were complaints that a Canadian missionary, Mr. Small, who was still on the WCUU campus was "talking too much and too freely, and very unadvisedly."[81] She also reported that his infant daughter was sick and there were grave concerns about her health.[82] Isabelle Miller, a Canadian missionary nurse still on campus at that point, was going to the hospital every day to help care for the child.[83] It is not clear whether the child survived or not.

Dr. Stewart Allen was imprisoned for ten months altogether – eight months in a tiny room in the Chongqing hospital with nightly interrogation, plus two more months in the common city jail after he signed a confession and was awaiting his exit permit.[84] Constance Ward was released, and arrived home on 25 August 1951.[85] By September 1951, only three WMS missionaries remained in West China: Katherine Hockin, Evelyn Ricker, and Canadian nurse Isabelle Miller.[86]

In March 1952, three months after Stewart Allen departed China, the last six Canadian missionaries left Chengdu: Earl and Katherine Willmott, William Small and his wife, and Drs. Leslie and Jean (Millar) Kilborn.[87] By that time, Isabelle Miller, was the last Canadian missionary nurse in China; she departed China sometime between September 1951 and March 1952.[88] Summing up their experience, one unidentified missionary wrote in 1952 that "we can think of the end of missions in China, at least for the time being, as the will of God, as the work of the Devil, as the result of political factors, as a tragedy, as a painful but necessary medicine, as a judgment; and in some or all of these ways taken together."[89]

Canadian missionary nurses came to China with the desire to give practical expression to their Christian faith. For some, the ultimate purpose of missionary nursing was to share the gospel of Jesus Christ with the Chinese and help them to come to Christianity. For others, nursing work itself was regarded as worship: regardless of whether those they came to serve were, or became, Christians, nursing was a calling. Helping to alleviate the suffering of others was a noble way to serve Christ. WCUU alumna Ho Jin-chin, a child of Christian parents, also viewed nursing this way. She said that she, like most of the students who entered nursing at the Canadian West China Mission, were Christian and went into nursing because this was what Christians did. "Nursing is noble," she noted in her interview with Janet Beaton in 2000.[90] For seventeen-year-old Ho Jin-chin, nursing was a way to serve Jesus. By 2000, however, she was no longer a Christian. Nor were her colleagues. As Chin Shu-wen noted in her 1995 interview with Janet Beaton, while most of the Chinese nurses in her program had been Christian, "none are Christian now."[91]

The baccalaureate program at the WCUU was closed in 1951, after graduating two classes totalling fifteen students (see Table 8.2). Over forty years later, in 1995, Canadian nurses returned to Chengdu, at the invitation of the renamed West China University. Together with the Canadian International Development Agency, these nurses, from the University of Manitoba and led by that university's dean of nursing, Janet Beaton, helped re-establish baccalaureate nursing at the WCUU.

The PUMC

Between 1924 and 1950, the PUMC School of Nursing graduated 238 nurses (Table 8.3). Of these, the largest proportion – over a third – worked in schools of nursing, as the principal of the school, superintendent of nurses, or director of studies, or in teaching and administration. A further 13 percent worked in public health nursing, and 17 percent worked

TABLE 8.2 Graduates from the WCUU School of Nursing, 1950–54

Year	Number of students	Type of degree	Total, by degree
1950	7	Baccalaureate	
1951	8	Baccalaureate	15 baccalaureates
1952	3	Associate degree	
1953	8	Associate degree	
1954	12	Associate degree	23 associate degrees
Total	38		

SOURCE: Ho Jin-chin, graduate of 1950, who supplied numbers to Beaton. October 2000, WMASC, A13-20, Janet Beaton fonds, box 12, file 2.

in hospitals. Of those in hospitals, the vast majority were in leadership positions, either as superintendent of nurses or in supervision and administration. Only 7 percent of PUMC graduates were "temporarily inactive." Taken together, an astonishing 80 percent of PUMC nursing graduates were in leadership positions or taking advanced study.[92] It was a remarkable legacy for a program that, within weeks of reporting these results, was, essentially, closed.

In 1953, after her position at the PUMC was taken over by a member of the Communist Party, Vera Nieh was posted as the assistant hospital superintendent in the new military hospital in Beijing, Number 103 Hospital. From 1954 to 1957, she was vice-director of the General Hospital of the People's Liberation Army, Number 1 Military Hospital.[93] Then, from 1956 to 1966, she was the superintendent of the Nursing Department of the Provincial Hospital of Anhui Province and executive director of the Anhui Branch of the Chinese Nurses Association. She struggled with the new Communist ideology. "To tell you personally," she told Anne Davis in 1985, "I am not political-minded, and I really didn't underst[and] ... know at all what Communist is." She continued:

Of course, I learned after the Liberation but, before that time I had no knowledge of Communist [ideology], I had no interest in that. But I think anyway, no matter what kind of a Party it is, why, they should mean well for their own country. Well, anyway, to work with this new officer, the Superintendent-so-called ([who] was an old Party Member), their thinking is very radical to me. I see him to be an enemy. They treat me, they do not trust me 'cause I was trained by the Americans. So, I was treated as an enemy. I couldn't do anything … I don't want to say too much. I had to be re-educated.[94]

Table 8.3 PUMC graduates, by professional position 1924–50

		Graduates	
Place of work	*Position*	#	%
Schools of nursing	Principal of school and superintendent of nurses	32	13.4
	Director of studies	4	1.7
	Teaching and administration	50	21.0
Public health nursing	Teaching and administration	30	12.6
	General	2	0.8
Hospitals	Superintendent of nurses	15	6.4
	Supervision and administration	24	10.0
	General	2	0.8
Other fields	General secretary of national nurses' organization	1	0.4
	Principal of midwifery school	1	0.4
	Director of studies in midwifery school	1	0.4
	Specialization in nutrition	1	0.4
	Specialization in child health	1	0.4
	Specialization in anesthesia	1	0.4
	Nursery work	3	1.2
	Changed to private practice in medicine (MD)	1	0.4
Others	Advanced study	32	13.4
	Temporarily inactive	16	6.7
	Unknown	9	3.7
	Sick	6	2.5
	Deceased	6	2.5
Total		238	100

SOURCE: Statistics on Medical and Nursing School Graduates of the PUMC, December 1950, Rockefeller Archive Center, Rockefeller Foundation, SG 1.1, series 601-China, box 37, folder 298.

For Nieh, the closure of the PUMC for the second time – this time by fellow Chinese – was heartbreaking. She retired in 1966.

In 1974, PUMC alumna Bernice Chu Chen immigrated to Canada. The next year, in a confidential letter written to the president of the Florence Nightingale Foundation in England, she noted that she was hoping to work as a registered nurse in Ontario but required proof of her former professional education. "I am sorry it is impossible for me [to obtain such proof] from mainland China," she wrote. "Therefore I beg you to help me out from this unfortunate situation."[95] She wondered if it would be possible for them to provide proof of her postgraduate study of public health nursing, at least. Bedford College in London dutifully responded with the required documents.[96] Two months later, Chu Chen wrote to thank the college for its response, noting that, in the past month, her and her husband's health "started to deteriorate quickly" and she decided against the idea of becoming a registered nurse in Canada.[97] It is just as well – Bernice Chu Chen was by then seventy-four years old.

In 1949, the International Council of Nurses (ICN) recognized the Republic of China in Taiwan as China's only legitimate government. As a result, the new People's Republic of China was removed from ICN membership, and remained an outsider for several decades.[98] In the 1980s, university-level education for nurses in China was reopened. Those who were foremost in getting baccalaureate nursing re-established were PUMC alumnae – including Lin Juying (PUMC 1941), who was president of the Chinese Nursing Association (CNA) from 1983 to 1991 and director of nursing and dean of the School of Nursing at Beijing Hospital for many years. (Lin Juying also received honorary doctorates from the University of Missouri and the University of Michigan.)[99] Although the CNA was reorganized in the 1980s, it was not readmitted into the ICN. China began working to rejoin the ICN. Finally, on 19 May 2013, the ICN announced the inclusion of the CNA, admitted by a unanimous vote of the assembled delegates at the meeting of the ICN's Council of National Representatives.[100]

In 1983, Vera Nieh was elected as an honorary member of the CNA, and in 1988 was appointed as the honorary director of the Department of Nursing at the PUMC, which, after thirty-five years, resumed its role as a site for higher learning. The department became a School of Nursing again in 1996. Reflecting on her role at the PUMC in her interview with Anne Davis in 1985, Nieh expressed satisfaction with what PUMC nursing had contributed to China – both in the years before the Communist victory and also in the ensuing years, as it provided nursing leadership in China. She noted that the current government had different policies than that of the government at the time of Liberation in 1949. The government of the mid-1980s understood that most of the PUMC graduates are "really doing good work all through China" – both graduates of the PUMC and nurses from other schools who took postgraduate programs at the PUMC. "There are always some outstanding people," she noted, "only if they had more education, they [could] do more. So, I mean the post-graduate work, I think it ... made a great contribution."[101] Deng Xiaoping, who became the leader of China after Mao Zedong's death in 1976, supported the notion of higher education for nurses. "We think that he is thinking on the right track," Nieh noted. "They understand that if you want to really raise the standard of medical education or medical work or service, that nursing also has to raise their standards."[102]

Throughout her years of service, Vera Nieh lived up to her father's teaching by helping to address some of what he considered to be China's four basic problems of poverty, ignorance, weak health, and selfishness. Not only did she herself work hard to counter these conditions in her own life, she managed to make a significant impact on the lives of others as well. Vera Nieh died of a heart attack on 22 August 1998. She was ninety-five.

Conclusion

The Rockefeller Effect: Nursing as a Liberating Movement for Women

Truly, nurses all over the world are of one family, one professional world. The leadership that the Rockefeller Foundation has shown in the fields of medicine and nursing has long demonstrated the international spirit.

— *Bernice Chu Chen, 1947*

Writing anonymously in the journal *African Affairs* in January 1952, a missionary who had worked in China commented on the "sociological failure" of Christian missions in China.[1] The article noted that "the various activities and institutions of the Christian Church and mission in China were at one time socially and culturally creative and revolutionary." However, it continued, "they have for the most part long ceased to be so."[2] Missionaries had built and maintained hospitals in which leading Chinese had been trained – and therefore depended on a certain technical standard, a supply of drugs and equipment, and an understanding of health and sickness that were lacking in China. However, "the Communist emphasis on public health," the writer noted, "and on the training to a lower level of very much larger numbers of medical personnel, is surely much more relevant to the actual needs of the country."[3] The article concluded that, in missions, educational, medical, and social service work should contribute creatively to the country and be part of the total state program, and should be genuinely capable of ultimate support and direction by the local church – or, it should be considered temporary and expendable. "Considering the vast amount of money, personnel, thought, and devotion that went into the Christian schools and colleges in China, our intellectual failure is remarkable."[4]

In a 1956 reflection on the same period, Hsu Ai-Chu, a Peking Union Medical College (PMUC) graduate who evacuated to Nationalist Taiwan after the Communist victory, contrasted nursing schools that had been started by missionaries and the PUMC, which had been founded by the Rockefeller Foundation (RF). She noted that, in the early days of missionary nursing, the idea of girls caring for sick strangers was not acceptable in China; for women to take care of male patients was considered indecent and immoral.[5] Moreover, educational resources were limited: the missionary nurses did their best translating their own English textbooks into Chinese. When the Nurses Association of China was established in 1909, its chief objective was to unify and upgrade nursing schools. Graduate nurses who passed a national examination were qualified to nurse professionally nation-wide in China. The establishment of the PUMC in 1920, she noted, was decisive in upgrading nursing education. That institution made senior high school graduation the minimum entrance requirement and offered a four-year nursing program, including a pre-nursing year. A degree program was instituted later, in co-operation with some of the leading universities in China. Significantly, Hsu Ai-Chu noted that old scholars and advanced education have always been highly respected by the Chinese. In this sense, whereas the missionary approach to nursing countered Chinese cultural values, the PUMC (elite) approach mirrored them.[6]

These two commentaries – by a missionary and a PUMC alumna, both writing from the standpoint of those who had recently departed from the People's Republic of China – capture the early ways in which "outside-insiders" tried to make sense of the missionary era, of which the Rockefeller Foundation was an anomalous part. They argued that Christian missions, while socially relevant early on, ultimately failed in their medical mission because of the emphasis on expensive curative rather than preventive care; they did not adapt well to changing times. Nor was their approach expandable. For example, although the founders of the West China Union University (WCUU) (and other Christian universities) viewed education as a key way to acculturate and spread Christian thinking and scientific progress, their focus on infrastructure (especially hospitals) ultimately limited their influence and impact. When the Woman's Missionary Society's (WMS) Women's Hospital in Chengdu burned down, nursing service and education were transferred to other buildings, but the quality of both suffered as a result. When provided the opportunity to take over the new University Hospital, WMS nurses and others declined, concerned about the financial and other costs involved. Although recognizing that the status quo was not working, they were not willing, or perhaps not able, to envision an alternative. For two generations, Canadian missionaries in West China had (successfully) worked to adapt local settings to Western ideals. However, eight years of war changed the landscape, demanding that missionaries adapt Western ideals to local realities and priorities. At this stage, having invested so much in teaching and providing curative medicine, it was difficult to change course.

Nor were missionaries as committed to the cause as they once had been. Those who, like Susie Kelsey and Margaret Prentice, viewed nursing as primarily an avenue to bring the Christian gospel to the Chinese populace, continued to be encouraged and fortified by a sense that God was at work among the people they came to serve, even through and after internment. Others, such as the displaced North China missionaries Clara Preston, Dorothy Boyd, and Margaret Gay, were unsettled (traumatized, in fact) by violence in Henan, and too depleted by the time they arrived in West China to adapt fully to the wartime conditions there. Long-serving missionary nurses Susan Haddock, Irene Harris, Alma Tallman, and Mary Crawley all departed before the end of the war in 1945, suggesting that the challenges of wartime conditions prevailed over intrinsic rewards of their religious vocation. Margaret Lee, whose Chinese ancestry and Montreal education gave her much in common with the PUMC nurses, was the most promising of the second-generation missionaries. However, she resigned to be married before having had the opportunity to make a lasting impact. China-born "mishkid" Cora Kilborn held on tenaciously but also lacked an ability to adapt to changing circumstances. In this sense, her tenacity was also her downfall; she held on to old approaches to education at Renji rather than fully embracing changes required for a successful baccalaureate program in Chengdu. Given Kilborn's deep knowledge of Chengdu and her status as the child of pioneering medical missionaries, one cannot imagine a more disappointing ending to her life's work in China than a literal slap in the face by a Chinese nursing colleague.

Although fear affected missionary nursing during wartime, fearsome conditions had always been part of missions in China. The first generation of Canadian missionaries (1890s–1920s) survived the anti-foreign movement (1890s), Boxer Rebellion (1900), Republican Revolution (1911), May Fourth Movement (1919), Warlord Era (1916–28), and Northern Expedition with its related great missionary exodus (1927). This generation was admired in Canada and could count on appreciative audiences back home to relay their triumphant tales. They were well supported, both financially and socially, their ideals reflecting Canada's dominant culture. In contrast, the second generation of Canadian missionaries (1930s–1940s) belonged to an era when Canadian and American Christians were rethinking the value and purpose of missionary work, re-framing Christian faith as a call to social reform rather than personal conversion. The emphasis was on serving, rather than saving, human-kind. While the social gospel, translated into public health approaches (concern for poverty, clean environments, and maternal mortality, for example), would have been a good fit for missionary nursing, the West China Mission (WCM) focus overall remained on a curative rather than preventive model for health. The curative model became increasingly problematic as costs skyrocketed and human and other resources dimin-ished over the course of the war.

The WCM's commitment to a curative model tied nursing practice to medical education at Chengdu. Medical students depended on a large and varied patient population in order to have the breadth of experience necessary for full learning. This, in turn, required a well-run hospital (or hospitals) with a range of medical and surgical services, and a well-qualified nursing staff to provide round-the-clock patient care. The most economical and reliable staffing source was nursing students, and a nursing school the most dependable manager of nursing services. Little wonder the WCUU was eager to have the Woman's Missionary Society (which hired missionary nurses) take over the University Hospital; it was the best guarantee for suitable clinical teaching for medical students.

The WMS, however, was not eager to take on that hospital's nursing service. Perhaps the society recognized the likelihood of losing its independence, as Canadian missionary nursing would then be subjugated to the priorities and desires of the WCUU Medical College.

Not so for the PUMC nurses. Having spent twenty years in a system where nursing students were *not* responsible for staffing – students were supernumerary; their first priority was learning, not nursing service – the refugee PUMC with Vera Nieh at the helm was not about to be subjugated to medicine or physicians. Instead, the PUMC School of Nursing disrupted missionary approaches to nursing, offering instead an innovative model that challenged medical authority, privileged nursing priorities, separated nursing education from practice, prioritized advanced education, and modelled nursing leadership. In this way, the PUMC unsettled traditional nursing (and medical) norms, positioning nursing as a liberating movement for women – in Chengdu, as in Beijing.

As the story of the last sustained period of transnational relationships (and knowledge flows) between China, Canada, and the United States, *Nursing Shifts in Sichuan* has demonstrated the extent to which a big idea initiated in one country – in this case, public health and advanced education for nurses as the future of health care – could reshape nursing and women's work in another. This particular big idea germinated first among American nursing leaders in the United States (as captured in the *Goldmark Report*), and was brought to life at the PUMC in Beijing. There it was translated and revised by Chinese nurses, who, living as a PUMC diaspora in West China during wartime, modelled a Chinese version of the big idea to Canadian and Chinese nurses, including those gathered as refugees in Chengdu. The big idea, and especially the part of it that emphasized the importance of university-level education for nurses, was taken up by Canadian nurses and the WCUU, who initiated a degree program for nurses just months after the refugee PUMC returned home. Although only offered for five years (1946–51), the Bachelor of Science degree for nurses at the WCUU made a lasting impression in Chengdu and on the nursing students able to take advantage of it. The effect of the Rockefeller Foundation's investment in nursing in China – the Rockefeller Effect – was nursing as a liberating movement for women. By promoting and supporting advanced education for nurses, the RF reframed an understanding of a health care system that placed nursing leaders at its core.

The significance of the Rockefeller Effect is best understood within the context of previous transnational knowledge flows. The prevailing model of nursing as a hospital-based vocation for unmarried, Christian women, as introduced in China in the late 1800s, was the product of mostly unidirectional knowledge flows from Europe to the "New World" to the colonies. More specifically, models for nursing followed colonial tracks from France (the Grey Nuns) to Canada in the 1700s; from Britain (Florence Nightingale) to Canada, the United States, and Australia in the 1800s; and from America and Canada to China and colonies in Asia and Africa in the 1900s. Such ideas were spread by Catholic and Christian missionaries acculturated in the belief that Western nations were divinely charged with civilizing others. In contrast, in wartime China, we see transnational nursing flows as iterative rather than unidirectional – something one can trace by examining the PUMC and the WCM under the same lens.

The PUMC School of Nursing differed from the WCM and other missionary schools of nursing in significant ways. First, influenced by the *Goldmark Report*, the PUMC emphasized public health and nursing leadership – that is, a commitment to strengthening the Chinese citizenry, including Chinese women who would now have access to advanced education and university degrees. While the PUMC could not have realized it at the time, this approach would particularly resonate during wartime, as it aligned with growing nationalism, allowing for an understanding in China of nursing as a patriotic act. In contrast, the WCM emphasized a well-established Christian approach to nursing dating back three hundred years in Canada to the time of Marguerite d'Youville and the Grey Nuns of Montreal – that is, the biblically mandated responsibility of the Christian church to care for ill and injured strangers, an altruistic response to human suffering. This approach explains the WMC emphasis on enrolling Christian students from Christian families, compared with the PUMC emphasis on enrolling bright and ambitious students from well-established families. In reality, both approaches were limited, since the pool of qualified candidates for both programs was relatively small.

Second, the PUMC emphasis on public health was an expandable model, in that a small cadre of nurses could have a wide impact. The Mass Education Movement and the Beijing First Health Station are prime examples of this, both emphasizing health education of families and districts as the best way to promote health and prevent disease. As John Watt has argued, during wartime it only took a small number of health care reformers to save tens of thousands of lives, promoting hygiene and sanitation, and bringing battlefield casualties, communicable diseases, and maternal mortality under control.[7] Although Canadian missionary nurses were also interested in public health (firmly established in Canada after the devastating 1918 Spanish influenza epidemic), those who worked in free-standing hospital training schools (for example, in Henan) had more opportunity to put public health into practice than those in Chengdu, where nursing education was linked closely to medical education – that is, as hospital-based care.

Third, the PUMC was well funded. In terms of foreign missions, there was (and is) little to compare to the support provided by the Rockefeller Foundation. John D. Rockefeller Jr., beneficiary of his father's vast Standard Oil fortunes, sought an opportunity in the second decade of the twentieth century to invest his wealth in something that would have an indelible impact. He invested millions of dollars to establish the finest medical school (and, by extension, nursing school) in Asia, one comparable to premier schools in the United States. In addition to establishing the landmark PUMC, the RF also established fellowships for promising individuals in nursing, giving scores of Chinese nurses, mostly PUMC alumnae, the opportunity to study in Canada, the United States, and Britain. Canadian medical missions, in comparison, relied primarily on modest funding by church members, along with government and private grants, including from the RF. The WMS had active chapters in Canada, with churchwomen across the country diligently raising funds through bake sales and teas. By the 1930s and 1940s, times of economic depression and war for Canadians, the United Church of Canada had started to question the costs involved with hospital-based missions in China. Combined with concerns that Western governments were indirectly supporting the Japanese military through sales of material used to manufacture armaments, the WCUU board of governors departed from the conventional tack in raising funds for the new University Hospital. Appealing to the collective Christian conscience, it suggested donations as a sort of penance for the atrocities in China allowed by passive Western governments. That departure from earlier fundraising, which had focused on evangelical aims, signalled a shift to a social gospel approach, which, ironically, aligned with the PUMC's focus on public health. In any case, the enormous costs of running a medical school, nursing school, and hospitals in wartime China weighed heavily on both the WCUU and PUMC.

Fourth, the PUMC had a strong alumnae base, whose graduates were firmly committed to the vision of nursing in China instilled and modelled at their alma mater. That PUMC alumnae comprised the entire nursing faculty when the refugee School of Nursing was opened in West China gives a sense of how deeply they believed in the value of their work. Reminiscent of the early days of missionary nursing in China, the PUMC alumnae formed a tightknit community that zealously protected the PUMC mission and its leaders, including Vera Nieh. While long-serving missionary nurses and their early graduates experienced and exuded a similar commitment to the Christian cause, wartime unsettled the ties between missionary nurses and their protégées. Based on interviews conducted in the 1980s, PUMC alumnae continued to embrace values that underpinned their nursing education, as nurses like Lin Juying, by then in her sixties, took up the cause to reinstate baccalaureate education at the PUMC. In contrast, and based on interviews conducted mostly in the 1990s, WCUU and Renji alumnae, while lamenting the loss of baccalaureate education, no longer espoused the Christian beliefs that underpinned and motivated Canadian missionary nursing.

Fifth, and this ties in with the previous point, by 1942, the staff of the PUMC School of Nursing was entirely Chinese, including a Chinese dean. After the United States and Canada declared war against Japan, all remaining American nurses were arrested and interned. Although Chinese nurses – and particularly Vera Nieh – still had access to mentors and advisers in the United States via cablegrams and letters, the PUMC was a de facto Chinese enterprise for its final ten years. In contrast, while the numbers of Canadian missionaries steadily decreased over the course of the war, Canadian missionary nurses still held leadership positions at the WCUU. Even after Chinese nurses, including PUMC alumnae, took on leadership roles in the United and University Hospitals in Chengdu during and after the departure of the refugee PUMC, positional power was still firmly held by Canadian missionaries. Although it is difficult to assess whether, and to what extent, Cora Kilborn deserved the criticism levelled at her by alumnae in the 1990s, there is enough evidence to conclude that, regardless of her sincere motivations and her affection for the Chinese community she was raised in, she was not, by the late 1940s, widely respected by Chinese students and staff.

Finally, as the "darling child" of the Rockefeller Foundation, the PUMC, both staff and alumnae, had unprecedented access to international networks of nursing's elite and the (mostly American) education institutions they belonged to. Garnering master's degrees in an era when even undergraduate degrees were still uncommon in nursing, PUMC nurses had access to career paths and nursing leaders not readily accessible to Canadian missionary nurses. What this did, in essence, was put Chinese, American, and Canadian nurses on a level playing field. For Western nurses, travelling to China provided them with adventure, broadened their understanding of the world, expanded their nursing experience, and increased their status among their peers back home. The same is true for Chinese nurses associated with the PUMC. In both cases, the nurses became bilingual and bicultural transporters of nursing knowledge. At the same time, both PUMC *and* WCM nurses held privileged positions that were in stark contrast to the vast majority of Chinese nurses. And both were purveyors, recipients, and translators of nursing knowledge.

The displacement of the PUMC School of Nursing to West China made obvious the difference between nursing approaches at the PUMC and the WCUU. Over the course of three years, PUMC nurses, all Chinese, influenced and changed the way nursing was practised and taught in Chengdu. Even after 1951, when the WCUU and PUMC were closed and Westerners expelled from the People's Republic of China, the PUMC diaspora continued to influence – most noticeably in Taiwan, where leading PUMC alumnae Hsu Ai-Chu and Chou Meiyu continued to instil PUMC values about public health and nursing leadership. Chou Meiyu, who was studying under her second Rockefeller fellowship at Columbia Teachers' College in New York when the Nationalist government (and army) relocated to Taiwan in the wake of the Communist victory in 1949, was eventually promoted to the rank of general, and continued as director of the Army Nursing School for the rest of her career.

Rana Mitter, writing on the reconstruction of postwar China, noted that one of the war's "principal ironies" was that it both weakened and strengthened China.[8] On the one hand, she argued, China's political centre and economy were thrown off balance, deprived of resources and undermined by massive corruption. On the other hand, war enabled the government to force a more centralized political culture and raised China's international profile. In a similar way, wartime both weakened and strengthened modern nursing in China. On the one hand, wartime challenged and devalued Western understandings of nursing as essentially an altruistic, Christian vocation, as Chinese nurses sought to reconcile the value of Western, scientific knowledge with China's desire to rid itself of foreign occupiers and influence. On the other hand, wartime strengthened Chinese nursing leadership and honed an understanding of nursing as a patriotic act as Chinese nurses embraced Western ideals of public health and advanced education for women. By the 1980s and 1990s when baccalaureate programs for nursing were reinstated at the PUMC and WCUU, certain elements of nursing introduced by Westerners prevailed against the odds of a half-century absence. These included a biomedical, hospital-based, physician-directed, compassionate approach to nursing practice. Furthermore, as baccalaureate education was closely followed by masters' and, in 2008, PhD programs in nursing, China embraced advanced education for nurses. Finally, having been excluded from the International Council of Nurses (ICN) in 1949, China looked again for opportunities to benefit from and contribute to transnational knowledge flows. This has been done, in part, through nursing exchanges and collaborative partnerships with Canadian and American (and other) universities. Perhaps most telling, in 2013 China was unanimously reinstated as a member of the ICN. Indeed, in 2019, China accounted for 500 of the 5,000 nursing delegates at the ICN Congress in Singapore.[9] After almost a century of war, revolution, and socio-political upheaval, nursing in China had come full circle to fully embrace an understanding of nurses first introduced by Elsie Mawfung Chung in 1914 – as *hushi*: caring scholars.

Acknowledgments

I became aware of Vera Nieh and the period when Canadian missionaries harboured the elite Peking Union Medical College (PUMC) School of Nursing through stories passed to me over mealtime conversations with seasoned scholars – particularly Janet Beaton, Anne Davis, Pierre-Yves Saunier, Sioban Nelson, John Watt, Mary Brown Bullock, and Bridie Andrews. One of my earliest exposures was in 2002 with Janet Beaton, then dean of nursing at the University of Manitoba. I had just started my doctoral research on Canadian missionary nursing in China, and she had recently published an article on Caroline Wellwood, a pioneer Canadian missionary nurse who worked at the Methodist (later United) Church West China Mission in Chengdu, Sichuan, from 1907 to 1942.[1] Janet Beaton's interest in the subject came out of her own work in China in the 1990s. In 1989, she had secured funding from the Canadian International Development Agency allowing University of Manitoba faculty to work with West China University faculty to develop an undergraduate program in nursing. During her visits to West China, she was surprised to learn that the nursing program there had originally been established by Canadians, and that they had started a baccalaureate program once before, in the 1940s. Beaton set about collecting related data from the West China Union University (WCUU) and the United Church of Canada Archives. Although my focus at that time was the history of nursing at the North China Mission (Henan), Beaton impressed upon me that there was also a significant Canadian-Chinese story in West China waiting to be written. Of particular interest to Beaton were two wartime events: the mysterious Women's Hospital fire (rumours attributing the blaze to arsonists who supported the Japanese invaders) and the start of a new baccalaureate program at the WCUU with the help of the PUMC, the latter one of five refugee institutions being supported by the WCUU, of which Canadian missionaries were a part. Janet Beaton has since reposited her substantial data collection at the University of Manitoba.

I also met with Anne Davis, professor emerita, University of California at San Francisco, and American Academy of Nursing "living legend."[2] Davis had asked me to join her for lunch after hearing my talk on Canadian missionary nurses in China at an American Association for the History of Nursing meeting in Atlanta. She had spent over thirty years travelling back and forth to China, helping to (re)establish nursing education there after China was reopened to the West in the late 1970s. In approximately 1985, Davis recorded interviews with Lin Juying, PUMC graduate and president of the Chinese Nurses Association, 1983 to 1991, and with Vera Nieh. Davis's recollection of the poignant and significant work done by Lin and Nieh in the establishment and re-establishment of nursing education in China suggested that there, too, was a story of historical significance awaiting attention. She encouraged me to take it on.

A third nudge came from Pierre-Yves Saunier, professor of history at Laval University in Quebec. Together with historians Sioban Nelson and Patricia D'Antonio, we spent a few days at the Rockefeller Archive Center in Tarrytown, New York, to work on "Nursing Activities of the Rockefeller Foundation, 1915–1965" – a project examining how the Rockefeller Foundation joined the world of nursing to support and expand the medical work of nursing personnel. Between 1919 and 1940, the Rockefeller Foundation awarded 489 fellowships to nurses in thirty-eight countries. Saunier directed me to the files of Rockefeller fellows Chou Meiyu (Zhou Meiyu) and Vera Nieh (Nieh Yuchan) in particular, as well as to Hsu Ai-Chu (Xu Aizhu) and Bernice Chu Chen (Zhu Bihui). Saunier and Nelson were both aware of the significant work of the RF in China, and encouraged me to dig further.

A final source of encouragement was a series of significant conversations with American and Chinese scholars who were members of the China Medical Board centenary book project, led by Mary Brown Bullock and Bridie Andrews. In particular John Watt, vice-president (and previous executive director) of the American Bureau of Medical Advancement in China Foundation, provided valuable insights. Watt's personal reminiscences of some of the PUMC graduates painted a story of larger-than-life personalities whose approach to wartime nursing included what he dubbed "guerrilla warfare" to change the view of physicians and others in authority to take the work of nurses more seriously. He noted the significance of the work of PUMC graduates, including Zhou Meiyu, Nieh Yuchan, and Xu Aizhu. The names were starting to sound familiar, and I became more curious.

In the years since then, I have received much support and encouragement. In addition to the persons noted above, I wish to acknowledge colleagues in China – particularly Yuhong Jiang (PUMC, Humanities and Social Sciences), Huaping Liu (PUMC past dean of Nursing), Zheng Li (PUMC dean of nursing), and Yingjuan Cao (Qilu, associate director of nursing), as well as PUMC archivist Zhang Xie. I am also grateful to my students and research assistants LuiXia Lee, Melody Pan, and Sharon Wang. Through my various projects, I have received much support from Canadian missionary children: Mary (Struthers) McKim has added new insights from the medical work in Qilu and Sichuan of her father, Ernest B. Struthers. History colleagues in Canada and the United States – including Geertje Boschma, Laurie Meijer Drees, Barbra Mann Wall, and Dominique Marshall – have kept me in the loop even as my growing responsibilities as dean of nursing at Trinity Western University (TWU) and president of the Canadian Association for Schools of Nursing kept me from participating as fully in history events. My colleagues in the TWU School of Nursing have also been unwavering in their encouragement, both for my ongoing preoccupation with nursing history and my interest in China. I am grateful to Sheryl Reimer Kirkham and Barbara Astle, who went so far as to accompany me on a visit to the Henan Peoples Provincial Hospital and Henan University in Zhengzhou. Much thanks to Yuming (David) and Yinong (Maria) Yang, who envisioned and organized this and the resultant visit of Henan nurses to TWU. Finally, I am grateful to TWU provost Bob Wood for supporting this research despite administrative pressures, and to TWU for providing a sabbatical to help me complete this manuscript. It is a particular joy to be part of a university that values missionary scholarship and Chinese scholarship in equal measure.

After almost twenty years of studying nursing history in China, my family has grown accustomed to my preoccupations with China; some have even accompanied me on trips there. I am most indebted to family members Jacoba (Cobi) Visser, Henk Visser, Janessa Warkentin, Luke Warkentin, Mike Grypma, Mike Visser, Nancy Visser, Sylvia Slagter, Lawrens (Lou) Slagter, Christi Nagel, Ellen Freestone, Martha Grypma, and Ron Grypma, and to my lifelong friend Allyson Julé (*oui*, aigu!). Their listening ears (or bemused curiosity) made me believe I was onto something significant. My deepest gratitude, however, is reserved for my husband of thirty years, Martin Grypma, my indefatigable cheerleader who has supported me every inch of the way.

Sonya (Visser) Grypma
Trinity Western University, July 2020

Appendix 1

List of Nurses at the West China Mission, 1895–1951

Name	Birthplace	Graduation place	Year of graduation	Dates as nurse WCM	# of years at WCM	Notes, including married names
Ford, Jennie	Ontario		1895	1895–97	2	Died: spinal meningitis
Foster, Mary A.				1896–08	12	Resigned (mental illness)
Forrest, Fannie	Ontario		1900	1900–06	6	Mrs. G. Franck
Dunfield, Lena M.				1904–05	2	Mrs. R.O. Joliffe
Service, Mrs. C.W.				1904–30?	26	Nee Robina M.I. Morgan?
Wilkins, Eleanor	Nova Scotia			1905–08	3	Mrs. Muir
Wellwood, Caroline	Ontario	Washington, DC	1902	1906–44	38	Nee Caramitta Gage
Allan, Mrs. F.F.	Kansas	Denver		1906–44	28	Nee L.E. Lawson
Small, Mrs. W.				1908–?		
Paton, I.P.	China	Guelph General Hospital	1907	1908–25	17	Mrs. A.T. Crutcher
Lawson, Lottie E.	PEI	Mt Allison		1908–11	3	Mrs. Walter Small
Switzer, M.E.	Ontario	Toronto General Hospital	1906	1908–21	13	
Asson, Margaret A.	Alberta	Missouri	1908	1909–30	21	
Bowles, Mrs. N.E.	Ontario	Elmira, NY	1909	1909–30	21	Nee Muriel O.B. Wood
McNaughton, B.G.	Quebec	Montreal	1902	1909–31	22	
Shuttleworth, Velettia				1910–12	2	
Smith, Mary Totten	Ontario?	Toronto?	1908	1910–19	9	
Morgan, Ada	Bella Bella, BC		1910	1912–32	20	Died: pneumonia

Name	Province/Country	City	Year	Period	No.	Notes
Kelly, Mrs. C.H.	Illinois			1912–27?	15	Nee Marion Miles
Dale, Elle	Ontario	Toronto?	1912	1913–32	18	
Best, Mrs. A.E.	Ontario			1914–?		Nee Gertrude J. Taylor
Haddock, Susan	Ireland	Ireland		1914–41	27	
Hartwell, Geraldine E.	China	Nanaimo?	1914	1914–?		Born in Chengdu
Wheeler, Myrtle M.	BC?	Brandon		1914–23	9	Died: gall bladder surgery
Beaton, Mrs. K.J.	Ontario?	Medicine Hat?		1914–30?	16	Nee Mary Borton
Birks, Mrs. W.H.	Ontario			1915–33	18	Nee Miss MacGregor
Bridgman, Mrs. C.A.	Ontario	Pittsburgh	1916	1916–?	3	Nee Margaret J. Modeland
Veals, Mrs. R.J.		Toronto		1917–20	6	Nee E.M. Bousfield
Barnett, Martha				1918–24	7	
Campbell, Florence M.			1917	1918–25		
McIntosh, Isobel K.	Ontario	Buffalo, NY	1916	1919	10	
Batstone, M.E.	India	Lindsay [?]	1916	1919–29	7	
Ross, K.D.	Nova Scotia	Winnipeg	1917	1919–26		
Reed, Mrs. F.J.	Ontario	Hamilton	1917	1920–?	24	Nee A.H. Male
Harris, Irene	Manitoba	Winnipeg	1919	1921–45	14	
Bedford, Grace	Manitoba	Winnipeg	1920	1921–35	8	
Sallery, Mrs. C.M.	Minnesota	Michigan		1921–29	24	Nee Gladys I. Taylor
Tallman, Alma	Ontario?	Detroit	1919	1921–45	5	
Imasen, Velma C.	Ontario	Vancouver	1921	1922–27	1	
Innis, Hattie B.				1924–25	6	
Taylor, Lana E.	Ontario	Bowmanville, ON	1918	1925–31	8	
Nicholls, P.B.	Ontario	Brandon	1925	1926–34	9	
Williams, Mrs. T.H. 2nd		Winnipeg		1926–35	24	Nee K.R. McKellar
Kilborn, Cora	Ontario?	Toronto General Hospital	1923	1926–50		Mishkid; Mrs. B. Cannell

Name	Birthplace	Graduation place	Year of graduation	Dates as nurse WCM	# of years at WCM	Notes, including married names
Crawley, Mary E.	England	Montreal		1929–42	13	
Allen, Mrs. A.S.	Nova Scotia	Cambridge [UK?]		1929–?		Nee Winnifred Griffin
Macleod, Marguerite	England	Montreal		1930–39	9	
Stanway, Mrs. F.R.	BC?	Vancouver		1931–?		Nee Elizabeth Higham
McIntosh, Janet M.	Ontario	Toronto	1931	1931–37	6	
Hoffman, Mrs. C.M.	England	Brandon and Moose Jaw		1932–?		Nee Jennie M. Scanlon
Dunkin, Hilda				1932–38	6	
Hinton, Lillian	England	St John's, Toronto		1933–36	3	Resigned: ill health
Owen, Mrs. A.E.	Manitoba	Winnipeg		1935–41	6	Nee Mary Vickers
Williams Mrs. T.H. 3rd	BC?	Toronto		1937–45 (r)	8	Nee M.E. Neil
Outerbridge, Mrs. R.E.	China	Toronto	193?	1938–45	7	Nee Mary E. Kergin
Boyd, Dorothy M.	China	Toronto	1929	1939–41	2	Born in Henan; from Henan (NCM)
Fox, Dorothy E.J.	Montreal	Montreal		1939–43	4	Later Canada
Lee, Margaret E.	Toronto	Vancouver		1939–44	5	Mrs. L. Lu
Gay, Margaret	Manitoba			1940–41	1	From Henan (NCM)
Preston, Clara	China	Toronto	1940	1940–43	3	From Henan (NCM)
Burwell, Eleanor E.				1944	1	Born in Zhengzhou, Henan
Julien, Bessie				1946–47	1	Mrs. A. Dayfoot
Alexander, Marjorie				1947–50	3	
Taylor, Lillian				1947–50	3	Later Angola
Turner, Helen				1947	0	Transferred to Henan (NCM); Mrs. P. Nelson
Miller, Isabelle E.				1948–52	4	Later Canada and Hong Kong

Appendix 2

PUMC Nursing Faculty, 1917–49

Year started	Year left	Number of years on faculty	Surname	Given Name	Additional information
1917	1923	6	Pai	Hsui-lan	
1918	1929	11	Ingram	Ruth	Superintendent of nurses, 1925–28; dean, 1925–29
1919	1920	1	Brown	Florence	
1919	1924	5	Beaty	Mary Louise	
1919	1924	5	Caulfield	Kathleen	
1919	1923	4	Goodman	Florence K.	
1919	1922	3	Lo	Yu-lin	Also 1929, 1949
1919	1924	5	McCoy	Mary	
1919	1922	3	Packer	Sophie	
1919	1920	1	Schaur	Martha	
1919	1922	3	Sutton	Bertha L.	
1919	1929	10	Sweet	Lula	
1919	1925	6	Wolf	Anna Dryden	Superintendent of nurses, 1919–25; dean, 1924–25
1920	1923	3	Abbott	Lucy	
1920	1922	2	Goforth	Helen R.	
1920	1921	1	Grayson	Mary L.	
1920	1921	1	Hall	Francis S.	
1920	1926	6	Harrell	Virginia	
1920	1921	1	Holland	Helen M.	Hospital anaesthetist, 1921–40
1920	1923	3	Jacobus	Dorothy	
1920	1924	4	Mooney	Winifred	
1920	1929	9	Purcell	Mary S.	Superintendent of nurses, 1928–29
1920	1942	22	Robinson	Ethel E.	
1920	1922	2	Rogers	Grace	
1920	1924	4	Sze	Li-sing (Elizabeth)	
1920	1921	1+	Tom	Mabel E.	Hospital admitting officer, 1921–32

Year started	Year left	Number of years on faculty	Surname	Given Name	Additional information
1920	1942	18	Whiteside	Faye	Superintendent of nurses, 1938–42
1921	1924	3	Banfield	Gertrude S.	
1921	1928	7	Dalrymple	Lila M.	Also 1933
1921	1922	1	Hackett	Elise M.	
1921	1938	17	Jen	Hsing-kuo	
1921	1925	4	Mooney	Mabel	
1921	1924	3	Moy-Orne	Pearl	
1922	1941	19	MacAlpine	Edith I.	
1922	1926	4	McIvor	Helen	
1922	1923	1	Moo	Mary Priscilla	
1922	1925	3	Tai	Zing-ling	
1923	1931	8	Chiu	Ding Ying	
1923	1928	5	Colver	Amanda	
1923	1927	4	Filandino	Elvira	
1923	1928	5	Godard	Winifred	
1923	1926	3	Loh	Anna	
1923	1925	2	Mitchell	Esther	
1923	1927	4	Rinell	Edith	
1923	1925	2	Rinell	Margaret	
1924	1926	2	Bray	Linda	
1924	1928	4	Downs	Ida M.	
1924	1927	3	Griswold	Laura	
1924	1928	4	Holland	Gladys Lemon	
1924	1938	14	Hao	Yu-hwa	
1924	1928	4	King	Lucile	
1925	1927	2	Dilworth	Jessie	
1925	1927	2	Josselyn	Marjorie	
1925	1930	5	Latimer	Helen F.	
1925	1930	5	Wang	Ia-fang (Hilda)	PUMC grad, 1925
1925	1932	7	Waung	E-tsung (Elsie)	PUMC grad, 1925
1925	1934	9	Yu	Kheng-eng (Kathleen)	PUMC grad, 1925
1926	1932	8	Chu	Pi-hui/Bi-hui (Bernice)	PUMC grad, 1926
1926	1929	3	Schott	Mary B.	
1926	1933	7	Tien	Tsai-lee (Ravenna)	PUMC grad, 1926
1927	1938	11	Kuo	Jung-hsun	
1927	1952	25	Nieh	Yuchan (Vera)	PUMC grad, 1927 Dean, 1940–52
1927	1942	15	Shao	Kuei-ying	Also 1948
1928	1937	8	Hirst	Elizabeth R.	
1928	1932	4	McCabe	Anne	
1928	1933	5	McCormick	Mildred	
1928	1930	2	Muller	Louise M.	

Year started	Year left	Number of years on faculty	Surname	Given Name	Additional information
1928	1929	1	Norelius	Jessie	
1928	1933	5	Sun	Tuan	PUMC grad, 1928
1928	1931	3	Taylor	Erma B.	Acting dean, 1929–30
1928	1942	14	Wyne	Margaret M.	Interned; repatriated to USA, 1943
1929	1932	3	Gorey	Margaret M.	
1929	1935	6	Hsu	Ai-Chu	PUMC grad, 1930
1929	1935	6	Hsueh	Yi	PUMC grad, 1929
1929	1942	13	Lo	Yu-lin	
1929	1935	6	Pao	Ai-ching	PUMC grad, 1929
1930	1936	6	Beaumont	Doris	
1930	1931	1	Chou (Zhou)	Meiyu	PUMC grad, 1930
1930	1934	4	Ellis	Ruth	
1930	1940	10	Hodgman	Gertrude E.	Dean, 1930–40; Superintendent of nurses, 1930–38
1930	1932	2	Holes	Clara A.	
1930	1933	3	Hu	Tun-wu	PUMC grad, 1930
1930	1940	10	Hsieh	Louise Tuttle	
1930	1938	8	Kunkel	Ruth H.	
1930	1939	9	Leach	Glyde M.	
1930	1931	1	Lurton	Corinne G.	
1930	1934	4	Stiles	Katherine L.	
1930	1936	6	Sun	Chin-feng	PUMC grad, 1930
1931	1933	2	Moylan	Mary B.	
1931	1933	2	Polanska	Zenaida	
1931	1935	4	Ch'en	Ch'i	PUMC grad, 1931 Also 1939, 1947
1931	1934	3	Ritchie	Mary A.	
1931	1946	15	Sia	Yun-hua (Mary)	PUMC grad, 1931
1932	1934	2	Parson	Maude	
1932	1936	4	Sheh	Yun-chu	PUMC grad, 1931
1932	1936	4	Sung	Pao-ti	PUMC grad, 1931
1932	1936	4	Tennent	Cornelia	
1932	1948	14+	Wang	Loh-loh (Wang Yi)	PUMC grad, 1932
1932	1939	7	Wong	Chien-chen (Margaret)	PUMC grad, 1932
1933	1938	5	Dalrymple	Lila M.	Also 1921
1933	1935	2	Wang	Su-yun	
1933	1940	7	Hsu	Yu-yung	PUMC grad, 1933
1934	1936	2+	Chen	Chun-hua	PUMC grad, 1934 Also 1949
1934	1937	3	Last	Ruth M.	
1934	1942	8	Lo	Kuei-chen	

Year started	Year left	Number of years on faculty	Surname	Given Name	Additional information
1934	1937	3	Wagner	Belle	
1934	1939	5	Zia	Ruth V.M.	PUMC grad, 1934
1935	1942	7	Chien	Chieh-hua	
1935	1942	9	Liu	Chieh-lan (Belle)	PUMC grad, 1934 Also 1948
1935	1938	3	Moser	Elizabeth	
1935	1936	1	Tao	Han-yen	PUMC grad, 1935
1936	1939	3	Blake	Florence	
1936	1942	6	Sia	Ming-be	PUMC grad, 1936
1937	1942	5	Liu	Chih-chen	PUMC grad, 1936
1937	1942	5	Liu	Ching-ho	PUMC grad, 1936
1937	1942	5+	Lo	Kuei-chen	PUMC grad, 1934 Also 1947
1937	1941	4	Uspensky	Margaret	PUMC grad, 1937 Also 1947
1937	?	?	Wang	Hsiu-ying	PUMC grad, 1936
1938	1942	4	Chen	Lu-teh	PUMC grad, 1937
1938	1940	2	Petchner	Miriam	
1938	1941	3+	Ts'ai	Heng-fang	PUMC Grad 1938 Also 1947
1939	1941	a/a	Chen	Ch'i	Also 1931, 1947
1939	1942	3	Ch'en	Shih-feng	PUMC Grad 1938
1940	1942	2	Chiang	Tsun-chun (Florence)	PUMC Grad 1934
1940	1942	2+	Wang	Mei-ying	Also 1946
1943	1947	a/a	Wang	Loh-loh	Also 1932, 1948
1946	?	?	Hsu	Yu-jung	Also 1933
1946	?	?	Wang	Mei-ying	Also 1940
1947	1949	a/a	Chen	Ch'i	Also 1931, 1939
1947	1949	2	Li	Mei-li	
1947	?	?	Lo	Kuei-chen	Also 1937
1947	?	?	Shen	Ch'ang-hui	
1947	?	?	Ts'ai	Heng-fang	Also 1938
1947	?	?	Uspensky	Margaret	Also 1937
1948	?	?	Huang	Wu-ch'ing	
1948	1949	1	Li	Han-ch'iang	
1948	?	?	Li	Yi-hsiu	
1948	1950	2	Liu	Chieh-lan (Belle)	Also 1935
1948	?	?	Lu	Pao-ch'i	
1948	?	?	Shao	Kuei-ying	Also 1927, possibly 1941
1948	?	?	Wang	Loh-loh	Also 1932, 1943
1949	?	?	Chen	Chun-hua	Also 1934
1949	?	?	Chen	Shu-chieh	
1949	?	?	Lo	Yu-lin	Also 1919, 1929
1949	?	?	Wang	Yi	

Appendix 3

List of Interned Nurses in China

	Name	Age	Nationality	Occupation	Professional or family affiliation	Dates in camp	Taken from	Event/destination on release
Ash Camp								
1	Back, Doris Hilda	35	British	Missionary nurse	Society for the Propagation of the Gospel	Apr. 43–Aug. 45		
2	Campbell, Amy Isabel	35	Canadian	Nurse	SM Nursing Service	Apr.–Sep. 43		Repatriated to Canada
3	Craine, Christian	50	British	Nurse		Apr. 43–Aug. 45		
4	Hayes, Anna Mary (Sr Constance)	61	American	Catholic nursing nun	American Church Mission, Wuhu	Jul. 43–Aug. 45		
5	Lewis, Georgina	38	Canadian	Married missionary nurse	Former UCC missionary nurse	Apr. 43–Aug. 45	Taiyuan	
6	Martin, Wilhelmina	35	British	Nurse	Shanghai General Hospital Xray dept	Apr. 43–Aug. 45		
7	Miles, Elizabeth Mary	42	British	Nurse	SMC[1] Isolation Hospital	Apr. 43–Aug. 45		
8	Parlane, Katherine Beatrice	60	British	Nursing sister	SMC Public Health Dept. Hospital Division	Apr. 43		Move Mot Lunghwa
9	Scott, Isabella Boyd	56	British	Hospital matron	SMC Public Health Dept. Hospital Division	Apr. 43–Aug. 45		

Name	Age	Nationality	Occupation	Professional or family affiliation	Dates in camp	Taken from	Event/destination on release
10 Scott, Marion Gibson Wallace	53	British	Hospital matron	SMC Public Health Dept. Hospital Division	Apr. 43–Aug. 45		

Canton Camp

Name	Age	Nationality	Occupation	Professional or family affiliation	Dates in camp	Taken from	Event/destination on release
11 Bischoff, Mary Wentz	n/a	American	Missionary nurse	Hackett Medical College	Feb.–Sep. 43	Canton	Repatriated to USA

Chapei Camp

Name	Age	Nationality	Occupation	Professional or family affiliation	Dates in camp	Taken from	Event/destination on release
12 Allen, Alice E.	67	American	Nurse		Mar. 43–Aug. 45		
13 Inch, Gladys Mabel	45	British	Nurse	Daughter of J.E. Inch	Sep. 43–Aug. 45	Yangchow A	Moved 1 AU 45 to Lincoln Ave
14 Jackson, Florence Mary	35	British	Nursing sister	Wife of Thomas Jackson	Mar. 43–Aug. 45		
14 Jorden, Ella Priscella	36	British	Missionary nurse	Methodist Missionary Society	Apr. 43–Aug. 45		
15 Lee, Ruth Irene	35	American	Nurse	Church by the Side of the Road	Mar.–Sep. 43		Repatriated to USA
16 Light, Constance Emily	29	British	Nurse	Wife of A.B. Light (birthed a son in camp)	Mar. 43–Aug. 45		
17 Nichols, Jessie Flech	42	American	Registered nurse		Mar.–Sep. 43		Repatriated to USA
18 Pollock, Elizabeth Morrison	46	American	Missionary nurse	Margaret Williamson Hospital	Mar.–Sep. 43		Repatriated to USA
19 Robinson, Ethel Estey	60	Canadian	Nurse		Mar.–Sep. 43		Repatriated to USA
20 Turner, Marie Yvonne	30	Canadian	Nurse	Wife of William G. Turner (police)	Apr. 43–Aug. 45		Repatriated to Canada

21	Worden, Leonie Liston	41	American	Nurse	Common law wife of T.G. Worden (physician)	Mar. 43–Aug. 45		Moved 1 AU 45 to Lincoln Ave
22	Wyne, Margaret R.	57	American	Nurse	Peking Union Medical College	Mar.–Sep. 43	Peking	Repatriated to USA

Great Western Road Camp

| 23 | Harris, Willie Pauline | 46 | American | Missionary nurse | American Baptist Foreign Missionary Society | Mar.–Sep. 43 | NIngpo | Repatriated to USA |

Lincoln Avenue Camp

24	Fletcher, Lilian Emma	43	Australian	Missionary nurse	China Inland Mission	Jun. 44–Aug. 45	Langchung	
25	Gedye, Nancy Marion	31	British	Missionary nurse	Methodist Missionary Society	Jun. 44–Aug. 45	Lunghwa	
*	Inch, Gladys Mabel	45	British	Nurse	Daughter of J.E. Inch	Jun. 44–Aug. 45	Chapei	
26	Kench, Elizabeth	48	British	Nurse	Wife of O.K. Kench	Jun. 44–Aug. 45	Country San	
27	Livessey, Lucy	56	British	Nurse		Aug. 44–Aug. 45	Country San	Died 27 Sep 44
28	Smith, Annie Gerhard S.	50	British	Missionary nurse	London Missionary Society Lester Chinese Hospital	Aug. 44–Aug. 45	Lunghwa	
29	Wilson, Helen Dickie	58	British	Nurse	Church of Scotland Mission	Jun. 44–Aug. 45	Ichang	
*	Worden, Leonie Liston	41	American	Nurse	Common law wife of T.G. Worden	Aug. 45	Chapei	

Name	Age	Nationality	Occupation	Professional or family affiliation	Dates in camp	Taken from	Event/destination on release
Lunghwa Camp							
30 Burgess, Myrtie Landon	50	Canadian	Nurse	Wife of J.C. Burgess	Apr.–Sep. 43		Repatriated to Canada
* Gedye, Nancy Marion	31	British	Missionary nurse	Methodist Missionary Society	Mar. 43–Jun. 44	Hankow	Moved to Lincoln Ave.
31 Martin, Mabel	62	British	Missionary nurse	London Missionary Society	Mar. 43–Aug. 45	Hankow	
32 Ozorio, Nadia Spencer	37	British	Nurse	Imperial Chemical Industries	Mar. 43–Jan. 44		Moved to Weihsien
33 Parker, Gladys Dorothy Spencer	44	British	Missionary nurse	London Missionary Society Lester Hospital	Mar. 43–Aug. 45		
* Parlane, Katherine Beatrice	60	British	Nursing sister	SMC Public Health Dept. Hospital Division	Aug. 45	Ash Camp	
34 Pearce, Valentia	34	British	Nurse	Wife of M. Pearce	Mar. 43–Aug. 45		
35 Ranson, Emily Elizabeth	45	British	Nurse anaesthesia	Wife of R.T. Ranson (physician)	Apr. 43–Aug. 45		
36 Rasey, Rose Sarah	49	Australian	Missionary nurse	China Inland Mission	Apr. 43–Aug. 45	Shunteh	
37 Rossiter, Emily Annie	63	British	Nurse	Baptist Missionary Society	Aug. 45	Ash Camp	
38 Stibee, Nina	47	British	Nurse		Jun. 43–Aug. 45		
39 Webb, May Lillian	41	British	Nurse	Church Missionary Society	Mar. 43–Aug. 45	Hangchow	
40 Williams, Nellie	44	Canadian	Nurse	Country Hospital	Apr. 43–Aug. 45		Repatriated to Canada
41 Wilson, Gladys Mary	45	Canadian	Nurse	Country Hospital	Apr. 43–Aug. 45		

Pootung Camp

#	Name	Age	Nationality	Occupation	Society / Notes	Dates	Camp	Moved
42	Davis, Sophia Vasiliena	53	British	Nurse		Mar. 43–Aug. 45	Yangchow A	Moved to Shanghai
43	Foster, Alice Mary	41	British	Nurse		Sep. 43–Aug. 45	Yangchow A	
44	Gale, Elizabeth Durie	33	British	Married missionary nurse	Former UCC missionary nurse	Sep. 43–Aug. 45	Yangchow B	
45	Gillison, Jean Brotch	44	British	Nurse	Sister of Dr G.H. Gillison	Sep. 43–Aug. 45	Yangchow B	
46	McIlroy, Hilda Elizabeth	37	Canadian	Missionary nurse	Church Missionary Society	Sep. 43–Aug. 45	Yangchow A	
47	Roberts, Lilian Grace	60	British	Missionary nurse	Society for the Propagation of the Gospel	Sep. 43–Aug. 45	Yangchow B	

Weihsien Camp

#	Name	Age	Nationality	Occupation	Society / Notes	Dates	Camp	Moved
48	Abbiss, Clara	41	British	Missionary nurse	Society for the Propagation of the Gospel	Nov. 43–Aug. 45	Hokien	
49	Alderson, Mary Marjory (Sr Julia)	41	British	Catholic nursing sister	St Francis of Assisi order	Mar. 43–Aug. 45	Tsinan	Moved to Peking Res.
50	Ball, Mary	50	S. African	Missionary nurse	Society for the Propagation of the Gospel	Mar. 43–Aug. 45	Tatung	
51	Beckman, Anna (Sr M Agnes)	43	American	Catholic nursing sister	Sisters St Francis Hospital	Mar.–Aug. 43	Tsinan	Moved to Peking Res.
52	Borghaus, Timothea	54	Dutch	Catholic nursing sister	Little Sisters of St Joseph	Mar.–Aug. 43	Luan	Moved to Peking Res.

	Name	Age	Nationality	Occupation	Professional or family affiliation	Dates in camp	Taken from	Event/destination on release
53	Bouckaert, Liberta.	41	Belgian	Catholic nursing sister	St Augustin St Pauls Hospital	Mar.–Aug. 43	Suiyuan	Moved to Peking Res.
54	Braspenning, Electa	42	Dutch	Catholic nursing sister	Little Sisters of St Joseph	Mar.–Aug. 43	Luan	Moved to Peking Res.
55	Braspenning, Wigarda	49	Dutch	Catholic nursing sister	Little Sisters of St Joseph	Mar.–Aug. 43	Luan	Moved to Peking Res.
56	Buchan, Anne Gray	49	British	Missionary nurse	London Missionary Society Mackenzie Hospital	Jul. 44–Aug. 45	Peking Emb	
57	Chan, May L.	43	Canadian	Nurse	Wife of G.H. Chan	Mar. 43–Aug. 45	Iltis Hydro	
58	Clements, Winifred Valentina	41	British	Nurse	Married W.B. Chilton in camp 10 Apr 44	Mar. 43–Aug. 45	Tongshan	
59	Danielsen, Inger W.	33	Norwegian	Missionary nurse	China Inland Mission	Mar. 43–Aug. 45	Iltis Hydro	
60	Declerq, Eudoxie	45	Belgian	Catholic nursing sister	St Augustin St Paul's Hospital	Mar.–Aug. 43	Suiyuan	Moved to Peking Res.
61	D'Houdt, Arnoldina	39	Belgian	Catholic nursing sister	St Augustin St Paul's Hospital	Mar.–Aug. 43	Suiyuan	Moved to Peking Res.
62	Fereman, Milburga	58	Dutch	Catholic nursing sister	Little Sisters of St Joseph	Mar.–Aug. 43	Sin Chang	Moved to Peking Res.
63	Friberg, Johanna Margaret	32	American	Missionary nurse	Augustana Synod Mission	Mar.–Sep. 43	Peking	Repatriated to USA
64	Gowland, S Louise G.	51	British	Nurse	Victoria Hospital Tientsin	Mar. 43–Aug. 45	Tientsin	
65	Griese, Maria (Sr Timothea)	58	American	Catholic nursing sister	Hospital Sisters of St Francis	Mar.–Aug. 43	Tsinan	Moved to Peking Res.

No.	Name	Age	Nationality	Role	Organization	Dates	Location	Fate
66	Hill-Murray, Grace Margaret	52	British	Senior staff nurse	Kailan Mining Admin	Mar. 43–Aug. 45	Tongshan Hospital	Repatriated to USA
67	Hirst, Elizabeth	53	American	Nurse	Peking Union Medical College	Mar.–Sep. 43	Peking	Repatriated to USA
68	Hochland, Flora	40	Dutch	Catholic nursing sister	Little Sisters of St Joseph	Mar.–Aug. 43	Sin Hang	Moved to Peking Res.
69	Hoffman, Ida (Sr M. Fridoline)	40	American	Catholic nursing sister	Hospital Sisters St Francis	Mar.–Aug. 43	Tsinan	Moved to Peking Res.
70	Kelsey, Susie		Canadian	Missionary nurse	Anglican Church	Apr 43?–Sep. 43		Repatriated to Canada
71	Kemball, Vera Flora	39	British	Nurse	Kailin Mining Admin	Mar. 43–Aug. 45	Tientsin	
72	Kunkel, Ruth H.	49	American	Nurse		Mar.–Aug. 43	Peking	Repatriated to?
73	Labeeuw, Flaviana	42	Belgian	Catholic nursing sister	St Augustins St Paul's Hospital	Mar.–Aug. 43	Siuyuan	Moved to Peking Res.
74	Labonte, Marie F. (Sr Mary Elaine)	36	American	Catholic nursing sister	St Francis of Assisi order	Mar.–Sep. 43	Tsinan	Repatriated to USA
75	Lovatt, Ethel Eileen	34	American	Nurse		Mar.–Sep. 43	Peking	Repatriated to USA
76	Luetkemeier, Anna (Sr Albertina)	57	American	Catholic nursing sister	Hospital Sisters St Francis	Mar.–Aug. 43	Tsinan	Moved to Peking Res.
77	Malycheff, Elena M.	52	Australian	Nurse		Mar. 43–Aug. 45	Tientsin	
78	Mann, May Caroline	26	British	Nurse Chefoo School	China Inland Mission	Mar. 43–Aug. 45	Chefoo	
79	McMillan, Elizabeth	53	British	Nurse	Peking Union Medical College	Mar. 43–Aug. 45	Peking	
80	Meer, Joseph	51	Dutch	Catholic nursing sister	Little Sisters of St Joseph	Mar.–Aug. 43	Sin Chang	Moved to Peking Res.

Name	Age	Nationality	Occupation	Professional or family affiliation	Dates in camp	Taken from	Event/destination on release
81 Mehl, Barbara (Sr Damascene)	43	American	Catholic nursing sister	Hospital Sisters St Francis	Mar.–Aug. 43	Tsinan	Moved to Peking Res.
82 Model, Miriam	43	British	Nurse		Mar. 43–Aug. 45	Tientsin	
83 Naeyeart, Cornelia	48	Belgian	Catholic nursing sister	St Augustins St Pauls Hospital	Mar.–Aug. 43	Suiyuan	Moved to Peking Res.
84 Ouwerkerk, Alexandra K.	46	Russian	Nurse	Wife of LCM Ouwerkerk	Mar. 43–Aug. 45	Tientsin	
* Ozorio, Nadia Spencer	37	British	Nurse	Imperial Chemical Industries	Feb. 44–Aug. 45	Lunghwa	
85 Pessina, Catherine (Sr M. Edward)	39	American	Catholic nursing sister	St Francis of Holy Family order			Moved
86 Quelch, Dorothy Tillie	56	British	Nurse		Mar. 43–Aug. 45	Chefoo	
87 Smith, Mary Janet	50	British	Nurse	Wife of D.H. Smith	Mar. 43–Aug. 45	Tientsin	
88 Stanley, Mary Boyd	31	Canadian	Married missionary nurse	Former UCC missionary nurse	Mar. 43–Aug. 45	Peking	
89 Stepanek, Marie (Sr Vitalia)	59	American	Catholic nursing sister	Hospital Sisters of St Francis	Mar. 43–Aug. 43	Tsinan	Moved to Peking Res.
90 Stickland, Gladys Mary	39	British	Nurse	London Missionary Society	Mar. 43–?	Tientsin	
91 Stienlet, Clemencia	43	Belgian	Catholic nursing sister	St Augustins St Paul's Hospital	Mar.–Aug. 43	Suiyuan	Moved to Peking Res.
92 Van Eisel, Viro	44	Dutch	Catholic nursing sister	Little Sisters of St Joseph	Mar.–Aug. 43	Sin Hang	Moved to Peking Res.

No.	Name	Age	Nationality	Role	Affiliation	Dates	Location	Movement
93	Whiteside, Faye	57	American	Nurse	Peking Union Medical College	Mar.–Sep. 43	Peking	Repatriated to USA
94	Wormann, Sophie (Sr M Otmara)	55	American	Catholic nursing sister	Hospital Sisters St Francis	Mar.–Sep. 43	Tsinan	Moved to Peking Res.

Yangchow A

No.	Name	Age	Nationality	Role	Affiliation	Dates	Location	Movement
95	Davis, Sophia Vasiliena	53	British	Nurse		Mar.–Sep. 43		Moved to Pootung
96	Edgar, Lillian	44	British	Nurse	Wife of J. Edgar	Mar.–Sep. 43		Moved to Pootung
97	Foster, Alice Mary	41	British	Nurse		Mar. 43–?	Yangchow B	Moved to Pootung
*	Inch, Gladys Mabel	45	British	Nurse	Daughter of J.E. Inch	Mar.–Sep. 43		Moved to Chapel
*	McIlroy, Hilda Elizabeth	37	Canadian	Missionary nurse	Church Missionary Society		Yangchow B	Moved to Pootung

Yangchow B

No.	Name	Age	Nationality	Role	Affiliation	Dates	Location	Movement
*	Foster, Alice Mary	41	British	Nurse		Mar. 43–?		Moved to Yangchow A
*	Gillison, Jean Brotch	44	British	Nurse	Sister of Dr G.H. Gillison	Mar.–Sep. 43		Moved to Pootung
98	Holmes, Hilda Mabel	45	British	Missionary nurse		Mar.–Sep. 43		Moved to Yangchow C
99	Holmes, Victoria Alice	44	British	Missionary nurse		Mar.–Sep. 43		Moved to Yangchow C
*	McIlroy, Hilda Elizabeth	37	Canadian	Missionary nurse	Church Missionary Society		Hankow	Moved to Yangchow A

Name	Age	Nationality	Occupation	Professional or family affiliation	Dates in camp	Taken from	Event/destination on release
Yangchow C							
100 Bunn, Winifred May	55	British	Missionary nurse	China Inland Mission	Mar. 43–Aug. 45		
101 Jagger, Amy	33	British	Missionary nurse	Baptist Missionary Society	Mar. 43–Aug. 45		
102 Shepherd, Hilda Esther	35	British	Missionary nurse	Methodist Missionary Society	Mar. 43–Aug. 45		
Yu Yuen Road							
103 Elders, Lily	33	British	Nurse	Wife of T. Elders (police)	Feb. 43–Apr. 45		Moved to Yangtzepoo
104 Hillhouse, Myfanwy	41	British	Nurse	Wife of J.Y. Hillhouse (police)	Feb. 43–Apr. 45		Moved to Yangtzepoo

* Listed more than once because of movement between camps

1 SMC: Possibly Shenyang Medical College.

Appendix 4

PUMC Nursing Graduates, 1924–39

Grad year	Name	Credential	Married names/Notes
1924	Tseng Hsien-tsang	CMB[1]	Mrs. Y.L. Ta
1925	Kong Kwai-laan	BA	Mrs. Y.L. Mei
	Perkins, Sara		
	Wang Ia-fang		Mrs. S.H. Liu
	Yu Kheng-eng	CMB	
1926	Chu Pi-hui		Mrs. H.I. Chen
	Lindberg, Svea A.		(Deceased 1931)
	Lin Sz-sing	CMB	
	Sinhanetra, Civili		
	Tien Tsai-lee	BS	
1927	Chao Hwei-ming		Mrs. K.I. Chung
	Cheo Chia-ih		
	Liu Su-chun		Mrs. Y.L. Cheng
	Nieh Yu-chan	MS	
1928	Chou Ssu-hsien		Mrs. C.M. Meng
	Liu Hsiao-tsent	CMB	Mrs. H. Chen
	Sun Tuan	BS	Mrs. C. Fan
1929	Chang Fei-cheng	CMB	
	Hsueh Yi	BS	Mrs. Y.E. Hsiao
	Pao Ai-ching		
	Shih Hung-yueh	BA, CMB	
	Tao Hui		Mrs. K.C. Wang
1930	Chao Nai-hsien		Mrs. T.H. Chang
	Chou Meiyu		
	Chu Mo-his		Mrs. F.S. Tsang
	Hsu Ai-Chu		
	Hu Tun-wu	MS	Mrs. Chen

Grad year	Name	Credential	Married names/Notes
	Huang Yu-kun		Mrs. Y.W. Frank
	Kuan Chung-hua		Mrs. S.E. Pai
	Kuan Pao-chen	CMB	Mrs. P.H. Li
	Sun Ching-feng	MA	(Deceased 1936)
1931	Chen Chi		
	Chu Chih-hao		Mrs. P.C. Ho
	Lao Yueh-chin		Mrs. S.F. Chung
	Sheh Yun-chu	BS	
	Sia Yun-hua	MA	
	Sung Pai-ti		Mrs. J.P. Li
	Wang Hsui-ying	MA	
1932	Chang Fang-hsiu	BS	
	Chu Shu-yu		
	Kuei Yu-the		
	Kung Ti-chen		
	Su Shu-yuan		
	Wang Loh Loh		
	Wang Chien-chen	BA	Mrs. F.T. Sung
	Wu Shun-chang		
1933	Chiang Chao-ai	BS	Mrs. I.B. Liong
	Hsu Yu-jung		Mrs. K.H. LI
	Li Hsueh-feng		
	Shih Mei-ying		Mrs. M. Cheng
1934	Chao Jung-en	BS	Mrs. H.C. Li
	Chen Chun-hua		
	Chiang Tsun-chun	BS	Mrs. C. Szuto
	Kuo Pei-cheng	BS	
	Lewis, Anna Mae	BA	Mrs. R.H.
	Liu Chieh-lan	BS	Mrs. C.L. Hsu
	Lo Kuei-chen	BS	
	Lu Chi-ying	BS	Mrs. W.P. Lei
	Wei Wen-chen	BS	Mrs. C.Y. Shih
	Zia, Ruth, VM	BS	Mrs. L.K. Hsu
1935	Chang Hsiu-chen	BS	Mrs. H.S. Fan
	Chen Liang-chiung	BA	
	Chu Lien-ching		Mrs. Y.K. Ko
	Hsiung Ai-hua		Mrs. G. Chao

Grad year	Name	Credential	Married names/Notes
	Li Chi-t.e.h.	BS	
	Li Huai-chin		Mrs. W.L. Chia
	Li Kuei-chen	BS	Mrs. H.F. Wu
	Pan Chin	BS	Mrs. T.M. Chang
	Tsao Hui-chen	BS	Mrs. H.A. Hsu
	Tso Han-yen	BA	
	Wang Su-chin	BS	Mrs. T.W. Chou
	Wang Su-jen		Mrs. Y.H. Hsu
1936	Chan Pao-chiu	BS	
	Chen Liang-you	BA	
	Chen Ti-yun		
	Chao Miao-lling	BS	
	Ho Chu-hsuau	BS	
	Huang Min-shan	BS	
	Li Shun-sheng		
	Liu Chih-chen	BS	Mrs. C.C. Tan
	Liu Ching-ho	BS	
	Sia Ming-be	BA	
	Wang Hui yin		
	Ying His-uing		Mrs. W.Y. Yu
1937	Chang Yn-fei	BS	
	Chen Jen-chien	BS	
	Chen Yu-the	BS	
	Chin Yuan-mei	BS	
	Chuan Ju-yu		
	Chu Jui-lin	BS	
	Ho Pei-fen		
	Ngai Shih-hua		
	Tuan Yung-chen		
	Uspensky, Margaret		
	Wen Lu-hsin	BS	Mrs. George Ouyang
	Yu Tao-chen	BS	
1938	Chang Tsai-yu		
	Chen Shih-feng		
	Chen Yu-wen		
	Cheng Yuan-hua	BA	
	Chu Pai-tien	BS	

Grad year	Name	Credential	Married names/Notes
	Fei Chao-yun		
	Huang The-hsing	BS	
	Ku Hsui-ling		
	Kuo Huan-wei	BS	Mrs. S.C. Wang
	Liu Pu-sheng	BS	
	Lu Hui-ching	BS	
	Lu Mei-yin		Mrs. S.C. Tang
	Tsai Heng-fang		
	Wy Yi-sheng	BS	
	Tsao Ching-hua		
1939	Chen Shao-chun	BS	
	Cheng Loh-the	BS	
	Fang Wen-pei		
	Huang, Pao-chu		
	Jen Chin-chih		
	Ku Tsai-kuang		
	Yang Yufeng	BS	Mrs. W.P. Wang

1 It is not clear what a CMB credential is. It might be a China Medical Board certificate.

Notes

Introduction | NURSING, SHIFTED

1 The missions that were part of this "union" were the General Board of Missions of the Methodist Church of Canada (Canada), the American Baptist Foreign Mission Society (United States), the Board of Missions of the Methodist Episcopal Church (United States), and the Friends Foreign Mission Association (Great Britain, Ireland).

2 Although arson was never definitely established, most medical and nursing personnel believed it was the work of Chinese who were collaborating with the Japanese.

3 The Canadian West China Mission had six nurses' training schools in Sichuan – at Chengdu (2), Rongxian, Zigong, Chongqing, and Fuzhou.

4 It is not clear whether there were any other high-grade nursing schools in China. From all of the evidence I have reviewed, it appears that the PUMC was the only one.

5 Charles Hodge Corbett, 1955. In Margaret Brown, *History of the Honan (North China) Mission of the United Church of Canada, Originally a Mission of the Presbyterian Church in Canada* (Unpublished manuscript, n.d.). Volume 4, Chapter 99, page 2.

6 According to Vera Nieh, her brother was killed by Guomindang (Chinese Nationalist Party) soldiers. Current PUMC faculty have told me that her brother was killed accidentally, by "friendly fire."

7 In 2005, when I completed a PhD at the University of Alberta, it was rare for universities to have active partnerships with China. Fifteen years later, it is rare to find a Canadian university without some connection to China. In 2004, for example, the University of Toronto initiated Green Path, an admissions pathway to support undergraduate Chinese students, who now number over 4,000; in 2005, the Alberta government gave a $35 million endowment to the University of Alberta's China Institute to, in part, promote linkages between that university and Chinese universities; in 2010, McMaster University signed an agreement with the China Scholarship Council to attract more doctoral students from China; in 2016, the University of British Columbia had ninety-five active agreements with fifty-two universities in China. Canada's interest in China today is as active as it was at the peak of the

missionary movement a century ago, when Canadian missionaries started nursing schools in Henan and Sichuan – and when the Rockefeller Foundation started China's most elite school of nursing at the Peking Union Medical College in Beijing, in 1920. Between completion and publication of this book, the world has been plunged into a global pandemic. COVID-19 has paralysed the movement of international students. At the time of this writing, the future of international educational partnerships is uncertain.

8 Xi Gao, "Chinese Perspectives on Medical Missionaries in the 19th Century: The Chinese Medical Missionary Journal," *Journal of Cultural Interaction in East Asia* 5 (2014): 97–118.

9 Jun Lu, Sonya Grypma, Yingjuan Cao, Lijuan Bu, Lin Shen, and Patricia Davidson, "Historically-Informed Nursing: A Transnational Case Study in China," *Nursing Inquiry* 25, 1 (2017).

10 This statement refers mostly to nursing education as introduced by missionary and other Western nurses in the early twentieth century in China. It does not include the establishment, for example, of army nursing or field nursing, and does not reflect myriad ways that nursing care was taught and practised less formally, especially during wartime.

11 Lu et al., "Historically-Informed Nursing," 3.

12 Sonya Grypma, *Healing Henan: Canadian Nurses at the North China Mission, 1888–1947* (Vancouver: UBC Press, 2008), 27.

13 Sonya Grypma and Cheng Zhen, "The Development of Modern Nursing in China," in *Medical Transitions in 20th Century China*, ed. Bridie Andrews and Mary Bullock, 298–99. (Bloomington: Indiana University Press, 2014).

14 Chung-tung Liu, "From San Gu Liu Po to 'Caring Scholar': The Chinese Nurse in Perspective," *International Journal of Nursing Studies* 28, 4 (1991): 321.

15 John Watt, "The Development of Nursing in Modern China, 1870–1949," *Nursing History Review* 12 (2004): 69.

16 Lu et al., "Historically-Informed Nursing," 5.

17 Watt, "Development of Nursing," 69.

18 Lu et al., "Historically-Informed Nursing," 6.

19 Ibid., 7.

20 Watt, "Development of Nursing," 75.

21 Ibid.

22 Ibid.

23 Ibid., 77.

24 The PUMC opened on 28 September 1920. The baccalaureate program started two years later. Gertrude Hodgman, School of Nursing, Peiping Union Medical College, Rockefeller Archive Center (RAC), China Medical Board Inc. (CMB), box

99, folder 711; Sarah E. Allison, "Anna Wolf's Dream: Establishment of a Collegiate Nursing Education Program," *Image: Journal of Nursing Scholarship* 25, 2 (1993): 127–31.

25 Nicole Elizabeth Barnes, *Intimate Communities: Wartime Healthcare and the Birth of Modern China, 1937–1945* (Oakland: University of California Press, 2018), 149.

26 "Nursing Education," *The Rockefeller Foundation: A Digital History*, https://rockfound.rockarch.org/nursing-education.

27 Christopher Maggs, "A History of Nursing: A History of Caring?," *Journal of Advanced Nursing* 23, 3 (1996): 632; Sioban Nelson, "The Fork in The Road: Nursing History vs the History of Nursing," *Nursing History Review* 10 (2002): 178.

28 Kathleen Cruickshank, "Education History and the Art of Biography," *American Journal of Education* 107, 3 (1999): 231–39.

29 Pamela Sugiman, "'Life Is Sweet': Vulnerability and Composure in the Wartime Narratives of Japanese Canadians," *Journal of Canadian Studies* 43, 1 (2009): 186–218.

30 Grypma, *Healing Henan*.

31 Sonya Grypma, *China Interrupted: Japanese Internment and the Reshaping of a Canadian Missionary Community* (Waterloo, ON: Wilfrid Laurier University Press, 2012).

32 Sonya Grypma, "Missionary Nursing: Internationalizing Religious Ideals," in *Religion, Religious Ethics, and Nursing*, ed. Marsha Fowler, Sheryl Reimer-Kirkham, Richard Sawatzky, and Elizabeth Johnston-Taylor, 129–50 (New York: Springer, 2011); Grypma and Zhen, "Development of Modern Nursing"; Lu et al. "Historically-Informed Nursing."

33 Evelyn Ricker, "Women's Missionary Society Appendices: Appendix A: Administrative History" United Church of Canada Woemn's Missionary Society Fonds, Records Relating to Overseas Missions: Honan" 1976: 3. United Church of Canada Archives (UCCA), United Church of Canada Woman's Missionary Society (WMS), 83.058C, series 3.

Chapter One | CHINA CALLING (1914–33): MISSIONARIES, WESTERN NURSING, AND THE ROCKEFELLERS

1 Karen Minden, *Bamboo Stone: The Evolution of a Chinese Medical Elite* (Toronto: University of Toronto Press, 1994), 45.

2 Ibid.

3 Sonya Grypma, "Missionary Nursing: Internationalizing Religious Ideals," in *Religion, Religious Ethics, and Nursing*, ed. Marsha Fowler, Sheryl Reimer-Kirkham,

Richard Sawatzky, and Elizabeth Johnston-Taylor (New York: Springer, 2011): 138.

4 Ibid., 129.

5 Chung-tung Liu, "From San Gu Liu Po to 'Caring Scholar': The Chinese Nurse in Perspective," *International Journal of Nursing Studies* 28, 4 (1991): 322.

6 J.G. Lutz, *China and the Christian Colleges, 1850–1950* (Ithaca, NY: Cornell University Press, 1971); Grypma "Missionary Nursing," 138.

7 Ibid.

8 Liu, "From San Gu Liu Po to 'Caring Scholar'," 316.

9 Sonya Grypma and Cheng Zhen, "The Development of Modern Nursing in China," in *Medical Transitions in 20th Century China*, ed. Bridie Andrews and Mary Bullock (Bloomington: Indiana University Press, 2014), 299.

10 Sonya Grypma, *Healing Henan: Canadian Nurses at the North China Mission, 1888–1947* (Vancouver: UBC Press, 2008).

11 Christoffer H. Grundmann, *Sent to Heal! Emergence and Development of Medical Missions* (Lanham, MD: University Press of America, 2005), 207.

12 Janet Beaton and Marion McKay, "Profile of a Leader: Caroline Wellwood, Pragmatic Visionary," *Canadian Journal of Nursing Leadership* 12, 4 (1999): 33.

13 Janet Beaton, "Caroline Wellwood: Founder of Modern Nursing in Southwest China," unpublished manuscript, UMASC A13-20, folder 8, box 11.

14 Ibid. 11.

15 Yuet-wah Cheung, *Missionary Medicine in China: A Study of Two Canadian Protestant Missions in China before 1937* (Lanham, MD: University Press of America, 1988); "The Central Stations of the West China Mission," *Vic in China*, 2015, Victoria University Library, http://library.vicu.utoronto.ca/exhibitions/vic_in_china/sections/missionaries_and_mission_stations/the_central_stations_of_the_west_china_mission.html.

16 Beaton, "Caroline Wellwood."

17 Cora Kilborn, "Chinese Leadership and Second-Generation Missionaries," *Missionary Monthly*, May 1942, UMASC, A13-20, box 15, file 7.

18 Cora Simpson, "Nursing in Mission Stations," *American Journal of Nursing* 14, 3 (1913): 191.

19 Ibid.

20 Cathy Green, *Canadian School in West China: Virgil Chittenden Hart*, blog. http://cschengdu.ca/?page_id=687. Accesssed May 20, 2019 [link no longer available].

21 Edward Bliss Jr., *Beyond the Stone Arches: An American Missionary Doctor in China, 1892–1932*. (New York: John Wiley and Sons, 2001), 138.

22 Alvyn Austin, *Saving China: Canadian Missionaries in the Middle Kingdom, 1888–1959* (Toronto: University of Toronto Press, 1986), 118.

23 Ibid.

24 Ibid., 119.

25 Alyvn Austin notes the name of the boy who was killed. Austin, *Saving China*, 119. Shulman notes that Lena Jolliffe did not report her son's death in a diary entry, but did note the anniversary of his birth after he had died. For example, in a 1915 entry she writes, "John's birthday. Would have been nine ..." Shulman also notes that Neil Semple reports in his book *The History of Canadian Methodism* (Montreal and Kingston: McGill-Queen's University Press, 1996) that John was killed by a stray bullet from the shore during the evacuation from the province to Shanghai at the time of the revolution. Deborah Shulman, "Prisms of China; Canadian Women Missionaries in China, 1904–1945" (PhD diss., Concordia University, 2008), 11, 38. https://spectrum.library.concordia.ca/975217/1/NR45679.pdf.

26 Bliss, *Beyond the Stone Arches*, 139.

27 Ibid.

28 Simpson, "Nursing in Mission Stations," 192.

29 Ibid.

30 Ibid.

31 Cheung, *Missionary Medicine in China*, 11.

32 Grypma, *Healing Henan*.

33 Austin, *Saving China*, 50–51

34 Minden, *Bamboo Stone*, 28–29.

35 The other founders were the Friends Foreign Mission Association (Great Britain and Ireland), the American Baptist Foreign Mission Society, and the Board of For-eign Missions of the Methodist Episcopal Church (United States). Cheung, *Missionary Medicine in China*, 49.

36 Ibid.

37 Ibid., 54.

38 Ibid., 54.

39 Ibid., 55.

40 "Our West China Mission" (n.d.), UCCA, Methodist Church (Canada) Woman's Missionary Society fonds, 78.079C, box 7, file 6.

41 "Our Mission Stations in Brief Review," (n.d.), UCCA, Methodist Church (Canada) Woman's Missionary Society fonds, 78.079C, box 7, file 6: 3.

42 Ibid.

43 Howard J. Veals, "China's Wartime Capital," (n.d.), UCCA, WMS, 83.058C series 5, box 62, file 23.

44 Cheung, *Missionary Medicine in China*.

45 West China Union University Collection, 1896–1950, Finding Aid 13, UCCA, fonds 14, series 3, subseries 2; Cheung, *Missionary Medicine in China*.

46 Cheung, *Missionary Medicine in China*, 43–44.

47 School of Nursing, The College of Medicine and Dentistry WCUU, 10 March 1943, box 158, folder 1154, CMB, RAC.

48 "1890s, Omar & Retta Kilborn and Family," *Vic in China*, 2015, Victoria University Library, http://library.vicu.utoronto.ca/exhibitions/vic_in_china/sections/missionaries_and_mission_stations/1890s_omar_retta_kilborn_and_family.html.

49 B. Hensman, "The Kilborn Family: A Record of a Canadian Family's Service to Medical Work and Education in China and Hong Kong," *Canadian Medical Association Journal* 97, 9 (1967): 471–75.

50 Ibid., 475

51 Ibid., 474.

52 Ibid., 476.

53 Ibid., 481.

54 Allison, "Anna Wolf's Dream," 128.

55 Mary E. Ferguson, *China Medical Board and Peking Union Medical College: A Chronicle of Fruitful Collaboration, 1914–1951* (New York: China Medical Board of New York, 1970), 23.

56 Ibid., 24.

57 Ibid., 25.

58 Ibid., 24, 25.

59 Michelle Renshaw, *Accommodating the Chinese: The American Hospital in China, 1880–1920* (New York: Routledge, 2005), 81.

60 Ibid., 84.

61 Bishop Logan H. Roots, letter to Roger S. Greene, 25 June 1915, cited in Renshaw, *Accommodating the Chinese*, 86.

62 Ibid.

63 Ferguson, *China Medical Board*, 34.

64 Ibid., 42.

65 Gertrude E. Hodgman, "School of Nursing, Peiping Union Medical College," Rockefeller Archive Center (RAC), China Medical Board, Inc. (CMB), box 99, folder 711.

66 The term "graduate nurses" is in keeping with the nomenclature of the period. Ferguson, *China Medical Board*, 240.

67 Ibid.

68 Anonymous Plan for Publicity, Peking University and Nurses Training School. 29 December, Peking Union Medical College Archives–School of Nursing Archives (PUMC-SNA), fonds 346, Old File Materials of Nursing School (A–G) 1932–1937: 49.

69 Ibid.

70 Anonymous report dated 21 September 1931, PUMC-SNA, fonds 346, Old File Materials of Nursing School (A-G) 1932–1937, 134.

71 "Why Not Nursing?," anonymous report date stamped 17 September 1931, PUMC-SNA, fonds 347, Old File Materials of Nursing School (P–R) 1931–1939.

72 Anonymous report dated 21 September 1931, PUMC-SNA, fonds 346, Old File Materials of Nursing School (A-G) 1932–1937, 133.

73 Ibid.

74 Ibid.

75 Note from Gertrude Hodgman to [F.S.?] Kiang, 17 December 1931, PUMC-SNA, fonds 347, Old File Materials of Nursing School (P–R) 1931–1939.

76 "Nursing Education."

77 Ibid.

78 "The Nursing Profession as a Preparation for Marriage," anonymous report dated 17 Septmber 1931, PUMC-SNA, fonds 347, Old File Materials of Nursing School (P–R) 1931–1939

79 Ibid.

80 Ibid.

81 Ibid.

82 Anonymous report dated 21 September 1931, PUMC-SNA fonds 346, Old File Materials of Nursing School (A-G) 1932–37.

83 "Nursing Education."

84 "China Needs Nurses." Anonymous report dated 25 July 1931, PUMC-SNA fonds 347, Old File Materials of Nursing School (P-R) 1931–1939.

85 Josephine Goldmark, *Nursing and Nursing Education in the United States: Report of the Committee for the Study of Nursing Education, and a Report of a Survey* (New York: Macmillan, 1923).

86 Jean Groft, "Everything Depends on Good Nursing," *Canadian Nurse* 102, 3 (2006): 19–22.

87 Ibid.

88 Ibid.

89 Anonymous report dated 21 September 1931, PUMC-SNA fonds 346, Old File Materials of Nursing School (A-G) 1932–37.

90 "Nursing Education," *The Rockefeller Foundation: A Digital History*, n.d., https://rockfound.rockarch.org/nursing-education.

91 Ibid.

92 Anonymous report dated 21 September 1931, PUMC-SNA fonds 346, Old File Materials of Nursing School (A-G) 1932–37, 137.

93 Ibid., 134.

94 According to her PUMC application, Vera Nieh was born on 15 April 1905: PUMC Training School for Nurses Application for Admission, Vera Nieh, ca. 1923,

PUMC-SNA, file 1927-2437-2024. According to an application to the Public Health Demonstration Metropolitan Police Department, Vera Nieh was born on 15 May 1905: PUMC-SNA, file 1927-2437.

95 Wang Yi, "Biography of Miss Vera Yu-chan Nieh," 28 June 1947, PUMC-SNA, file 1927-2437.

96 Interview by Anne Davis, 1985 (audiotape in author's possession).

97 Nieh, interview. Her father died at age sixty-one of arteriosclerosis: Vera Nieh Yu-Chan, Peiping Union Medical College Personal History Record, 1 February 1932, PUMC-SNA, file 1927-2437.

98 Hsun Yuan Yao, "The First Year of the Rural Health Experiment in Ting Hsien, China," *Milbank Memorial Fund Quarterly Bulletin* 9, 3 (1931): 61.

99 Nieh, interview.

100 Miss Nieh Yu-Ch'an, nursing interview, 1923, PUMC-SNA, file 1927-2437.

101 Letter from Maude Mueler (?) (Tianjin) to Mrs. T.D. Macmillan (Beijing), 21 May 1923, PUMC-SNA, file 1927-2437.

102 PUMC Nurses Application for Admission, PUMC-SNA, file 2437.

103 PUMC School of Nursing Efficiency Record from 8 December 1926 to 28 January 1927, PUMC-SNA, file 1927-2437.

104 Wang, "Biography of Vera Nieh."

105 Ibid.

106 Ibid.

107 PUMC School of Nursing Efficiency Record of Vera Nieh by K. Yu, from 26 April to 13 May 1926, PUMC-SNA, file 1927-2437.

108 PUMC School of Nursing Efficiency Record of Vera Nieh from 8 December 1926 to 28 January 1927, PUMC-SNA, file, 1927-2437.

109 Appointment of Miss Nieh Yu Chan as Staff Nurse (minutes) 23 May 1927, PUMC-SNA, file 1927-2437.

110 The term "Hong Kong foot" originated from the stationing of the British army in Hong Kong, where the humid climate resulted in ringworm of the foot. "Kulat Air – Tinea Pedis – Athlete Foot – Hong Kong Foot," *Do What I Want* (blog), 8 March 2011, http://dowhatiwant-amin.blogspot.com/2011/03/kulat-air-tinea-pedis-athlete-foot-hong.html.

111 Note from Joyce Walker (Tianjin) to "Ruth" [Ingram], 15 March 1928, PUMC-SNA, file 1927-2437.

112 Letter from [Ruth Ingram] to "Joyce" [Walker], 16 March 1928, PUMC-SNA, file 1927-2437.

113 Ibid.

114 Interdepartmental note from Miss [Anne] McCabe to Mary S. Purcell, 22 November 1928; excerpt from note from Miss Ingram to Dr. Grant, 14 June 1928; note from Dr. Grant to Miss Ingram, 15 June 1928, all PUMC-SNA, file 1927-2437.

115 R. Tien, PUMC School of Nursing Efficiency Record for Vera Nieh, 4 November 1928 to 1 December 1928, PUMC-SNA, file 1927-2437.
116 Ibid.
117 J. Martin [?], PUMC School of Nursing Efficiency Record for Vera Nieh, 4 November 1928 to 1 December 1928, PUMC-SNA, file 1927-2437.
118 M.S. Purcell, note on PUMC School of Nursing Efficiency Record for Vera Nieh, n.d., PUMC-SNA, file 1927-2437.
119 Liping Bu and Elizabeth Fee, "John B. Grant International Statesman of Public Health," *American Journal of Public Health* 98, 4 (2008): 628–29.
120 Minutes of the Peking Union Medical College Board of Trustees Executive Committee, 22 August 1929, PUMC-SNA, file 1927-2437.
121 Since the Rockefeller Fellowship funds for 1929 were already exhausted, Vera Nieh's expenses while abroad were paid from her salary and maintenance allowance, and supplemented by the PUMC Department of Hygiene and Public Health.
122 Note from Anne McCabe to Roger Greene, 13 September 1929, PUMC-SNA, file 1927-2437.
123 Ibid.
124 The International House was started by John D. Rockefeller and others in 1924. The idea was to have a house that fostered relationships between students from different countries. It is still in existence as a private, non-profit residence for graduate students, scholars, trainees, and interns attending schools in New York. "International House of New York," Wikipedia, https://en.wikipedia.org/wiki/International_House_of_New_York.
125 Letter from M.K. Eggleston to R.S. Greene, 10 October 1929, PUMC-SNA, file 1927-2437.
126 Letter from Anne McCabe (Beijing) to Mary Beard (New York), 24 September 1929, PUMC-SNA, file 1927-2437.
127 Copy of interdepartmental correspondence between JBG [John B Grant] and CHH, 18 August 1929, PUMC-SNA, file 1927-2437.
128 Memo from H.S. Houghton (Beijing) to R.S. Greene (Beijing), 11 March 1927, UMASC, A13-20, box 17, file 16.
129 The course was arranged by the League of Red Cross Societies at Bedford College. International Course in Public Health Nursing Application Form for Bernice Pu-Hui Chu, Royal Holloway Archives and Special Collections (RHASC) Bedford College Papers (BC).
130 Memo from H.S. Houghton to R.S. Greene, 11 March 1927.
131 Ibid.; Memo from Miss Eggleston (New York) to Miss McCabe and R.S. Greene (Beijing), 23 August 1929, PUMC-SNA, file 1927-2437.
132 "Nursing Education," Rockefeller Foundation.

133 Letter from Anne McCabe (Beijing) to Vera Nieh (New York), 29 January 1931, PUMC-SNA, file 1927-2437.
134 Ibid.
135 Note from Vera Nieh (New York) to Miss Beard (New York), 11 November 1930, RAC, CMB, box 104, folder 747A.
136 Letter from Anne McCabe (Beijing) to Vera (Nieh) (Toronto?), 21 February 1930, PUMC-SNA, file 1927-2437.
137 Liping Bu, "John B. Grant: Public Health and State Medicine," in *Medical Transitions in Twentieth-Century China*, ed. Bridie Andrews and Mary Brown Bullock (Bloomington: Indiana University Press, 2014), 212–26.
138 Ibid.
139 The 1919 May Fourth Movement was a political, cultural, and anti-imperialist movement that began with a series of demonstrations by students in Beijing; they were objecting to what they saw as their government's ineffective response to the Treaty of Versailles, especially in allowing Japan to receive territories in Shandong. "May Fourth Movement," Wikipedia, https://en.wikipedia.org/wiki/May_Fourth_Movement.
140 Confidential letter from R.S. Greene (Beijing) to M.K. Eggleston (New York), 7 August 1933, RAC, CMB, box 104, folder 747A.
141 Ibid.
142 Ibid.
143 Ibid.
144 John B. Grant, "Nursing," undated report, PUMC-SNA, fonds 346, Old File Materials of Nursing School (A-G) 1932–37, 96–97.
145 Ibid.
146 Ibid.
147 Yao, "The First Year of the Rural Health Experiment," 63.
148 Ibid.
149 Ibid.
150 Ibid. To compare, the 2014 mortality rate in China was 0.7 percent.
151 "Tetanus neonatorum," *Medical Dictionary*, 2019, https://medical-dictionary.the freedictionary.com/tetanus+neonatorum.
152 Ibid.
153 Yao, "Rural Health," 61
154 Ibid.
155 Hu Tun-wu, address delivered at the "Lady of the Lamp" ceremony at the School of Nursing of Peiping Union Medical College, 12 June 1929, PUMC-SNA, fonds 347.
156 Ibid.
157 Ibid.
158 See "The Gospel of Soap and Water," Grypma, *Healing Henan*, 25–50.

159 Hu Tun-wu, "Lady of the Lamp" Address.

160 Report Re: Conference with Miss Nieh and Miss Parson, 23 February 1933, PUMC-SNA, file 1927-2437, RSG (R.S. Greene) file.

161 Ibid.

162 Letter from Vera Nieh to Miss Maude Parsons, 5 June 1933, PUMC-SNA, file 1927-2437.

163 Confidential letter from R.S. Greene (Beijing) to M.K. Eggleston (New York), 7 August 1933, RAC CMB, box 104, folder 747A.

164 Ibid.

165 Rockefeller Foundation Inter-Office Correspondence, memorandum from Dr. Heiser re: Conference with Miss Beard and Miss Hodgman, 3 August 1933, RAC, Rockefeller Foundation (RF), SG 1.1, series 601-China, box 37, folder 298.

166 Confidential letter from R.S. Greene (Beijing) to M.K. Eggleston, 7 August 1933.

167 Ibid.

168 Ibid.

169 Ibid.

170 Ibid.

171 Ibid.

172 Letter from Gertrude Hodgman (New Haven?) to Mary Beard (New York), 12 August 1933, PUMC-SNA, fonds 346.

173 Ibid.

174 Letter from Gertrude Hodgman (Beijing) to Mary Beard (New York), 27 September 1933, PUMC-SNA, fonds 346.

Chapter Two | UNSETTLING NURSING (1932–40): JAPANESE INVASION
AND THE SHIFT TO CHINESE LEADERSHIP

1 Letter from Roger S. Greene (Beijing) to Selskar Gunn (Shanghai), 17 March 1933, Peking Union Medical College Archives–School of Nursing Archives (PUMC-SNA), fonds 346.

2 Ibid.

3 Letter from Gertrude Hodgman (Beijing) to Mary Beard (New York), 7 February 1936, PUMC-SNA, fonds 346.

4 PUMC Medical Corps, Announcement for All Chinese Staff Members, Professional & Non-Professional, 26 February 1932, PUMC-SNA, fonds 347.

5 Ibid.

6 Letter from Vera Nieh (Health Station, Beijing) to Roger Greene (Beijing), 3 March 1932, PUMC-SNA, file 1927-2437.

7 PUMC Medical Corps, Announcement for All Chinese Staff Members.

8 Ibid.

9   Letter from Gladys Stephenson (Hankou) to Gertrude Hodgman (Beijing), 27 February 1932, PUMC-SNA, fonds 347.

10 "Stephenson, Gladys," *Mundus: Gateway to Missionary Collections in the United Kingdom*, n.d., http://www.mundus.ac.uk/cats/4/961.htm.

11 Letter from Gladys Stephenson (Hankou) to Gertrude Hodgman (Beijing), 24 February 1932, PUMC-SNA, fonds 347.

12 Letter from Gertrude Hodgman (Beijing) to Gladys Stephenson (Hankou), 2 March 1932, PUMC-SNA, fonds 347.

13 Ibid.

14 Letter from Gladys Stephenson (Hankou) to Gertrude Hodgman (Beijing), 7 March 1932, PUMC-SNA, fonds 347.

15 Ibid.

16 Ibid.

17 Evelyn Lin, "Nurses Association of China Report," October 1936, PUMC-SNA, fonds 833.

18 Ibid.

19 Kaiyi Chen, "Missionaries and the Early Development of Nursing in China," *Nursing History Review* 4 (1996): 133.

20 Ibid., 134.

21 Harold Balme, *China and Modern Medicine: A Study in Medical Missionary Development* (London: United Council for Missionary Education, 1921), 153.

22 Cora Simpson, *A Joy Ride through China for the N.A.C.* (Shanghai: Kwang Hsueh Publishing, 1926).

23 Chen, "Missionaries and the Early Development of Nursing."

24 A. Clark, "The Nurses Association of China, Fifth Annual Conference, Shanghai, 1914," *British Journal of Nursing*, 12 September 1914, 211–12.

25 Simpson, *Joy Ride*, 11.

26 Balme, *China and Modern Medicine*, 150.

27 Evelyn Lin, "Nurses Association of China Report," October 1936.

28 The committee members were Yu Chih Suai Lan, Victoria Pen Yen, James Liu, and Bernice Chu Chen. Letter from Cora Simpson (Nanjing) to Gertrude Hodgman (Beijing), 17 November 1936, PUMC-SNA, fonds 833.

29 Caroline Maddock Hart was the second wife to Dr. Edgerton H. Hart, and the head of a mission hospital in Wuhu from 1905 to 1913. Her husband was the son of Virgil Hart, who had been the superintendent of the first Canadian Methodist Mission in the late nineteenth century. He and his wife, Adeline Gilland Hart, were among the first group of eight Canadian Methodist missionaries in West China, departing for China in 1891. Green, *Canadian School*; "The Central Stations of the West China Mission," *Vic in China*, 2015, Victoria University Library, http://library.

vicu.utoronto.ca/exhibitions/vic_in_china/sections/missionaries_and_mission_stations/the_central_stations_of_the_west_china_mission.html.

30 Yuhong Jiang, "Shaping Modern Nursing Development in China before 1949," *International Journal of Nursing Sciences* 4, 1 (2017): 19–23.

31 Ibid.

32 Letter from Cora Simpson (Nanjing) to Gertrude Hodgman (Beijing), 17 November 1936, PUMC-SNA, fonds 833.

33 *Annual Report of the WMS of the UCC*, 1936–37, UMASC, Janet Beaton fonds, box 15, folder 5, A13-15.

34 Ibid.

35 Ibid.

36 Jeanette Radcliffe [sic], "War in Weihwei," *Canadian Nurse* 34, 7 (1938): 356–58.

37 Nicole Elizabeth Barnes, *Intimate Communities: Wartime Healthcare and the Birth of Modern China, 1937–1945* (Oakland: University of California Press, 2018), 134.

38 Gladys Stephenson, "The Nurses Association of China," *American Journal of Nursing* 46, 9 (1946): 612.

39 Ibid.

40 Ibid.

41 Ibid.

42 Ibid.

43 Gertrude Hodgman, "Nursing in Formosa," *American Journal of Nursing* 53, 7 (1953): 838–40.

44 Gertrude Hodgman, "The Teaching of Public Health Nursing at Yale," *American Journal of Nursing* 29, 11 (1929): 1354–60.

45 "Nursing Education," *Rockefeller Foundation: A Digital History*, n.d., https://rockfound.rockarch.org/nursing-education.

46 Steve Kemper, "C-E.A. Winslow, Who Launched Public Health at Yale a Century Ago, Still Influential Today," *Yale News*, 2 June 2015, https://news.yale.edu/2015/06/02/public-health-giant-c-ea-winslow-who-launched-public-health-yale-century-ago-still-influe.

47 Hodgman, "Teaching of Public Health Nursing."

48 Ibid.

49 Letter from Gertrude Hodgman (Beijing) to Selskar M. Gunn (Shanghai), 6 February 1936, PUMC-SNA, fonds 346.

50 Ibid.

51 Ibid.

52 Letter from Gertrude Hodgman (Beijing) to Mary Beard (New York), 7 February 1936, PUMC-SNA, fonds 346.

53 Ibid.

54 On this night, shots were fired between Japanese and Chinese forces near the Marco Polo Bridge outside Beijing. This is considered the trigger that developed into warfare between Japan and China.

55 Letter from Henry Houghton (Beijing) to Dr. Wilber A. Sawyer (New York), 18 March 1937, Rockefeller Archive Center (RAC), Rockefeller Foundation (RF), RB 1.1, series 601-China, box 37, folder 298.

56 Ibid.

57 Letter from W.A. Sawyer (New York) to Henry S. Houghton (Beijing), 3 May 1937, RAC RF, RB 1.1, series 601-China, box 37, folder 298.

58 Letter from John B. Grant (Shanghai) to Dr. Sawyer (New York), 26 May 1937, RAC RF, RB 1.1, series 601-China, box 37, folder 298.

59 Letter from Henry Houghton (Beijing) to Dr. W.A. Sawyer (New York), 29 September 1937, RAC RF, RB 1.1, series 601-China, box 37, folder 298.

60 Ibid.

61 Ibid.

62 Ibid.

63 Ibid.

64 Ibid.

65 Letter from W.A. Sawyer (New York) to Dr. Henry S. Houghton (Beijing), 25 October 1937, RAC, RF, RB 1.1, series 601-China, box 37, folder 298.

66 Ibid.

67 PUMC Governing Council Educational Division Minutes, 14 December 1937, RAC, China Medical Board Inc. (CMB), box 60, folder 422.

68 Ibid.

69 Sonya Grypma and Cheng Zhen, "The Development of Modern Nursing in China," in *Medical Transitions in 20th Century China*, ed. Mary Bullock and Bridie Andrews (Bloomington: Indiana University Press, 2014).

70 Ibid.

71 Minutes of the PUMC Governing Council Educational Division, 13 December 1938, PUMC-SNA, file 1937-2437.

72 PUMC Governing Council Educational Division Minutes, 14 December 1937, RAC, CMB, box 60, folder 422.

73 Minutes of the PUMC Governing Council Educational Division, 13 December 1938, PUMC-SNA, file 1937-2437.

74 Letter from Roger S. Greene to G.E. Hodgman, 25 February 1935, PUMC-SNA, file 1937-2437.

75 Vera Nieh, interview by Anne Davis, 1985 (audiotape in author's possession).

76 Ibid.

77 Letter from F. Oldt (Guangzhou) to Miss Hodgman (Beijing), 25 March 1936, PUMC-SNA, file 1937-2437.

78 Ibid.
79 Letter from Gertrude Hodgman (Beijing) to F. Oldt (Guangzhou), 8 April 1936, PUMC-SNA, file 1937-2437.
80 Ibid.
81 Letter from Vera Nieh (Jinan) to Miss Hodgman (Beijing), 12 October 1936 PUMC-SNA, file 1937-2437.
82 Ibid.
83 Copy of note from Secretary (PUMC) to American Consul General (Tianjin), 22 October 1936, PUMC-SNA, file 1937-2437.
84 Ibid.
85 Ibid.
86 Letter from Gertrude E. Hodgman (Beijing) to Dean of the Graduate School, University of Cincinnati (Cincinnati), 20 October 1936, PUMC-SNA, file 1937-2437.
87 Nieh interview.
88 Ibid.
89 Ibid.
90 Ibid.
91 Ibid.
92 Excerpt of letter from H.S. Houghton to E.C. Lobenstine, 9 December 1938, RAC, CMB, box 104, folder 747A.
93 Ibid.
94 Circular Docket, Governing Council, Medical Services Division, 19 August 1938, PUMC-SNA, file 1937-2437.
95 Interdepartmental correspondence from F. Whiteside to Dr. C.E. Lim and Dr. S.T. Wang, 18 August 1938, PUMC-SNA, file 1937-2437.
96 Nieh interview.
97 Minutes of the Peiping Union Medical College, Governing Council Educational Division, 12 March 1940, PUMC-SNA, file 1937-2437.
98 Minutes of the Peiping Union Medical College, Board of Trustees Adjourned Annual Meeting, 27 March 1940, PUMC-SNA, file 1937-2437.
99 Ibid.

Chapter Three | SHIFTING MISSIONS (1936–40): THE EROSION
OF MISSIONARY NURSING IN WEST CHINA

1 Grypma, "Missionary Nursing: Internationalizing Religious Ideals," in *Religion, Religious Ethics, and Nursing*, ed. Marsha Fowler, Sheryl Reimer-Kirkham, Richard Sawatzky, and Elizabeth Johnston-Taylor (New York: Springer, 2011), 141.
2 Dr. Stephen Chang, for example, played the organ and was able to play hymns for the Japanese soldiers at the PUMC on demand. "Letter from Stephen Chang to

Claude E. Forkner, 1943 July," *The Rockefeller Foundation: A Digital History*, n.d., https://rockfound.rockarch.org/digital-library-listing/-/asset_publisher/yYxp-feI4W8N/content/letter-from-stephen-chang-to-claude-e-forkner-1943-july.

3 Vera Nieh, "A Brief Account of the PUMC School of Nursing During and After World War II: A Message to Its Alumnae," unpublished report, 25 September 1948, Peking Union Medical College Archives–School of Nursing Archives (PUMC-SNA), fonds 732.

4 "China," *The Rockefeller Foundation: A Digital History*, n.d., https://rockfound.rockarch.org/china.

5 John Z. Bowers, *Western Medicine in a Chinese Palace: Peking Union Medical College, 1917–1951* (Philadelphia: Josiah Macy Jr. Foundation, 1972).

6 John S. Baick, "Cracks in the Foundation: Frederick T. Gates, the Rockefeller Foundation, and the China Medical Board," *Journal of the Guilded Age and Progressive Era* 3, 1 (2004): 59–89.

7 "China," *Rockefeller Foundation, Digital History*.

8 Geo J. Bond, *Our Share in China and What We Are Doing with It* (Toronto: Missionary Society of the Methodist Church, 1909), 57.

9 Quoted in Munroe Scott, *McClure: The China Years* (Markham, ON: Penguin Books, 1977), 106.

10 William Earnest Hocking, *Re-Thinking Missions: A Layman's Inquiry after One Hundred Years* (New York: Harper & Brothers, 1932), 201.

11 Ibid., v–vi

12 Ibid., 201.

13 Ibid., 326; emphasis in original.

14 Ibid., 201.

15 Margaret Brown, "History of the Honan (North China) Mission of the United Church of Canada, Originally a Mission of the Presbyterian Church in Canada" (unpublished manuscript, n.d.), vol.3, ch 66, 13.

16 Sonya Grypma, *Healing Henan: Canadian Nurses at the North China Mission, 1888–1947* (Vancouver: UBC Press, 2008), 113.

17 Helen Vandenberg, "Race, Hospital Development and the Power of Community: The History of Japanese and Chinese Hospitals in British Columbia, 1880–1920" (PhD diss., University of British Columbia, 2014).

18 Kathryn McPherson, *Bedside Matters: The Transformation of Canadian Nursing, 1900–1990* (Toronto: Oxford University Press, 1996), 118.

19 Trudy Harrold, *On Highest Mission Sent: The Story of Health Care in Lamont, Alberta* (Lamont, AB: Lamont Health Care Centre, 1999), 25.

20 Sonya Grypma, *China Interrupted: Japanese Internment and the Reshaping of a Canadian Missionary Community* (Waterloo, ON: Wilfrid Laurier University Press, 2012), 30.

21 Helen Vandenberg, "Canadian Nursing History Stories: Canada's First Chinese Nurse," *Canadian Association for the History of Nursing Newsletter* 25, 1 (2012): 13.

22 Ibid.

23 Ibid.

24 Muriel McIntosh, "Nursing in China," *Canadian Nurse* 37, 1 (1941): 18.

25 Hocking, *Re-Thinking Missions*.

26 Grypma, *Healing Henan*, 117–18.

27 Ibid.

28 Mary E. Ferguson, *China Medical Board and Peking Union Medical College: A Chronicle of Fruitful Collaboration, 1914–1951* (New York: China Medical Board of New York, 1970), 24.

29 Ibid.

30 Ibid.

31 Letter from Adelaide Harrison (Pengxian?) to Miss Buck (Toronto?), 23 October 1937, United Church of Canada Archives (UCCA), United Church of Canada Woman's Missionary Society (WMS), 83.058C, series 5, box 36, file 36.

32 Ibid.

33 "The West China Union University," 1939, UCCA, Methodist Church (Canada) Woman's Missionary Society fonds, 78.097C7, box 7, file 17.

34 Ibid.

35 Memorandum from John B. Grant to Selskar Gunn, 11 November 1938, Rockefeller Archive Centre (RAC), RG1, series 601, box 3, folder 26.

36 Ibid.

37 Ibid.

38 "The West China Union University," 1939.

39 Alvyn Austin, *Saving China: Canadian Missionaries in the Middle Kingdom, 1888–1959* (Toronto: University of Toronto Press, 1986), 259.

40 "Morale in China: Dr. Kilborn's Address," newspaper clipping, 4 February 1944, UMASC, A13020, box 15, folder 6.

41 Ibid.

42 L. Clara Preston, *Flowers amongst the Debris: A Canadian Nurse in Wartorn China* (Brockville, ON: Preston Robb, n.d.), 99.

43 Ibid.

44 Austin, *Saving China*, 260.

45 Marnie Copland, *Mooncakes and Maple Sugar* (Burlington, ON: G.R. Welch, 1980), 61.

46 Ibid., 62.

47 Ibid.

48 Austin, *Saving China*, 260.

49 Copland, *Mooncakes*, 62.

50   Ibid.

51   Ibid., 63.

52   Ibid., 68.

53   Ibid., 67–68.

54   Austin, *Saving China*, 260.

55   Ibid.

56   "The West China Union University," 1939.

57   Ibid.

58   Ibid.

59   Ibid.

60   Ibid.

61   Letter from Assistant Treasurer to Miss Kilborn, 7 May 1938, UCCA, WMS, 83.058C, series 5, box 64, file 42.

62   Letter from Adelaide Harrison (Chengdu) to Mrs. Taylor (Toronto), 9 December 1942, UCCA, WMS, 83.058C, box 61, file 82.

63   Copland, *Mooncakes*, 61.

64   Ibid.

65   Gerald A. Bell, "The Present Situation," n.d., UCCA, WMS, 83.058C, series 3, box 62, file 22.

66   Margaret Outerbridge, Chengdu, 26 March 1939, quoted in John Munro, *Beyond the Moon Gate: A China Odyssey, 1938–1950* (Vancouver: Douglas & McIntyre, 1990), 28.

67   Ibid.

68   Ibid.

69   *Chungking – China's War Capital*, China Handbook Series No. 21, Chinese Ministry of Information (Chungking, July 1943), 27, http://www.cbi-theater.com/chungking/chungking.html.

70   Ibid.

71   Bell, *The Present Situation*.

72   Ibid.

73   Cited by W.E. Smith from a report of "one of our missionaries." W.E. Smith, *A Canadian Doctor in West China: Forty Years under Three Flags* (Toronto: Ryerson Press, 1939), 274–75.

74   Ibid., 275.

75   Copy of China Information Committee News Release No. 409, Chungking, 5 May 1939, copy by Frank Price, UCCA, WMS, 83-058C, series 5, box 61, file 27.

76   Ibid.

77   Ibid.

78 Quoted in Munro, *Beyond the Moon Gate*, 39.

79 Mrs. Gerald S. Bell, "They Come – The Japanese," article based on letter sent to relatives after 11 June 1939, UCCA, WMS, 83-058C, series 5, box 61, file 31:1.

80 Ibid., 2.

81 Ibid., 4.

82 Ibid., 6.

83 Ibid., 8.

84 Ibid.

85 Ibid., 11.

86 Quoted in Munro, *Beyond the Moon Gate*, 40.

87 Letter from Winifred Harris (Chengdu) to Myrtle M. Buck (Toronto), 25 August 1939, UCCA, 83.058C, series 5, box 62, file 43.

88 Ibid.

89 Quoted in Munro, *Beyond the Moon Gate*, 49.

90 Ibid.

91 Ibid., 50.

92 Ibid.

93 Ibid.

94 Copland, *Mooncakes*, 26, 51. The term "coolie" referred to unskilled labourers, who, for example, acted as carriers of persons and belongings. According to Marnie Copland, the term is actually two Chinese words, *k'u li*, meaning bitter strength. It signified that the man made his living by the strength or energy of his body. It was not considered a derogatory term at the time but is now.

95 Gordon R. Jones, "The Bombing of Luchow, Szechwan, China," 11 September 1939, UCCA, WMS, 83.058C, series 5, box 62, file 31.

96 James G. Endicott, "The Bombing of Luchow, Szechwan, China," 11 September 1939, UCCA, WMS, 83.058C, series 5, box 62, file 31.

97 Ibid.

98 Smith, *Canadian Doctor in West China*, 275.

99 Letter from Adelaide Harrison (Pengxian?) to Miss Buck (Toronto?), 7 March 1938, UCCA, WMS, 83.058C, series 5, box 62, file 38.

100 Letter from Adelaide Harrison (Pengxian?) to Mrs. Taylor (Toronto), 21 February 1938, UCCA, WMS, 83.058C, series 5, box 61, file 19.

101 "News from the Air," 18 February 1938, UCCA, WMS, 83.058C, series 5, box 61, file 25.

102 Ibid.

103 Letter from Adelaide Harrison (Pengxian?) to Miss Buck (Toronto?), 7 March 1938, UCCA, WMS, 83.058C, series 5, box 62, file 38.

104 Grypma, *China Interrupted.*

105 Letter from Winifred Harris (Chengdu) to Mrs. H.D. Taylor (Toronto), 6 April 1940, UCCA, WMS, 83.058C, series 5, box 61, file 55.

106 Letter from Winifred Harris (Chengdu) to Mrs. H.D. Taylor (Toronto), 20 April 1940, UCCA, WMS, 83.058C, series 5, box 62, file 49.

107 Qilu was part of the Shandong Christian University, a union university that, like the WCUU, was started by Canadian, American, and British missionaries. The Canadian North China Mission had been involved in the medical school there since 1918, when Dr. William McClure transferred there from Henan.

108 Quoted in Mary McKim, "Called to Serve: A Memoir" (unpublished manuscript, 2017), chap. 25.

109 Ibid.

110 Grypma, *China Interrupted.*

111 Grypma, *Healing Henan*, 169.

112 Preston, *Flowers amongst the Debris*, 104.

113 Ibid.

114 Ibid.

115 Preston, *Flowers amongst the Debris*, 103.

116 Grypma, *Healing Henan.*

117 "Missionary Tells about War in China" *Kingston Whig-Standard*, 16 March [no year], private collection, courtesy Ward Skinner.

118 Nicole Elizabeth Barnes, *Intimate Communities: Wartime Healthcare and the Birth of Modern China, 1937–1945* (Oakland: University of California Press, 2018), 136.

119 Grypma, *Healing Henan.*

120 Ibid., 150.

121 Ibid.

122 Ibid., 172.

123 Ibid.

124 Ibid.

125 Ibid., 173.

126 Letter from Adelaide Harrison (Chengdu) to Mrs. Taylor (Toronto), 25 March 1941, UMASC A13-20, box 15, file 6.

127 Ibid.

128 Grypma, *Healing Henan*, 175.

129 Letter from Mrs. Ruth Taylor to G.K. King, 5 May 1941. UCCA 83.058C, series 3, box 56, file 10.

130 Grypma, *Healing Henan*, 175

131 Ibid., 176.

132 Letter from Adelaide Harrison (Chengdu) to Mrs. Taylor (Toronto), 26 July 1941, UMASC A13-20, box 15, file 6.

133 Letter from Winifred Harris (Chengdu?) to Mrs. H.D. Taylor (Toronto), 19 September 1939, UCCA, WMS, 83.058C, series 5, box 61, file 44.

134 Letter from MMB (Toronto?) to Margaret Lee (Montreal), 29 July 1940, UCCA, WMS, 83.058C, series 5, box 64, file 84.

135 Letter from Margaret Lee (Montreal) to Canadian Girls in Training, n.d., UCCA, WMS, 83.058C, series 5, box 64, file 89.

136 Mabel Carroll, "Margaret Lee Goes to China," n.d., UCCA, WMS, 83.058C, series 5, box 64, file 90.

137 Ibid.

138 Letter from Margaret Lee (Montreal) to Canadian Girls in Training, n.d., UCCA, WMS, 83.058C, series 5, box 64, file 89.

139 Letter from Margaret Lee (Chengdu) to A1, 21 February 1941, Margaret Scaia Private Collection.

140 Ibid.

141 Ibid.

142 Ibid.

143 Ibid.

144 Margaret Lee to AI.

145 *United Church Observer*, 15 August 1940, UMASC, A13-20, box 15, file 7. Geraldine Hartwell started at the WCM in 1914, but there is nothing about her in the archival records after that; she is not included in WMS lists except for 1914. In addition to an RN, Hartwell also had a "PhN," which might have been a designation in pharmacy. It is possible, therefore, that Hartwell was in China since 1914, but worked primarily in pharmacy.

146 Letter from Winifred Harris (Chengdu) to Mrs. H.D. Taylor (Toronto), 2 May 1940, UCCA, WMS, 83.058c, series 5, box 61, file 56.

147 Ibid.

148 Ibid.

149 Letter from Harris to Taylor, 2 May 1940.

150 Ibid. Given the dates on file 73, it seems that this was not part of the February 1941 letter, but one written subsequently.

151 Ibid.

152 "Hospitals Wrecked Carry On," newspaper clipping from Toronto (?), n.d., UCCA, WMS, 83.058C, series 5, box 62, file 2.

153 Letter from Winifred Harris (Chengdu) to Mrs. H.D. Taylor (Toronto), 2 May 1940, UCCA, WMS, 83.058C, series 5, box 61, file 56.

154 Ibid.

155 Hazel Heffren, *Letters from Old China: Letters and Diary Entries from 1901 to 1943 by Laura Hambley* (Asquith, SK: author, 1989), diary entry for 14 July 1940.

156 Ibid.

157 Letter from Winifred Harris (Chengdu) to Mrs. H.D. Taylor (Toronto), 2 May 1940, UCCA, WMS, 83.058C, series 5, box 61, file 56.

158 "WMS Hospital," *United Church Observer*, 18 May 1940, UMASC, A13-30, box 15, file 7.

159 Ibid.

160 *Sixteenth Annual Report of the WMS of the United Church of Canada, 1940–41*, UMASC, A13-20, box 15, file 7.

161 *Eighteenth Annual Report of the WMS of the United Church of Canada, 1942–43*, UMASC, A13-20, box 15, file 7.

162 Ibid.

163 Letter from Adelaide Harrison (Chengdu) to Mrs. Taylor (Toronto), 7 February 1941, UCCA, WMS, 83.058C, series 5, box 61, file 73.

164 Ibid.

165 Letter from Adelaide Harrison (Chengdu) to Mrs. Taylor (Toronto), 23 February 1942, UMASC, A13-20, box 15, file 6.

166 Letter from Adelaide Harrison (Chengdu) to Mrs. Taylor (Toronto), 7 February 1941, UCCA, WMS, 83.058C, series 5, box 61, file 73.

167 Barnes, *Intimate Communities*, 136.

168 Irene Harris, 1943 Work Report from Chongqing, cited in ibid., 136.

169 Ibid., 138.

Chapter Four | WAITING TO EXHALE (1940–42): UNCERTAINTY, INTERNMENT, AND THE JAPANESE TAKEOVER OF THE PUMC

1 Letter from Winifred Harris (Chengdu) to Mrs. H.D. Taylor, August 1940, United Church of Canada Archives (UCCA), United Church of Canada Woman's Missionary Society (WMS), 83.058C, series 5, box 61, file 61.

2 Letter from William G. Sewell (Chengdu) to Friends, 18 May 1941, Rockefeller Archive Center (RAC), Rockefeller Foundation (RF), SG 1.1, series 601-China, box 22, folder 196.

3 Letter from Winifred Harris (Chengdu) to Mrs. H.D. Taylor, 20 August 1940, UCCA, WMS, 83.058C, series 5, box 61, file 59.

4 Ibid.

5 Letter from Winifred Harris (Chengdu) to Mrs. H.D. Taylor, 21 September 1940, UCCA, WMS, 83.058C, series 5, box 61, file 61.

6 Ibid.

7 Letter from Ernest B. Struthers (Chengdu) to Friends, 26 September 1940, UCCA, WMS, 83.058C, series 5, box 62, file 26.

8 Ibid.

9 Ibid.

10 "A Call to Good Samaritans: An Appeal for Medical Aid in Free China – Robert E. Brown Fund for the University Hospital, West China Union University, Chengtu, Szechwan, China" (brochure, n.d.), RAC, RF, SG 1.1, series 601-China, box 37, folder 298.

11 Letter from Adelaide Harrison (Chengdu) to Mrs. Taylor (Toronto), 7 February 1941, UCCA, WMS, 83.058C, series 5, box 61, file 70. Although the hospital was now considered a General Hospital, it was still referred to by its long-standing characteristic as the "Men's" Hospital.

12 Ibid.

13 Ibid.

14 Letter from Adelaide Harrison (Chengdu) to Mrs. Taylor (Toronto), 1942?, UCCA, WMS, 83.058C, series 5, box 61, file 74.

15 "A Call to Good Samaritans."

16 Ibid.

17 Ibid.

18 The New Life Movement was an education campaign launched by Chiang Kai-shek to mobilize the population in China to improve hygienic and behavioural standards. This was expected to lead the moral regeneration of the Chinese people, and increase public awareness of and concern for China's problems. Arif Dirlik, "The Ideological Foundations of the New Life Movement: A Study in Counterrevolution." *Journal of Asian Studies* 34, 4: 946.

19 Stephen Endicott, *James G. Endicott: Rebel Out of China* (Toronto: University of Toronto Press, 1980), 159.

20 Munroe Scott, *McClure: The China Years* (Markham, ON: Penguin Books, 1977), 284–85.

21 Ibid.

22 "A Call to Good Samaritans."

23 Ibid.

24 Ibid.

25 Lillian Bertha Craigie, "Woman's Missionary Society Notes," 1926, Glenbow Museum and Archives, M 285, box 3, file 25.

26 Ibid., 7.

27 Hocking, *Re-Thinking Missions*

28 Sonya Grypma, *Healing Henan: Canadian Nurses at the North China Mission, 1888–1947* (Vancouver: UBC Press, 2008).

29 "A Call to Good Samaritans."

30 Letter from William G. Sewell (Chengdu) to Friends, 18 May 1941, RAC, RF, SG 1.1, series 601-China, box 22, folder 196.

31 Ibid.

32 Robert E. Brown, Statement Regarding the University Hospital Needs of the West China Union University Medical College, RAC, RF, SG 1.1, series 601-China, box 22, folder 196.

33 Ibid.

34 Ibid.

35 Ibid.

36 Ibid.

37 Ibid. The Burma Road was a road linking Lashio in Burma with Kunming in China. Construction of the road started with the outbreak of the Sino-Japanese War, while Burma was still a British colony. It was used to transport goods and supplies to China.

38 Letter from Dr. Robert Brown (San Francisco?) to Dr. Allen Gregg (New York), 15 March 1941, RAC, RF, SG 1.1, series 601-China, box 22, folder 196.

39 Brown, Statement Regarding the University Hospital Needs.

40 Ibid.

41 Ibid.

42 Letter from Alan Gregg to Doctor Brown, 17 March 1941, RAC, RF, SG 1.1, series 601-China, box 22, folder 196.

43 Alan Gregg Diary, 24 March 1941, RAC, RF, SG 1.1, series 601-China, box 22, folder 196.

44 Ibid. It is not clear what the China Foundation is.

45 The controversial Boxer Indemnity dated back to 1900, when, as a result of damages that resulted from the Boxer Rebellion, China was forced to make reparation payments to the British.

46 Letter from Adelaide Harrison (Chengdu) to Mrs. Taylor (Toronto), 11 June 1942, UCCA, WMS, 83.058C, series 5, box 61, file 78.

47 Letter from Gertrude Hodgman (Beijing) to Annie Tittman (Chicago), 10 November 1938, Peking Union Medical College Archives–School of Nursing Archives (PUMC-SNA), fonds 347.

48 Sonya Grypma, *China Interrupted: Japanese Internment and the Reshaping of a Canadian Missionary Community* (Waterloo, ON: Wilfrid Laurier University Press, 2012).

49 Letter from Gertrude Hodgman (Beijing) to Anne [Anna] Tittman (Chicago), 10 November 1938, PUMC-SNA, fonds 347.

50 Letter from Anna Tittman (Chicago) to Gertrude Hodgman (Beijing), 6 March 1939, PUMC-SNA, fonds 347.

51 Letter from Gertrude Hodgman (Beijing) to Anne [Anna] Tittman (Chicago), 23 November 1939, PUMC-SNA, fonds 347.

52 Ibid.

53 Ibid.

54 Mary E. Ferguson, *China Medical Board and Peking Union Medical College: A Chronicle of Fruitful Collaboration, 1914–1951* (New York: China Medical Board of New York, 1970), 152.

55 Ibid.

56 Ibid.

57 Ibid., 154.

58 Ibid., 161.

59 Ibid., 162.

60 Peking Union Medical College, "The School of Nursing Annual Announcement, 1939–1940," 1 July 1939, Peking, China, PUMC-SNA, fonds 377.

61 Faye Whiteside Records, RAC, China Medical Board Inc. (CMB), box 106, folder 165.

62 According to camp records of Robinson's internment, she was Canadian. Greg Leck, *Captives of Empire: The Japanese Internment of Allied Civilians in China, 1941–1945* (Bangor, PA: Shandy Press, 2006), 543.

63 Ferguson, *China Medical Board*, 161.

64 Ibid.

65 Ibid., 165.

66 Minutes: Nursing Faculty Committee, 1938–1940, 27 February 1941, PUMC-SNA, fonds 340.

67 Ibid.

68 Ibid.

69 Bernice Chu [Chen], "Confidential Plans that the Technical Committee on Nursing Education Aims to Accomplish during the Years 1940–1943," 20 October 1940, RAC, RF, SG 10.1, series 601-China, subseries 601L, box 22, Fellowship Files.

70 Ibid., 1

71 Ibid.

72 Ibid.

73 Ibid.

74 Ibid., 1–4.

75 Ibid.

76 Note that the report uses the initials "$LC" to denote currency. It is not clear whether this is Chinese or other currency.

77 The others were the Methodist Mission School of Nursing in Fuling and the Mission Huitien School of Nursing in Kunming. Ibid.

78 Letter from M.C. Balfour (New York) to Miss Chu (Chongqing), 15 January 1941, RAC, RF, SG 10.1, series 601-China, subseries 601L, box 22, Fellowship Files.

79 Ibid.

80 Ibid. Although Balfour identified this only as the "Chengdu School," I presume he was referring to the Canadian Mission School of Nursing in Chengdu, since that was the only one listed in Chengdu in Chu Chen's Confidential Plans.

81 Ibid.

82 Letter from M.C. Balfour (New York) to Dr. Y.C. Wang (Chongqing), 1 May 1941, RAC RF, SG 10.1, series 601-China, subseries 601L, box 22, Fellowship Files.

83 Ibid.

84 Ibid.

85 Note from M.C. Balfour (New York) to Mary E. Tennant (New York), 27 October 1941, RAC, RF, SG 10.1, series 601-China, subseries 601L, box 22, Fellowship Files.

86 Letter from M.C. Balfour (New York) to Dr. Wang (Chongqing), 1 May 1941, RAC RF, SG 10.1, series 601-China, subseries 601L, box 22, Fellowship Files.

87 Ferguson, *China Medical Board*, 166.

88 Ibid., 168.

89 Ibid.

90 Ibid., 169.

91 Ibid., 171.

92 Ibid.

93 Vera Nieh interview with Anne Davis, ca. 1985 (audiotape in author's possession).

94 Margaret May Prentice was a missionary with the Woman's Foreign Missionary Society of the Methodist Church, who had been at the Isabella Fisher Hospital in Tianjin since 1924. Chao Pei-chen was a graduate of the Peking Presbyterian Hospital nursing program; the Douw Hospital was also in Beijing. Margaret May Prentice, *Unwelcome at the Northeast Gate* (Mission, KS: Inter-Collegiate Press, 1966).

95 Ferguson, *China Medical Board*, 174.

96 Margaret May Prentice, *Unwelcome at the Northeast Gate* (Mission, KS: Inter-Collegiate Press, 1966), 83.

97 Vera Nieh, "A Brief Account of the PUMC School of Nursing during and after World War II: A Message to Its Alumnae," unpublished report, 25 September 1948, PUMC-SNA, fonds 742.

98 Nieh, interview.

99 Prentice, *Unwelcome at the Northeast Gate*, 83.

100 Ibid.

101 Ibid., 84.

102 Ibid., 84.

103 Nieh, interview.

104 Ferguson, *China Medical Board*, 174.

105 Nieh, "A Brief Account of the PUMC School of Nursing."

106 Prentice, *Unwelcome at the Northeast Gate*, 85.

107 Letter from Stephen Chang to Claude E. Forkner, July 1943, RAC, Office of the Messrs. Rockefeller records, serios O, box 13, folder 111.
108 Ibid.
109 May [Mary?] Ferguson, "Report on the Peking Union Medical College," 15 May 1942, PUMC-SNA, fonds 806.
110 Ibid., 1.
111 Ibid., 1.
112 Vera Nieh, *A Brief Account.*
113 Ibid.
114 Ferguson, *China Medical Board,* 175.
115 Leck, *Captives of Empire,* 543.
116 In January 1942, China, the United States, and Britain formalized their agreement as allies. The Second World War was primarily fought between the Axis Powers (Germany, Italy, Japan) and the Allies. The Allies included Britain, France, Australia, Canada, New Zealand, India, the Soviet Union, and the United States.
117 Grypma, *China Interrupted.*
118 Prentice, *Unwelcome at the Northeast Gate,* 122–24.
119 "Winnipeg Nurse Moved by Japs," newspaper clipping, 30 May 1942, Winnipeg General Hospital / Health Sciences Center Archives.
120 Prentice, *Unwelcome at the Northeast Gate,* 78–80.
121 Ibid., 79.
122 Ibid.
123 Ibid., 80.
124 Letter from Chang to Forkner.
125 Ferguson, *China Medical Board,* 175.
126 Ibid., 173.
127 Letter from Chang to Forkner.
128 Mary Ferguson, "Peking, China, December 8, 1941–September 15, 1943," n.d., RAC, CMB, box 57, folder 397.
129 Ibid.
130 Ibid.
131 May [Mary?] Ferguson, "Report on the Peking Union Medical College," 15 May 1942, PUMC-SNA, fonds 806, 2.
132 Ibid.
133 Letter from Chang to Forkner.
134 Ibid.
135 Ibid.
136 Dr. Harold Loucks, a surgeon, was interned at Weixian Camp in March 1943 and repatriated in September 1943. It is not clear whether Dr. Fortuyn was interned.
137 Letter from Chang to Forkner.

138 Ibid. A civilian Japanese physician, Dr. Mashuhashi, was well known at the PUMC (spending many mornings, as he did, at the PUMC medical library). He was appointed immediately by the Japanese to take charge of the PUMC and its library.

139 Ibid.

140 Ibid.

141 Ibid.

142 Ibid.

143 Ferguson, *China Medical Board*, 175.

144 Ferguson, "Report on the Peking Union Medical College."

145 Letter from Chang to Forkner.

146 Ibid.

147 Ferguson, "Report on the Peking Union Medical College."

148 Ibid.

149 Letter from Chang to Forkner.

150 Ibid.

151 Ferguson, *China Medical Board*, 175.

152 Ibid.

153 Ferguson, "Report on the Peking Union Medical College."

154 Letter from Chang to Forkner.

155 Ibid.

156 Ibid.

157 Ibid.

158 Nieh, interview.

159 Ibid.

160 Ferguson, "Report on the Peking Union Medical College."

161 Letter from Chang to Forkner

162 Ferguson, *China Medical Board*, 176.

163 Letter from Chang to Forkner.

164 Ibid.

165 Ibid.

166 Ibid.

167 Ibid.

168 Ibid.

169 Ibid.

170 Ferguson, *China Medical Board*, 176.

171 Ibid.

172 Letter from Chang to Forkner.

173 Ibid.

174 Ibid.

175 Ferguson, *China Medical Board*, 176.

176 Nieh, "A Brief Account of the PUMC School of Nursing."
177 Ferguson, *China Medical Board*, 177.
178 Nieh, "A Brief Account of the PUMC School of Nursing."
179 Ibid.
180 Letter from Chang to Forkner.
181 Ibid.
182 Ferguson, "Report on the Peking Union Medical College."
183 Letter from Chang to Forkner; Ferguson, "Report on the Peking Union Medical College."
184 Letter from Chang to Forkner. Unless otherwise noted, quotations and other information in this section are taken from this document.
185 Ferguson, "Peking, China, December 8, 1941–September 15, 1943."
186 Hamish Ion, "Much Ado about Too Few: Aspects of the Treatment of Canadian and Commonwealth POWs and Civilian Internees in Metropolitan Japan, 1941–1945," *Defence Studies* 6, 3 (2006): 293.
187 Counts taken from Camp Nominal Rolls in Leck, *Captives of Empire*.
188 The numbers are difficult to calculate for certain. Of the 245 American missionaries, 107 were single women who may have also been nurses but are listed primarily as missionaries. Similarly, in the Canadian list I have included three Canadian nurses whom I know through my previous studies, but, since they were all married to British husbands, they are not listed as Canadian or as nurses. Undoubtedly there are other married nurses whose roles and nationality are subsumed under their husbands' and therefore are impossible to include in the calculations. Also, I did not include Yangzhou Camps in the calculation, as these internees were all transferred there from other camps, and were therefore already accounted for.
189 Mary Ferguson, "Peking, China, December 8, 1941–September 15, 1943."
190 Ibid.
191 Ibid.
192 Leck, *Captives of Empire*, 488.
193 Grypma, *China Interrupted*, 141–42.
194 Brigette C. Kamsler, "The Gripsholm Exchange and Repatriation Voyages," 17 September 2012, Burke Library Blog, Columbia University Libraries, https://blogs.cul.columbia.edu/burke/2012/09/17/the-gripsholm-exchange-and-repatriation-voyages-2/.
195 Ferguson, "Peking, China, December 8, 1941–September 15, 1943"; In the list of internees at the Peking British Embassy Camp, only these three had the additional note "held in detention." Leck, *Captives of Empire*, 488 and 592–93.
196 "Peking Union Medical College, Yenching University Abolished: Japanese Army Authorities Get Proofs of Their Pro-Chungking Activities," 13 or 14 February 1942, RAC CMB box 125, folder 910.

197 Ibid.
198 Ibid.
199 Ferguson, "Report on the Peking Union Medical College."
200 Ibid.
201 Letter from Chang to Forkner.
202 Ibid.
203 Ibid.
204 Ferguson, "Report on the Peking Union Medical College."
205 Ibid.
206 Ibid.
207 Letter from Chang to Forkner.
208 Ferguson, "Report on the Peking Union Medical College."
209 Leck, *Captives of Empire*, 543.
210 Ferguson, "Peking, China, December 8, 1941–September 15, 1943."
211 The distance between these two points is uncertain, but presumably a distance normally not taken on foot, and likely the equivalent of a few city blocks.
212 Leck, *Captives of Empire*, 587.
213 Ibid.
214 Ibid.
215 Ferguson, "Peking, China, December 8, 1941–September 15, 1943."
216 Ibid.
217 Grypma, *China Interrupted*, 182.
218 Leck, *Captives of Empire*, 592, 593.
219 Letter from Chang to Forkner.
220 Ibid.
221 Ferguson, *China Medical Board*, 179.
222 According to Ferguson, these included Dr. H.H. Anderson, Dr. J.L. Boots, Miss M.E. Ferguson, Miss E.H. Hirst, Dr. H.H. Loucks, Miss M. McMillan, Mrs. M.I. Pratt, Miss. E.E. Robinson, Dr F.E. Whitaker, Miss F. Whiteside, and Miss M. Wyne. Ibid., 185. However, there is no record of Whitaker in the camp nominal roll lists. Leck, *Captives of Empire*.
223 Ibid.
224 Letter from Chang to Forkner.
225 Cited in Leck, *Captives of Empire*, 488.
226 In Stephen Chang's letter, Miss McMillan is described as a physiotherapist. In the Weishien Camp Nominal Rolls, she is listed as a nurse.
227 Letter from Chang to Forkner.
228 Ibid.
229 Ibid.

230 Ibid.
231 Ibid.

Chapter Five | STARTING OVER IN WEST CHINA (1943–45):
DISPLACEMENT AND REIMAGINING ELITE NURSING IN FREE CHINA

1 "Educational Progress in Wartime China," *Timely Topics*, no. 5 (Chinese News Service), 1943(?).
2 Ibid.
3 Memorandum, West China Union University Medical School, 8 April 1943, Rockefeller Archive Center (RAC), China Medical Board Inc. (CMB), box 158, folder 1154.
4 Ibid.; emphasis in original.
5 Nicole Elizabeth Barnes, *Intimate Communities: Wartime Healthcare and the Birth of Modern China, 1937–1945* (Oakland: University of California Press, 2018), 138.
6 Here I am estimating the number of nursing students at Chongqing as 100, since the Chengdu nursing school, which also took in 40 students, had 95 students in 1942. The figure of 50 out-of-province students comes from Barnes, *Intimate Communities*, 140.
7 Minutes, College of Medicine and Dentistry, WCUU, 4 June 1942, UMASC, A13-20, box 15, file 6.
8 *Eighteenth Annual Report of the WMS of the United Church of Canada, 1942–43*, UMASC, A13-20, box 15, file 7.
9 "University Hospital Building Situation, the College of Medicine and Dentistry WCUU," 10 March 1943, RAC, CMB, box 158, folder 1154.
10 Kilborn, "School of Nursing, The College of Medicine and Dentistry."
11 Ibid.
12 *Seventeenth Annual Report of the WMS of the United Church of Canada, 1941–42*, UMASC, A13-20, box 15, file 7.
13 Ibid.
14 Letter from Adelaide Harrison (Chengdu) to Miss Buck (Toronto?), 12 November 1942, United Church of Canada Archives (UCCA), United Church of Canada Woman's Missionary Society (WMS), 83.058C, series 5, box 62, file 63.
15 Letter from Jesse H. Arnup (Toronto) to Dr. Bell (Chengdu), 30 November 1942, UMASC, A13-20, box 15, file 6.
16 B. Hensman, "Kilborn Family: A Record of a Canadian Family's Service to Medical Work and Education in China and Hong Kong," *Canadian Medical Association Journal* 97, 9 (1967): 471–83.
17 Ibid.

18 Letter from Adelaide Harrison (Chengdu) to Mrs. Taylor (Toronto), 9 December 1942, UCCA, WMS, 83.058C, series 5, box 61, file 82.

19 Letter from Caroline Wellwood (Bombay) to Mrs. Taylor (Toronto), 26 March 1943, UCCA, WMS, 83.058C, series 5, box 65, file 37.

20 Letter from Caroline Wellwood (Lingham?), 5 July 1943, UCCA, WMS, 83-058C, series 5, box 65, file 39.

21 *Eighteenth Annual Report of the WMS of the United Church of Canada, 1942–43,* UMASC, A13-20, box 15, file 7.

22 Ibid.

23 *Nineteenth Annual Report of the WMS of the United Church of Canada, 1943–44,* UMASC, A13-20, box 15, file 7.

24 Letter from Adelaide Harrison? (Chengdu) to Mrs. Taylor (Toronto), 18 January 1943, UCCA, WMS, 83-058C, series 5, box 61, file 90.

25 Ibid.

26 Letter from Adelaide Harrison (Chengdu) to Miss Buck (Toronto), 6 April 1943, UCCA, WMS, 83-058C, series 5, box 63, file 1.

27 Letter from Assistant Treasurer (Toronto?) to Inspector of Income Tax (Toronto), 28 April 1945, UCCA, WMS, 83.058C, series 5, box 64, file 43.

28 Letter from Adelaide Harrison (Chengdu) to Mrs. Taylor (Toronto), 23 May 1943, UCCA, WMS, 83,058C, series 5, box 61, file 98.

29 Ibid.

30 Ibid.

31 Ibid.

32 Ibid.

33 Letter from L. Kilborn (Chengdu) to Dr. T. Harry Williams (Chongqing), 21 April 1943, UMASC, A13-20, box 15, file 6.

34 Letter from Adelaide Harrison (Chengdu) to Mrs. Taylor (Toronto), 23 May 1943, UCCA, WMS, 83.058C, series 5, box 61, file 98.

35 Letter from Adelaide Harrison (Chengdu) to Mrs. Taylor (Toronto), 1 May 1943, UMASC, A13-20, box 15, file 6.

36 Letter from Adelaide Harrison (Chengdu) to Mrs. Taylor (Toronto), 7 June 1943, UCCA, WMS, 83.58C, box 63, file 4.

37 Letter from Dr. A.E. Best (Chengtu) to "Friends of Centennial," 26 December 1943, UMASC, A13-30, box 15, folder 6.

38 Telegram from Wong Wen-hao (Chongqing) to E. Lobenstine (New York), 9 September 1942, RAC, CMB, box 143, folder 1038.

39 Letter from Wang Hsui-ying (Chengdu) to Misses Hodgman and Tennant (New York), 5 April 1944, RAC, RF, SG 1.1, series 601-China, box 37, folder 298.

40 Report from MCB [M.C. Balfour, Chengdu] to Mr. Lobenstine, 30 January 1943, RAC, CMB, box 143, folder 1038.

41 Report from MCB [M.C. Balfour, Chengdu] to Mr. Lobenstine, 30 January 1943, RAC, CMB, box 143, folder 1038; excerpt ECL [Edwin C. Lobenstine] to CEF [Claude E. Forkner], 27 May 1943, RAC, CMB, box 143, folder 1038.

42 Ibid.

43 Report from MCB [M.C. Balfour, Chengdu] to Mr. Lobenstine, 30 January 1943, RAC, CMB, box 143, folder 1038.

44 Ibid.

45 Ibid.

46 Ibid.

47 Ibid.

48 Minutes of the Meeting on the Subcommittee on the School of Nursing, 22 February 1943, Chongqing, RAC, CMB, box 143, folder 1038.

49 Ibid.

50 Letter from Marshall Balfour (India) to Mr. Lobenstine (New York), 19 April 1943, RAC, CMB, box 143, folder 1038; letter from the Director of the CMB [Claude Forkner] and Steve [Chang] to "All the teaching staff and graduates of the PUMC," RAC, CMB, box 143, folder 1038.

51 Claude Forkner, Letter to CMB National Institute of Health, Koloshan, Chongqing, 23 May 1943RAC, CMB, box 143, folder 1038.

52 Ibid.

53 Ibid.

54 Ibid.

55 Ibid.

56 Letter from the Director of the CMB [Claude Forkner] and Steve [Chang] to "All the teaching staff and graduates of the PUMC," 26 June 1943, RAC, CMB, box 143, folder 1038.

57 Ibid.

58 Ibid.

59 Letter from Claude Forkner (Chongqing) to Mr. Lobenstine and Miss Pearce (New York), 3 July 1943, RAC, CMB, box 143, folder 1038.

60 Ibid.

61 Ibid.

62 Ibid.

63 Ibid.

64 Telegram from Wong Wen-Hao and [Claude] Forkner to Edwin Lobenstine, 10 July 1943, RAC, CMB, box 143, folder 1038.

65 Excerpt from letter from Claude Forkner to Leslie Kilborn, 3 July 1943, RAC, CMB, box 143, folder 1038.

66 Ibid.

67 Ibid.

68 Memorandum on Recent Developments in the Wartime Program of the China Medical Board That Are of Special Interest to the West China Union University, 2 September 1943, RAC, CMB, box 158, folder 1154.

69 Ibid.

70 Excerpt from letter from Claude Forkner to Leslie Kilborn, 3 July 1943, RAC, CMB, box 143, folder 1038.

71 Ibid.

72 Confidential letter from Claude Forkner (Koloshan) to Mr. Lobenstine and Miss Pearce (New York), 11 July 1943, RAC, CMB, box 143, folder 1038.

73 Telegram from Edwin Lobenstine (New York?) to Claude Forkner (Chongqing), 15 July 1943, RAC, CMB, box 143, folder 1038.

74 Telegram from Vera Nieh (Chongqing) to Edwin Lobenstine (New York), 16 July 1943, RAC, CMB, box 143, folder 1038.

75 Confidential letter from Claude Forkner (Koloshan) to Mr. Lobenstine and Miss Pearce (New York), 11 July 1943, RAC, CMB, box 143, folder 1038.

76 Ibid.

77 Ibid.

78 Memorandum on Recent Developments in the Wartime Program of the China Medical Board.

79 Confidential letter from Claude Forkner (Koloshan) to Mr. Lobenstine and Miss Pearce (New York), RAC, CMB, box 143, folder 1038.

80 Excerpt letter from ECL [Edwin Lobenstine] to CEF [Claude Forkner], 15 July 1943, RAC, CMB, box 143, folder 1038.

81 Letter from "Three Branch Party" to "Lady Members," 22 July 1943, RAC, CMB, box 143, folder 1038.

82 Ibid.

83 Letter from Claude Forkner to Chang Wen-po, 28 July 1943, RAC, CMB, box 143, folder 1038.

84 Letter from M.C. Balfour (Delhi) to Claude [Forkner] (Koloshan), 29 July 1943, RAC, CMB, box 143, folder 1038.

85 Ibid.

86 Ibid.

87 Ibid.

88 Ibid.

89 Letter from Edwin C. Lobenstine (New York?) to Miss Nieh (Chengdu), 28 July 1943, RAC, CMB, box 104, folder 747A.

90 Ibid.

91 Vera Nieh, interview by Anne Davis, ca. 1985 (audiotape in author's possession).

92 Ibid.

93 Ibid.

94 Excerpt from CEF [Claude E. Forkner] to ECL [Edwin C. Lobenstine] Memo #34 21 October 1943, RAC, CMB, box 104, folder 747A.

95 Nieh, interview.

96 Ibid.

97 Letter from Wang Hsui-ying (Chengdu) to Misses Hodgman and Tennant (New York), 5 April 1944, RAC, RF, SG 1.1, series 601-China, box 37, folder 298.

98 Ibid.

99 Letter from [Ed Cunningham?] (Chengdu?) to Dr. T.H. Williams (Chongqing), 27 August 1943, UMASC, A13-20, box 15, file 6.

100 Report by Preliminary Committee on School of Nursing, 5 August 1943, Peking Union Medical College Archives–School of Nursing Archives (PUMC-SNA), fonds 337.

101 "Faculty Meeting II" PUMC School of Nursing. 13 October 1943, PUMC-SNA, fonds 343.

102 UCC WMS DB Foreign Missions Committee, 13 April 1944, UMASC, A13-20, box 15, file 6.

103 Minutes, Seventh Joint Council, West China Mission, United Church of Canada, Chengdu, January 1945, UMASC, A13-20, box 15, file 6.

104 Ibid.

105 Vera Nieh, "A Brief Account of the PUMC School of Nursing during and after World War II: A Message to Its Alumnae," unpublished report, 25 September 1948, PUMC-SNA, fonds 742.

106 Ibid.

107 "Faculty Meeting I," Minutes, 24 September 1943, PUMC-SNA, fonds 343.

108 Letter from Adelaide Harrison (Chengdu) to Mrs. Taylor (Toronto), 9 November 1943, UMASC, A13-20, box 15, file 6.

109 UCC WMS DB Foreign Missions Committee, 14 September 1944, UMASC, A13-20, box 15, file 6. Margaret Lee became Mrs. Margaret Lee Lu.

110 "News about Nursing, New School in Chengtu, China," *American Journal of Nursing* 44, 1 (1944): 82

111 "News from China," *American Journal of Nursing* 44, 5 (1944): 504.

112 "News about Nursing," 82.

113 Ibid.

114 Nieh, "A Brief Account of the PUMC School of Nursing."

115 Preliminary Committee on School of Nursing, 5 August 1943, PUMC-SNA, fonds 337.

116 Letter from Wang Hsui-ying (Chengdu) to Misses Hodgman and Tennant (New York), 5 April 1944, RAC, RF, SG 1.1, series 601-China, box 37, folder 298.

117 Nieh, interview.

118 Letter from Wang Hsui-ying (Chengdu) to Misses Hodgman and Tennant (New York), 5 April 1944, RAC, RF, SG 1.1, series 601-China, box 37, folder 298.

119 Minutes of the Committee on Students' Standing, 14 September 1943, PUMC-SNA, fonds 337.

120 Letter from Roger S. Greene (Beijing) to Mary Beard (New York), 9 December 1936, RAC, RF, SG 1.1, series 601-China, box 37, folder 298.

121 Ibid.

122 Mary Bullock, *An American Transplant: The Rockefeller Foundation and Peking Union Medical College* (Berkeley: University of California Press, 1980), 196.

123 Faculty Committee Meetings Minutes, 27 September 1945, PUMC-SNA, fonds 340.

124 Bullock, *American Transplant*, 196.

125 Ibid.

126 Margaret Lee, "Annual Report of the West China Mission, Chengdu Hospital," in *Nineteenth Annual Report of the WMS of the United Church of Canada, 1943–44*.

127 Ibid.

128 Ibid.

129 Faculty Committee Meeting Minutes, 8 December 1943, PUMC-SNA, fonds 340.

130 *Faculty of Medicine Report of Progress, 1944*, 28 December 1944, UMASC A13-2, box 15, file 6.

131 Excerpt from letter from C.R. Cunningham, Committee Chair, to President Edgar Tang of Qilu and Dean S.H. Fong, Acting President of WCUU, 15 October 1944. The letter also noted that Dr. A.E. Best was nominated as the superintendent of the United Hospital. UMASC, A113-20, box 12, file 1.

132 Letter from Wang Hsui-ying (Chengdu) to Misses Hodgman and Tennant (New York), 5 April 1944, RAC, RF, SG 1.1, series 601-China, box 37, folder 298.

133 Faculty Committee Meeting Minutes, 13 October 1943, PUMC-SNA, fonds 340.

134 Faculty Committee Meeting Minutes, 10 November 1943, PUMC-SNA, fonds 340.

135 Faculty Committee Meeting Minutes, 31 January 1944, PUMC-SNA, fonds 340.

136 Faculty Committee Meeting Minutes, 16 February 1944, PUMC-SNA, fonds 340.

137 Letter from Wang Hsui-ying (Chengdu) to Misses Hodgman and Tennant (New York), 5 April 1944, RAC, RF, SG 1.1, series 601-China, box 37, folder 298.

138 Ibid.

139 Faculty Committee Meeting Minutes, 29 March 1944, PUMC-SNA, fonds 340.

140 Faculty Committee Meeting Minutes, 25 July 1944, PUMC-SNA, fonds 340.

141 Faculty Committee Meeting Minutes, 7 February 1945, PUMC-SNA, fonds 340.

142 Faculty Committee Meeting Minutes, 14 May 1945, PUMC-SNA, fonds 340.

143 Sonya Grypma, "In Retrospect: The Value of Feisty Students," *Journal of Christian Nursing* 28, 2 (2011): 71.

144   Faculty Committee Meeting Minutes, 12 June 1945, PUMC-SNA, fonds 340.

Chapter Six | FIGHTING THE FOUNDATION'S "DARLING CHILD"
(1943–46): CONFLICTS WITH PUMC

1   Excerpt from CEF [Claude E. Forkner] to ECL [Edwin C. Lobenstine]. Memo #34, 21 October 1943, Rockefeller Archive Center (RAC) China Medical Board Inc. (CMB), box 104, folder 747A.

2   Ibid.

3   Letter from Dr. A.E. Best (Chengdu) to "Friends of Centennial," 26 December 1943, UMASC, A13-20, box 15, file 6.

4   Ibid. It is not clear who Friends of Centennial are, but presumably a group of prospective donors in Canada and the USA.

5   Ibid.

6   Ibid.

7   Nicole Elizabeth Barnes, *Intimate Communities: Wartime Healthcare and the Birth of Modern China, 1937–1945* (Oakland: University of California Press, 2018), 153.

8   Letter from Dr. Gerald Bell (Chengdu) to Jessie Arnup, 31 March 1944, UMASC, A13-20, box 15, file 6.

9   Ibid.

10   Excerpt from MCB [Marshall C. Balfour] diary, 23 May [1947?], RAC, CMB, box 104, folder 747A.

11   Ibid.

12   Ibid.

13   Yuhong Jiang, "Shaping Modern Nursing Development in China before 1949," *International Journal of Nursing Sciences* 4, 1 (2017): 19–23.

14   Faculty Committee Meeting Minutes, 25 February 1944, PUMC-SNA, fonds 340.

15   Minutes of First Meeting of PUMC Trustees in Free China, 17 January 1944, RAC, Rockefeller Foundation (RF), SG 1.1, series 601-China, box 37, folder 298.

16   Ibid.

17   "CN" stands for Chinese currency, not Canadian currency (which is "CAD"). Chinese currency was also referred to as "dollars" and written using a "$", likely a colonial approach influenced by the fact that English keyboards only had "$" as a currency symbol.

18   Ibid.

19   Ibid.

20   Letter from Vera Nieh (Chengdu) to Dr. Claude E. Forkner (Chongqing?), 23 February 1944, RAC, RF, SG 1.1, series 601-China, box 37, folder 298.

21   Ibid.

22 Cablegram from Vera Nieh (Chengdu) to Edwin Lobenstine (New York), 23 February 1944, RAC, CMB, box 104, folder 747A.

23 Cablegram from Edwin Lobenstine (New York) to Y.T. Tsur (Guiyang), 26 February 1944, RAC, CMB, box 104, folder 747A.

24 Cablegram from Claude Forkner (Chengdu) to China Medical Board (New York), 3 March 1944, RAC, CMB, box 104, folder 747A.

25 Cablegram from Li Ting-an (Chengdu) to China Medical Board (New York), 3 March 1944, RAC, CMB, box 104, folder 747A.

26 Earle Ballou had been a missionary in China since 1916. After being repatriated to the USA on the MS Gripsholm in Septebmer 1943, he became Executive Secretary for the United Board for Christian Colleges in China. Presumably he was working in this capacity when responding to the telegram from Li Ting-an. Earle and Thelma Ballou Papers description, Archives at Yale RG 165, https://archives.yale.edu/repositories/4/resources/122.

27 Cablegram from Earle Ballou (New York) to Li Ting-an (Chengdu), 6 March 1944, RAC, CMB, box 104, folder 747A.

28 Letter from Claude Forkner (Chengdu) to Dr. Y.T. Tsur (Guiyang), 10 March 1944, RAC, CMB, box 104, folder 747A.

29 Ibid.

30 Ibid.

31 Ibid.

32 Letter from Stephen Chang (Chengdu) to Edwin Lobenstine (New York), 18 March 1944, RAC CMB, Inc., box 104, folder 747A.

33 Ibid.

34 Ibid.

35 Ibid.

36 Ibid.

37 Ibid.

38 Ibid.

39 Letter from Li Ting-an (Chengdu) to Y.T. Tsur (Guiyang), 19 March 1944, RAC, CMB, box 104, folder 747A; letter from Li Ting-an (Chengdu?) to Vera Nieh (Chengdu), 19 March 1944, RAC, CMB, box 104, folder 747A.

40 Dr. Y.T. Tsur, Outline of Regulations Governing the Administration of the PUMC School of Nursing, 1 March 1944, RAC, RF, SG 1.1, series 601-China, box 37, folder 298.

41 Ibid.

42 Letter from Faculty, PUMC School of Nursing (Chengdu) to Dr. Y.T. Tsur (Guiyang), 20 March 1944, RAC, RF, SG 1.1, series 601-China, box 37, folder 298.

43 Ibid.

44 Ibid.

45 Letter from Li Ting-an (Chengdu) to Y.T. Tsur (Guiyang), 19 March 1944, RAC, CMB, box 104, folder 747A.

46 Ibid.

47 Excerpt of letter from ECL (New York?) to Dr. Wong Wen-hao (Chengdu?), 21 March 1944, RAC, CMB, box 104, folder 747A.

48 Ibid.

49 Letter from Wang Hsui-ying (Chengdu) to Misses Hodgman and Tennant (New York), 5 April 1944, RAC, RF, SG 1.1, series 601-China, box 37, folder 298.

50 Ibid.

51 Ibid.

52 Ibid.

53 Ibid.

54 Letter from Gertrude Hodgman (Brazil) to Vera Nieh, Wang Hsui-ying, Mary Sia, "and others," RAC, RF, SG 1.1, series 601-China, box 37, folder 298.

55 Ibid.

56 Letter from Kathleen King (New York) to Gertrude Hodgman (New York?), 6 July 1944, RAC, CMB, box 102, folder 730.

57 Excerpt of Minutes, Trustees, PUMC, 13 October 1944, RAC, CMB, box 104, folder 747A.

58 Excerpt of letter from Dr. C.C. Chen to Dr. Forkner, 12 March 1945, RAC, CMB, box 104, folder 747A.

59 Ibid.

60 Executive Committee, PUMC Trustees (Chengdu?), 1 March 1945, RAC, CMB, box 104, folder 747A.

61 Excerpt of letter from Dr. C.C. Chen to Dr. Forkner, 12 March 1945, RAC, CMB, box 104, folder 747A.

62 Ibid.

63 Letter from Dr. Claude Forkner (Chengdu) to Dr. C.C. Chen (Chengdu), 13 March 1945, RAC, CMB, box 104, folder 747A.

64 Ibid.

65 Letter from M.C. Balfour (New York?) to Agnes M. Pearce (New York), 7 June 1945, RAC, CMB, box 104, folder 747A.

66 Ibid.

67 Minutes, Executive Committee, PUMC Trustees, 26 July 1945, RAC, CMB, box 104, folder 747A.

68 Letter from Dr. Y.T. Tsur to Dr. Sao-ke Alfred Sze, 25 August 1945, RAC, CMB, box 104, folder 747A.

69 Ibid.

70 Excerpt from MCB diary, 23 May [1947?], RAC, CMB, box 104, folder 747A.

71 Faculty Committee Meeting Minutes, 21 August 1945, PUMC-SNA, fonds 340.

72 Ibid.

73 Note regarding PUMC Nursing School meeting, 25 July 1945, UMASC, A13-20, box 17, file 16.

74 Letter from Mary Elizabeth Tennant (Beijing) to Mrs. Henrietta A. Loughran (Colorado), 25 February 1947, PUMC-SNA, file 1937-2437.

75 Ibid.

76 College of Medicine and Dentistry Minutes, 27 January 1944, UMASC, A13-20, box 15, file 6.

77 College of Medicine and Dentistry Minutes, 16 March 1944, UMASC, A13-20, box 15, file 6.

78 It is not clear when in 1944 this tentative plan was proposed, or whether before or after the College of Medicine and Dentistry resolution.

79 Eva Liu (?), "A College Grade Nursing School: Presentation of a Tentative Plan" (1944?), UMASC, A13-20, box 12, file 1.

80 Ibid.

81 Ibid.

82 Note regarding PUMC Nursing School meeting, 25 July 1945, UMASC, A13-20, box 17, file 16.

83 Letter from E.R. Cunningham (Chengdu) to M.E. Streeter (Chengdu), 18 March 1944, UMASC, A13-20, box 12, file 1.

84 Ibid.

85 Letter from E.R. Cunningham (Chengdu) to T.A. Li (Chengdu), 21 March 1944, UMASC, A13-20, box 12, file 1.

86 Letter from E.R. Cunningham (Chengdu) to S.H. Fong (Chengdu), 21 March 1944, UMASC, A13-20, box 12, file 1.

87 Letter from Connie Ward (Chengdu) to Dr. Cunningham (Chengdu), 10 April 1944, UMASC, A13-20, box 12, file 1.

88 Letter from Li Ting-an (Chengdu) to Dr. E.R. Cunningham (Chengdu), 28 April 1944, UMASC, A13-20, box 12, file 1.

89 Table included in letter from Vera Nieh (Chengdu) to T.A. Li (Chengdu), 30 April 1945, UMASC, A13-20, box 12, file 1.

90 Letter from Vera Nieh (Chengdu) to T.A. Li (Chengdu), 30 April 1945, UMASC, A13-20, box 12, file 1.

91 Ibid.

92 Ibid.

93 Ibid.

94 Cited in Mary Bullock, *American Transplant: The Rockefeller Foundation and Peking Union Medical College* (Berkeley: University of California Press, 1980), 195.

Chapter Seven | "OUR TRIUMPHANT RETURN" (1946–49):
POSTWAR DREAMS AND DASHED HOPES

1 Sonya Grypma, *China Interrupted: Japanese Internment and the Reshaping of a Canadian Missionary Community* (Waterloo, ON: Wilfrid Laurier University Press, 2012), 219.

2 Sonya Grypma, *Healing Henan: Canadian Nurses at the North China Mission, 1888–1947* (Vancouver: UBC Press, 2008), 215–16.

3 Letter from General Secretary (Toronto?) to Commissioner of Immigration, Department of Mines and Resources (Ottawa), 12 February 1945, Anglican Church of Canada / General Synod Archives (ACC/GSA) Missionary Society of the Church of England in Canada (MSCC), GS75-103/3, series 3.3, box 78, file 104. Interestingly Kelsey would be working under the auspices of the Qilu University rather than the WCUU, likely because the request was initiated by Dr. Ernest Struthers, a Canadian missionary with the North China Mission who was refugeeing with Qilu in Chengdu.

4 Letter from (Canon) L.A. Dixon to Mrs. Taylor, 3 February 1945 and from Foreign Mission Executive Secretary to Canon L.A. Dixon, 9 February 1945, United Church of Canada Archives (UCCA), United Church of Canada Woman's Missionary Society (WMS), 83.058C, series 3, box 56, file 17.

5 Susie Kelsey, Class of 1923 graduation photo, and Irene Harris, notations in records that she was from Class of 1919. Winnipeg General Hospital/Health Sciences Center Archives.

6 Grypma, *China Interrupted*, 244–45.

7 Letter from Susie S. Kelsey (Chungking) to Miss Watts (Henan), 28 October 1945, ACC/GSA, MSCC, GS75-103/3, series 3.3, box 78, file 104.

8 Ibid.

9 Ibid.

10 Ibid.

11 Ibid.

12 Letter from Susie Kelsey (Sanqui) to Canon L.A. Dixon, 4 February 1946, ACC/GSA, MSCC, GS75-103/3, series 3.3, box 78, file 104.

13 Letter from [member of Anglican Office, Toronto?] to Mrs. R.E. Wodehouse (Ottawa), 29 January 1946, ACC/GSA, MSCC, GS75-103/3, series 3.3, box 78, file 104.

14 S.S. Kelsey, letter to the editor, 28 January 1946, *Living Message* 57 (April 1946): 128–29, ACC/GSA, MSCC, GS75-103/3, series 3.3, box 78, file 104.

15 Letter from Susie Kelsey (Sanqui) to Rev. Canon L.A. Dixon (Toronto), 17 March 1946, ACC/GSA, MSCC, GS75-103/3, series 3.3, box 78, file 104.

16 Kelsey, Letter to the Editor, *Living Message*.

17 Ibid.

18 Susie Kelsey, *Report for the Year Ending March 15, 1948*, ACC/GSA, MSCC, GS75-103/3, series 3.3, box 78, file 104.

19 Ibid.

20 Grypma, *Healing Henan*.

21 Ibid.

22 Ibid.

23 Minutes of Planning Committee on Nursing Education, 2 October to 6 November 1945, UMASCA13-20, box 12, file 1.

24 Ibid.

25 It is not clear who R. Westra was. She is not in any of the personnel lists of the Woman's Missionary Society I was able to review, as either a nurse or other missionary.

26 Minutes of Planning Committee on Nursing Education, 2 October to 6 November 1945.

27 Ibid.

28 Ibid.

29 Ibid.

30 Letter to Sir or Madame from H.D. Robertson (Chengdu), 20 December 1945, UMASC, A13-20, box 12, file 1.

31 Letter from S.H. Fong to Leslie G. Kilborn, 28 February 1946, UMASC, A13-20, box 12, file 1.

32 Letter from Leslie Kilborn to Mr. Fong, 8 March 1946, UMASC, A13-20, box 12, file 1.

33 Minutes of the WCUU College of Medicine and Dentistry, 19 April 1946, UMASC, A13-20, box 12, file 1.

34 Ibid.

35 WCUU Minutes of General Faculty, 4 May 1946, UMASC, A13-20, box 12, file 2.

36 Extract from WCCU Associate Board of Directors *Planning Committee Report* (1945 edition), UMASC, A13-20, box 12, file 1.

37 Ibid.

38 Nursing Education reply from Ministry of Education, 17 May 1946, UMASC, A13-20, box 12, file 2.

39 Ibid.

40 Ibid.

41 Ibid.

42 Letter from Dr. Y.T. Tsur to Dr. Sao-ke Alfred Sze, 25 August 1945, RAC, CMB, box 104, folder 747A.

43 Ibid.

44 Ibid.

45 Ibid.

46 Excerpt of letter from Dr. Kilborn (Chengdu) to Dr. Balfour (New York?), RAC, CMB, box 144, folder 1042.

47 Ibid.

48 Ibid.

49 Minutes, PUMC Trustees, Executive Committee, 26 February 1946, RAC, CMB, box 158, folder 1042, folder 1154; minutes, Executive Committee Meeting, 26 February 1946, RAC, CMB, box 144, folder 1042.

50 Minutes, PUMC, Trustees, Executive Committee, 26 February 1946.

51 Minutes, Executive Committee Meeting, 26 February 1946.

52 Minutes, PUMC, Trustees, Executive Committee, 26 February 1946.

53 Ibid.

54 Letter from MEF (Chongqing) to Miss Nieh (Chengdu), 17 February 1946, RAC, CMB, box 144, folder 1042.

55 Excerpt of letter from Vera Nieh to M.E. Ferguson, 16 April 1946, RAC, CMB, box 104, folder 747A.

56 Ibid.

57 Ibid.

58 Letter from Vera [Nieh] (Chengdu) to Mary [Ferguson] (New York?), 16 April 1946, RAC, CMB, box 144, folder 1042.

59 Letter from Vera Nieh (Chengdu) to Dr. Tsur (Chongqing), 13 April 1946, RAC, CMB, box 144, folder 1042.

60 Letter from Bernice Chu Chen to Dr. Balfour, 20 April 1946, UMASC, A13-20, box 17, file 16.

61 Letter from Elsie M. Priest (Chengdu) to Mary Ferguson (New York), 19 May 1946, RAC, CMB, box 144, folder 1042.

62 Ibid.

63 Ibid.

64 Letter from Leslie Kilborn (Chengdu) to Dr. M.C. Balfour (Delhi), 24 April 1946, RAC, CMB, box 144, folder 1042.

65 Ibid.

66 Ibid.

67 Letter from MCB (Delhi) to Dr. L.G. Kilborn (Chengdu), 9 May 1946, RAC, CMB, box 144, folder 1042.

68 Ibid.

69 Letter from MF [Mary Ferguson?] to Bal [M.C. Balfour] (Shanghai), 24 May 1946. RAC, CMB, box 144, folder 1042.

70 Ibid.

71 Ibid.

72 Ibid.; emphasis in original.

73   Ibid.

74   Letter from Elsie M. Priest (Chengdu) to Mary Ferguson (New York), 19 May 1946, RAC, CMB, box 144, folder 1042.

75   Ibid.

76   Ibid.

77   Ibid.

78   Vera Nieh, "A Brief Account of the PUMC School of Nursing during and after World War II: A Message to Its Alumnae," unpublished report, 25 September 1948, PUMC-SNA, fonds 742: 1–9.

79   Letter from I.C. Yuan to Dr. Alan Gregg, 31 May 1946, RAC, CMB, box 104, folder 747A. It is unclear what "the Commission" refers to.

80   Ibid.

81   Ibid.

82   Ibid.

83   Ibid.

84   Nieh, "A Brief Account of the PUMC School of Nursing," 2.

85   Ibid., 3.

86   Vera Nieh, interview by Anne Davis, ca. 1985 (audiotape in author's possession).

87   Nieh, "A Brief Account of the PUMC School of Nursing," 3

88   Ibid.

89   Ibid.,

90   Ibid., 4.

91   Faculty Committee Meeting Minutes, 14 July 1947, PUMC-SNA, fonds 340.

92   Nieh, "A Brief Account of the PUMC School of Nursing," 5.

93   Ibid., 6

94   Ibid., 3.

95   Ibid.

96   Ibid., 7.

97   Ibid.

98   Ibid.

99   Ibid.

100 Ibid.

101 Letter from Assistant Treasurer (Toronto?) to Winifred Harris (Chengdu), 5 September 1947, UCCA, WMS, 83.058C, series 5, box 63, file 15; Letter from Assistant Treasurer (Toronto?) to Winifred Harris (Chengdu), 12 September 1947, UCCA, WMS, 83.058C, series 5, box 63, file 18; List of West China Missionary Nurses, UMASC A13-20, box 18, folder 9.

102 Letter from Leslie Kilborn (Chengdu) to Ed and Gladys Cunningham, 6 January 1946, UMASC, A13-20, box 15, file 6.

103 Ibid.
104 Letter from Leslie Kilborn (Chengdu) to Ed and Gladys Cunningham, 25 February 1946, UMASC, A13-20, box 15, file 6.
105 Ibid.
106 Letter from Leslie Kilborn to President Fong, 25 July 1947, UMASC, A13-20, box 12, file 2.
107 Letter from S.H. Fong to Cora Kilborn, 26 July 1947, UMASC, A13-20, box 12, file 2. Wang Hui-yin was the head of the Renji Nursing School on the West China Chengdu campus. She was also called Xiao Zhang of Renji Nursing School (principal of the school) – the same title Vera Nieh held. Personal communication with Yuhong Jiang, 31 August 2020.
108 Ho Jin-chin, interview by Janet Beaton, 6 October 2000. UMASC, A13-20, box 12, file 2.
109 Ibid.
110 Ibid.
111 Chin Shu-wen, interview by Janet Beaton, 11 June 1995, UMASC, A13-20, box 12, file 2.
112 Deng Shi pu, interview by Janet Beaton, 6 October 2000, UMASC, A13-20, box 12, file 2.
113 Shu-wen, interview.
114 Pu, interview.
115 Luo Don xiu, interview by Janet Beaton, 6 October 2000, UMASC, A13-20, box 12, file 2.
116 Ho Jin-chin, interview.
117 Letter from Leslie Kilborn to President Fong, 6 October 1947, UMASC, A13-20, box 12, file 2.
118 "Ideas and Opinions and Petition from 2nd Year Students of the Department of Nursing," Notes from Janet Beaton Fonds, UMASC, A13-20, box 12, file 2.
119 Ibid.
120 Letter from Leslie Kilborn to Liu Chwan-ih, 1 December 1947, UMASC, A13-20, box 12, file 2.
121 Ibid.
122 Ibid.
123 Letter from Leslie Kilborn to President Fong, 1 December 1947, UMASC, A13-20, box 12, file 2.
124 Ibid.
125 Letter from S.H. Fong to Dr. Kilborn, 10 December 1947, UMASC, A13-20, box 12, file 2.
126 Jin-chin, interview.

127 Letter from Chang Fang-Hsiu to Dr. Kilborn, 5 June 1948, UMASC, A13-20, box 12, file 2.

Chapter Eight | THE LAST CHAPTER (1949–51):
MISSIONS, THE PUMC, AND THE END OF MODERN NURSING IN CHINA

1 "Red Cross Society of China," Wikipedia, https://en.wikipedia.org/wiki/Red_Cross_Society_of_China.

2 Sonya Grypma and Cheng Zhen, "The Development of Modern Nursing in China," in *Medical Transitions in 20th Century China*, ed. Bridie Andrews and Mary Bullock (Bloomington: Indiana University Press, 2014), 297–317.

3 Nicole Elizabeth Barnes, *Intimate Communities: Wartime Healthcare and the Birth of Modern China, 1937–1945* (Oakland: University of California Press, 2018), 200–1.

4 Susan Armstrong-Reid, *China Gadabouts: New Frontiers of Humanitarian Nursing, 1941–1951* (Vancouver: UBC Press, 2018).

5 Ibid.

6 Rana Mitter, "Imperialism, Transnationalism, and the Reconstruction of Post-War China: UNRRA in China, 1944–7," *Past and Present* 218, 8 (2013): 51–69.

7 Watt, "Development of Nursing in Modern China, 1870–1949," *Nursing History Review* 12 (2004): 71–72.

8 Ibid.

9 Letter from MET [Mary Tennant] (New York) to Dr. Hu Shih (Shanghai), 7 March 1947, Rockefeller Archive Center (RAC), Rockefeller Foundation (RF), SG 1.1, series 601-China, box 37, folder 298. While specifics of the RF Commission Report are not identified, the focus was on postwar medicine and public health.

10 Ibid.

11 Ibid.

12 Letter from Vera Nieh to Dr. Hu Shih, 21 January 1947, Peking Union Medical College Archives–School of Nursing Archives (PUMC-SNA), file 1937-2437.

13 Ibid.

14 Letter from Vera Nieh (Carmel, CA) to Dr. Lee (Beijing), 19 August 1947, PUMC-SNA, file 1937-2437.

15 Vera Nieh, interview by Anne Davis, ca. 1985 (audiotape in author's possession).

16 Y.C. Nieh, "Report of the School of Nursing," 4 November 1950, PUMC-SNA, fonds 826, 1.

17 Ibid., 1.

18 Ibid., 2.

19 Ibid., 2.

20 Ibid., 5.

21 Faculty Committee Meeting Minutes, 18 January 1951, PUMC-SNA, fonds 340.

22 Ibid.

23 Nieh, interview.

24 Immanuel C.Y. Hsu, "The Reorganisation of Higher Education in Communist China, 1949–61," *China Quarterly* 19 (1964): 138.

25 The interview is undated, but, based on the contents of this and another interview Davis completed at the same time with Madame Lin Juying, my best estimate is that this was in 1985.

26 Nieh, interview.

27 Letter from [Canadian Ambassador?] (Nanjing) to Dr. Cunningham (Chengdu), 29 November 1948, UCCA, WMS, 83.058C, series 5, box 63, file 36.

28 Ibid.

29 Letter dated 1 October 1948 from F.H. Chang to Dr. Kilborn. UMASC, A13-20, Janet Beaton fonds, box 15, file 6.

30 Excerpt from unindentified letter dated 2 December 1948 transcribed by Janet Beaton from "WMS DB Foreign Missions Committee" A13-20, Janet Beaton fonds, box 15, file 6.

31 Ibid.

32 Letter from Winifred Harris (Chengdu) to Edith McKenzie (Toronto), 7 December 1948, UCCA, WMS, 83.058C, box 63, file 44.

33 Letter from Violet Stewart (Chengdu) to Mrs. Taylor (Toronto), 28 December 1948, UCCA, WMS, 83.058C, series 5, box 64, file 236.

34 Ibid.

35 Letter from Assistant Treasurer (Toronto) to Winifred Harris (Chengdu), 23 March 1949, UCCA, WMS, 83.058C, series 5, box 63, file 47.

36 Notes, 1948, UMASC, A13-20, Janet Beaton fonds, box 15, file 6.

37 Ibid.

38 Ibid.

39 Ibid.

40 Ibid.

41 Ho Jin-chin, interview by Janet Beaton, 22 October 2000 UMASC Janet Beaton fonds, box 18, file 1.

42 Letter from Gladys S. Cunningham to Dr. Kilborn, 11 February 1950, UMASC, A13-20, box 12, file 2.

43 Letter from Leslie Kilborn to President Fong, 18 March 1950, UMASC, A13-20, box 12, file 2.

44 Excerpt of letter from Leslie Kilborn to President Fong, 21 November 1950, UMASC, A13-20, box 12, file 2.

45 Letter from Leslie Kilborn (Chengdu) to Robert J. McMullen (New York), 9 October 1950, UMASC, A13-20, box 12, file 2.

46 Ibid.

47 Ibid.

48 Excerpt from "West China Mission Executive" dated 8 December 1949 transcribed by Janet Beaton from "WMS DB Overseas Missions Committee," UMSAC, A13-20, Janet Beaton fonds, box 15, file 6.

49 Ibid.

50 Ibid.

51 Ibid.

52 Lewis C. Walmsley, *West China Union University* (New York: United Board for Christian Education in Asia, 1974), 149.

53 Ibid.

54 Cited in Alvyn Austin, *Saving China: Canadian Missionaries in the Middle Kingdom, 1888–1959* (Toronto: University of Toronto Press, 1986), 322.

55 Letter from VS (Violet Stewart) to Mrs. Taylor, 10 April 1950 (date stamped), UCCA, WMS, 83.058C, series 5, box 64, file 239.

56 Letter from Mrs. Hugh D. Taylor (Toronto) to Violet Stewart (Chengdu), 20 April 1950, UCCA, WMS, 83.058C, series 5, box 64, file 240.

57 Letter from Assistant Treasurer (Toronto) to Winifred Harris (Chengdu), 13 June 1950, UCCA, WMS, 83.058C, series 5, box 63, file 49.

58 Walmsley's *West China Union University*, 150.

59 Letter from Assistant Treasurer (Toronto) to Cora Kilborn (Toronto), 27 October 1950, UCCA, WMS, 83.058C, series 5, box 62, file 52.

60 Letter from Lillian Taylor (Toronto) to Edith McKenzie (Toronto), 5 January 1951, UCCA, WMS, 83.058C, series 5, box 65, file 33.

61 It is not clear when Burwell left, but in May 1951, she requested retirement information from the WMS, which confirmed that she had paid into the fund for 6.5 years, which suggests she was in West China from 1944 to 1950 or 1951. UCCA, WMS, 83.058C, series 5, box 64, file 4.

62 Ho Jin-chin (Chengdu), interview by Janet Beaton, Ho Jin-chin, 22 October 2000. UMASC, A13-20, box 12, file 2.

63 Ibid.

64 Walmsley's *West China Union University*, 153.

65 Ibid.

66 Ibid.

67 Ibid.

68 Letter from Winifred Harris (Hong Kong) to Edith MacKenzie (Toronto), 10 July 1951, UMASC, A13-20, box 12, file 6.

69 Ibid.

70 UCC WMS DB [?] Overseas Missions Committee, 8 March 1951, UMASC, A13-20, Janet Beaton fonds, 1950s, box 12, file 26.

71   Ibid.

72   Austin, *Saving China*, 292.

73   Ibid., 319.

74   Ibid.

75   Letter from Violet Stewart (Hong Kong) to Mrs. Taylor (Toronto), 27 February 1951, UCCA, WMS, 83.058C, series 5, box 64, file 241.

76   Ibid.

77   Ibid.

78   Letter from V [Violet Stewart] (Hong Kong?) to unknown (missing first page), n.d. (sometime between 23 March and 5 April 1951), UCCC, WMS, 83.058C, series 5, box 64, file 248.

79   Letter from Mrs. Taylor (Toronto) to Violet Stewart (Hong Kong), 16 March 1951, UCCA, WMS, 83.058C, series 5, box 64, file 243.

80   Ibid.

81   Letter from Violet Stewart (Hong Kong) to Mrs. Taylor (Toronto), 23 March 1951, UCCA, WMS, 83.058C, series 5, box 64, file 247.

82   Letter from V [Violet Stewart] (Hong Kong?) to unknown, n.d., UCCA, WMS, 83.058C, series 5, box 64, file 248.

83   Letter from Violet Stewart (Hong Kong) to Mrs. H.D. Taylor (Toronto), 18 March 1951, UCCA, WMS, 83.058C, series 5, box 64, file 245.

84   Austin, *Saving China*, 319.

85   Letter from Mrs. Hugh D. Taylor (Toronto) to Jean Stewart (Glasgow), 25 September 1951, UCCA, WMS, 83.058C, series 5, box 64, file 212.

86   Ibid.

87   Austin, *Saving China*, 320. Leslie and Jean Kilborn moved to Hong Kong, where they taught at Chung Chi College until 1963.

88   List of Missionaries of the Woman's Missionary Society, West China Mission A13-20, box 18, file 9. Some sources list Isabelle Miller as a missionary until 1951; it is possible that she arrived in Canada in 1952, having departed China after September 1951. She is listed as working later in Canada and Hong Kong.

89   China Missionary, "First Thoughts on the Debacle of Christian Missions in China," *African Affairs*, January 1952, 33–41.

90   Ho, interview.

91   Janet Beaton interview with Chin Shu-wen, 11 June 1995, UMASC, A13-20, box 12, file 2.

92   Statistics on Medical and Nursing School Graduates of the PUMC, December 1950, RAC RF, SG 1.1, series 601-China, box 37, folder 298.

93   Personal communication with Yuhong Jiang, PUMC, 15 July 2020.

94   Nieh, interview.

95 Confidential Letter from Chu Pi-hui (Willowdale, ON) to President of the Florence Nightingale Foundation (London), 10 April 1975, Royal Holloway Archives and Special Collections (RHASC), Bedford College Papers (BC).

96 Certification of Bernice Chu Pi-hui as full-time student at Bedford College from 1927 to 1928, RHASC, BC.

97 Letter from Chu Pi-hui (Willowdale, ON) to L.P. Turnball (London), 21 June 1975, RHASC, BC.

98 Sally Chan and Francis Wong, "Development of Basic Nursing Education in China and Hong Kong," *Journal of Advanced Nursing* 29, 6 (1999): 1300–7.

99 Anne Davis, "Interview with Madam Lin Ju Ying," *Nursing Ethics* 8, 4 (2001): 484–86.

100 Grypma and Zhen, "Development of Modern Nursing," 315.

101 Nieh, interview.

102 Ibid.

Conclusion | THE ROCKEFELLER EFFECT: NURSING AS A LIBERATING MOVEMENT FOR WOMEN

1 China Missionary, "First Thoughts on the Debacle of Christian Missions in China," *African Affairs*, January 1952, 33.

2 Ibid.

3 Ibid., 36.

4 Ibid., 36.

5 Ai-chu Hsu, "Nursing Education in China," *American Journal of Nursing* 56, 8 (1956): 991.

6 Ibid.

7 John Watt, *Saving Lives in Wartime China: How Medical Reformers Built Modern Healthcare Systems amid War and Epidemics, 1928–1945* (Boston: Brill, 2014).

8 Rana Mitter, "Imperialism, Transnationalism, and the Reconstruction of Post-War China: UNRRA in China, 1944–7," *Past and Present* 218, 8 (2013): 57.

9 As announced at the ICN Congress in Singapore, which I attended from 27 June to 1 July 2019.

Acknowledgments

1 Janet Beaton and Marion McKay, "Profile of a Leader: Caroline Wellwood: Pragmatic Visionary," *Canadian Journal of Nursing Leadership* 12, 4 (1999): 30–33.

2 "Anne Davis Named 'Living Legend' by AAN," *UCSF School of Nursing*, 27 June 2012, https://nursing.ucsf.edu/news/anne-davis-named-living-legend-aan.

Bibliography

ARCHIVAL SOURCES

Anglican Church of Canada / General Synod Archives (ACC/GSA)
Missionary Society of the Church of England in Canada (MSCC) fonds, series 3,
  General Secretary's Records, 1897–1975.

Glenbow Museum Archives
Lillian Bertha Craigie collection; Woman's Missionary Society Minutes and
  Reports, 1926–29

Peking Union Medical College Archives – School of Nursing Archives (PUMC-SNA)
Fonds 337, 340–47, 377, 721, 806, 826, 833, 2437; files 1927-2437-2001 to 1927-
  3427-2203 and 1937-2437-3001 to 1937-2437-3225

Rockefeller Archive Center (RAC)
China Medical Board Inc. (CBA) records, 1914–2012, FA 065
Rockefeller Foundation (RF) records, Projects FA 386b, SG 1.1, series 601-China;
  Fellowship Files (1917–1979), A 244, SG 10.1, series 601-China

Royal Holloway Archives and Special Collections (RHASC)
Bedford College for Women Papers (BC), University of London

United Church of Canada Archives (UCCA)
Methodist Church (Canada) Woman's Missionary Society fonds, accession no.
  78.079C, fonds F15, FA 14, Series 3: West China Mission Collection, 1891–1931
United Church of Canada Woman's Missionary Society (WMS), accession no.
  83.058C, fonds 505, FA 90, series 3: China (Honan) 1925–55
United Church of Canada Woman's Missionary Society (WMS), accession no.
  83.058C, fonds 505, FA 90, series 5: China (West) 1935– 52

University of Manitoba Archives and Special Collection (UMASC)
Janet Beaton Collection, Research on China Mission, Mss 413 (A13-20), boxes 11, 12, 15–18.

Winnipeg General Hospital / Health Sciences Center Archives
WGH Yearbook Blue and White; Alumnae Scrapbook; *Alumnae Journal*, 1914–42

OTHER SOURCES

"1890s, Omar & Retta Kilborn and Family." *Vic in China*, 2015. Victoria University Library, University of Toronto. http://library.vicu.utoronto.ca/exhibitions/vic_in_china/sections/missionaries_and_mission_stations/1890s_omar_retta_kilborn_and_family.html.

"1890s, Virgil & Adeline Hart and Family." *Vic in China*, 2015. Victoria University Library, University of Toronto. http://library.vicu.utoronto.ca/exhibitions/vic_in_china/sections/missionaries_and_mission_stations/1890s_virgil_adeline_hart_and_family.html.

Allison, Sarah E. "Anna Wolf's Dream: Establishment of a Collegiate Nursing Education Program." *Image: Journal of Nursing Scholarship* 25, 2 (1993): 127–31.

Andrews, Bridie, and Mary Brown Bullock, eds. *Medical Transitions in Twentieth-Century China*. Indianapolis: Indiana University Press, 2014.

Armstrong-Reid, Susan. *China Gadabouts: New Frontiers of Humanitarian Nursing, 1941–1951*. Vancouver: UBC Press, 2018.

Austin, Alvyn. *Saving China: Canadian Missionaries in the Middle Kingdom, 1888–1959*. Toronto: University of Toronto Press, 1986.

Baick, John S. "Cracks in the Foundation: Frederick T. Gates, the Rockefeller Foundation, and the China Medical Board." *Journal of the Guilded Age and Progressive Era* 3, 1 (2004): 59–89.

Balme, Harold. *China and Modern Medicine: A Study in Medical Missionary Development*. London: United Council for Missionary Education, 1921.

Barnes, Nicole Elizabeth. *Intimate Communities: Wartime Healthcare and the Birth of Modern China, 1937–1945*. Oakland: University of California Press, 2018.

Beaton, Janet, and Marion McKay. "Profile of a Leader: Caroline Wellwood, Pragmatic Visionary." *Canadian Journal of Nursing Leadership* 12, 4 (1999): 30–33.

Beaton, Kenneth J. *West of the Gorges*. Toronto: United Church of Canada, 1948.

Bliss Edward, Jr. *Beyond the Stone Arches: An American Missionary Doctor in China, 1892–1932*. New York: John Wiley and Sons, 2001.

Bond, Geo J. *Our Share in China and What We Are Doing with It*. Toronto: Missionary Society of the Methodist Church, 1909.

Bowers, John Z. *Western Medicine in a Chinese Palace: Peking Union Medical College, 1917–1951*. Philadelphia: Josiah Macy Jr. Foundation, 1972.

Bu, Liping. "John B. Grant: Public Health and State Medicine." In *Medical Transitions in Twentieth-Century China*, ed. Bridie Andrews and Mary Brown Bullock, 212–26. Bloomington: Indiana University Press, 2014.

Bu, Liping, and Elizabeth Fee. "John B. Grant International Statesman of Public Health." *American Journal of Public Health* 98, 4 (2008): 628–29.

Bullock, Mary. *An American Transplant: The Rockefeller Foundation and Peking Union Medical College*. Berkeley: University of California Press, 1980.

"The Central Stations of the West China Mission." *Vic in China*, 2015. Victoria University Library, University of Toronto. http://library.vicu.utoronto.ca/exhibitions/vic_in_china/sections/missionaries_and_mission_stations/the_central_stations_of_the_west_china_mission.html.

Chan, Sally, and Francis Wong. "Development of Basic Nursing Education in China and Hong Kong." *Journal of Advanced Nursing* 29, 6 (1999): 1300–7.

Chen, Kaiyi. "Missionaries and the Early Development of Nursing in China." *Nursing History Review* 4 (1996): 129–49.

Cheung, Yuet-wah. *Missionary Medicine in China: A Study of Two Canadian Protestant Missions in China before 1937*. Lanham, MD: University Press of America, 1988.

China Missionary. "First Thoughts on the Debacle of Christian Missions in China." *African Affairs*, January 1952, 33–41.

Chung, E. "How Can the Nurses Association Help China?" *China Medical Journal* (1914): 416–18.

Clark, A. "The Nurses Association of China, Fifth Annual Conference, Shanghai, 1914." *British Journal of Nursing*, 12 September 1914, 211–12.

Copland, Marnie. *Mooncakes and Maple Sugar*. Burlington, ON: G.R. Welch, 1980.

Cruickshank, Kathleen. "Education History and the Art of Biography." *American Journal of Education* 107, 3 (1999): 231–39.

Davis, Anne. 2001. "Interview with Madam Lin Ju Ying." *Nursing Ethics* 8, 4 (2001): 484–86.

Dirlik, Arif. "The Ideological Foundations of the New Life Movement: A Study in Counterrevolution." *Journal of Asian Studies* 34, 4 (1975): 945–80.

"Educational Progress in Wartime China." *Timely Topics No. 5* (Chinese News Service) (1943?).

Endicott, Stephen. *James G. Endicott: Rebel Out of China*. Toronto: University of Toronto Press, 1980.

Ferguson, Mary E. *China Medical Board and Peking Union Medical College: A Chronicle of Fruitful Collaboration, 1914–1951*. New York: China Medical Board of New York, 1970.

Gao, Xi. "Chinese Perspectives on Medical Missionaries in the 19th Century: The Chinese Medical Missionary Journal." *Journal of Cultural Interaction in East Asia* 5 (2014): 97–118.

Goldmark, Josephine. *Nursing and Nursing Education in the United States: Report of the Committee for the Study of Nursing Education, and a Report of a Survey.* New York: Macmillan, 1923.

Green, Cathy. Canadian School in West China: Virgil Chittenden Hart. Accessed 20 May 2019. http://cschengdu.ca/?page_id=687 [no longer accessible].

Groft, Jean. "Everything Depends on Good Nursing." *Canadian Nurse* 102, 3 (2006): 19–22.

Grundmann, Christoffer H. *Sent to Heal! Emergence and Development of Medical Missions.* Lanham, MD: University Press of America, 2005.

Grypma, Sonya. *China Interrupted: Japanese Internment and the Reshaping of a Canadian Missionary Community.* Waterloo, ON: Wilfrid Laurier University Press, 2012.

–. *Healing Henan: Canadian Nurses at the North China Mission, 1888–1947.* Vancouver: UBC Press, 2008.

–. "In Retrospect: The Value of Feisty Students." *Journal of Christian Nursing* 28, 2 (2011): 71.

–. "Missionary Nursing: Internationalizing Religious Ideals." In *Religion, Religious Ethics, and Nursing,* ed. Marsha Fowler, Sheryl Reimer-Kirkham, Richard Sawatzky, and Elizabeth Johnston-Taylor, 129–50. New York: Springer, 2011.

Grypma, Sonya, and Cheng Zhen. "The Development of Modern Nursing in China." In *Medical Transitions in 20th Century China,* ed. Mary Bullock and Bridie Andrews, 297–317. Bloomington: Indiana University Press, 2014.

Hampton Robb, Isabel Adams. *Nursing Ethics: For Hospital and Private Use.* Cleveland: J.B. Savage, 1901.

Harrold, Trudy A. *On Highest Mission Sent: The Story of Health Care in Lamont, Alberta.* Lamont, AB: Lamont Health Care Centre, 1999.

Heffren, Hazel. *Letters from Old China: Letters and Diary Entries from 1901 to 1943 by Laura Hambley.* Asquith, SK: Author, 1989.

Hensman, B. "The Kilborn Family: A Record of a Canadian Family's Service to Medical Work and Education in China and Hong Kong." *Canadian Medical Association Journal* 97, 9 (1967): 471–83.

Hocking, William Ernest. *Re-Thinking Missions: A Layman's Inquiry after One Hundred Years.* New York: Harper & Brothers, 1932.

Hodgman, Gertrude. "Nursing in Formosa." *American Journal of Nursing* 53, 7 (1952): 838–40.

–. "The Teaching of Public Health Nursing at Yale." *American Journal of Nursing* 29, 11 (1929): 1354–60.

Hsu, Ai-Chu. "Nursing Education in China." *American Journal of Nursing* 56, 8 (1956): 991–94.

Hsu, Immanuel C.Y. "The Reorganisation of Higher Education in Communist China, 1949–61." *China Quarterly* 19 (1964): 128–60.

Ion, Hamish. "Much Ado about Too Few: Aspects of the Treatment of Canadian and Commonwealth POWs and Civilian Internees in Metropolitan Japan, 1941–1945." *Defence Studies* 6, 3 (2006): 292–317.

Jiang, Yuhong. "Shaping Modern Nursing Development in China before 1949." *International Journal of Nursing Sciences* 4, 1 (2017): 19–23.

Kamsler, Brigette C. "The Gripsholm Exchange and Repatriation Voyages." *Burke Library Blog*, 17 September 2012. https://blogs.cul.columbia.edu/burke/2012/09/17/the-gripsholm-exchange-and-repatriation-voyages-2/.

Kemper, Steve. "C-E.A. Winslow, Who Launched Public Health at Yale a Century Ago, Still Influential Today." *Yale News*, 2 June 2015. https://news.yale.edu/2015/06/02/public-health-giant-c-ea-winslow-who-launched-public-health-yale-century-ago-still-influe.

Leck, Greg. *Captives of Empire: The Japanese Internment of Allied Civilians in China, 1941–1945*. Bangor, PA: Shandy Press, 2006.

Lin, Evelyn. "Nursing in China," *American Journal of Nursing* 38, 1 (1938): 1–8.

Liu, Chung-tung. "From San Gu Liu Po to 'Caring Scholar': The Chinese Nurse in Perspective." *International Journal of Nursing Studies* 28, 4 (1991): 315–24.

Lu, Jun, Sonya Grypma, Yingjuan Cao, Lijuan Bu, Lin Shen, and Patricia Davidson. "Historically-Informed Nursing: A Transnational Case Study in China." *Nursing Inquiry* 25, 1 (2017): doi:10.1111/nin.12205.

Lutz, J.G. *China and the Christian Colleges, 1850–1950*. Ithaca, NY: Cornell University Press, 1971.

Maggs, Christopher. "A History of Nursing: A History of Caring?" *Journal of Advanced Nursing* 23, 3 (1996): 630–35. https://doi.org/10.1111/j.1365-2648.1996.tb00028.x.

McIntosh, Muriel. "Nursing in China." *Canadian Nurse* 37, 1 (1941): 17–20.

McKim, Mary. "Called to Serve: A Memoir." Unpublished manuscript, 2017.

McPherson, Kathryn. *Bedside Matters: The Transformation of Canadian Nursing, 1900–1990*. Toronto: Oxford University Press, 1996.

Minden, Karen. *Bamboo Stone: The Evolution of a Chinese Medical Elite*. Toronto: University of Toronto Press, 1994.

Mitter, Rana. "Imperialism, Transnationalism, and the Reconstruction of Post-War China: UNRRA in China, 1944–7." *Past and Present* 218, 8 (2013): 51–69.

Munro, John. *Beyond the Moon Gate: A China Odyssey, 1938–1950*. Vancouver: Douglas & McIntyre, 1990.

Nelson, Siobhan. "The Fork in the Road: Nursing History vs the History of Nursing." *Nursing History Review* 10 (2002): 175–88.

"News about Nursing: New School in Chengtu, China." *American Journal of Nursing* 44, 1 (1944): 81–82.

"News from China." *American Journal of Nursing* 44, 5 (1944): 504.

Prentice, Margaret May. *Unwelcome at the Northeast Gate*. Mission, KS: Inter-Collegiate Press, 1966.

Preston, L. Clara. *Flowers amongst the Debris: A Canadian Nurse in Wartorn China*. Brockville, ON: Preston Robb, n.d.

Radcliffe [sic], Jeanette. "War in Weihwei." *Canadian Nurse* 34, 7 (1938): 356–58.

Renshaw, Michelle. *Accommodating the Chinese: The American Hospital in China, 1880–1920*. New York: Routledge, 2005.

Scott, Munroe. *McClure: The China Years*. Markham, ON: Penguin Books, 1977.

Shulman, Deborah. "Prisms of China: Canadian Women Missionaries in China, 1904–1945." PhD diss., Concordia University, 2008.

Simpson, Cora. *A Joy Ride through China for the N.A.C.* Shanghai: Kwang Hsueh Publishing, 1926.

–. "Nursing in Mission Stations." *American Journal of Nursing* 14, 3 (1913): 191–94.

Smith, W.E. *A Canadian Doctor in West China: Forty Years under Three Flags*. Toronto: Ryerson Press, 1939.

Stephenson, Gladys. "The Nurses Association of China." *American Journal of Nursing* 46, 9 (1946): 612.

Sugiman, Pamela. "'Life Is Sweet': Vulnerability and Composure in the Wartime Narratives of Japanese Canadians." *Journal of Canadian Studies* 43, 1 (2009): 186–218.

Vandenberg, Helen. "Canadian Nursing History Stories: Canada's First Chinese Nurse." *Canadian Association for the History of Nursing Newsletter* (2012): 13.

–. "Race, Hospital Development and the Power of Community: The History of Japanese and Chinese Hospitals in British Columbia, 1880–1920." PhD diss., University of British Columbia, 2014.

Walmsley, Lewis Calvin. *West China Union University*. New York: United Board for Christian Education in Asia, 1974.

Watt, John. "The Development of Nursing in Modern China, 1870–1949." *Nursing History Review* 12 (2004): 67–96.

–. *Saving Lives in Wartime China: How Medical Reformers Built Modern Healthcare Systems amid War and Epidemics, 1928–1945*. Boston: Brill, 2014.

Yao, Hsun Yuan. "The First Year of the Rural Health Experiment in Ting Hsien, China." *Milbank Memorial Fund Quarterly Bulletin* 9, 3 (1931): 61–93.

Index

Note: Figures are indicated by an (f) appended to page numbers, and tables are indicated by a (t)

Incident, 62–64, 79; unease prior to Japanese occupation, 60–61; wartime challenges, 116–17, 128

Peking Union Medical College, School of Nursing: about, 4, 10, 317n4; alumnae, 249–50, 261(t), 288; alumnae leadership in Nurses Association of China, 51, 66–67, 67(t); attempts to continue as normal during war, 133–34; and Beijing Health Station conflict, 55–57; challenges finding Hodgman's successor, 72–75; Chinese leadership and staff, 155–56, 155(f), 288–89; Class of 1943 graduation, 265–66; closure by Communists, 231, 266–67, 277; comparison to missionary nursing, 286–89; comparison to WCUU, 12–13; conflict between Nieh and administrators, 209–12, 212–15, 215–16, 217–18, 220–22; departure from WCUU, 239–45; establishment, 37–38, 318n24; faculty concerns prior to Japanese occupation, 129–30; faculty while at WCUU, 189, 190(t), 191–92, 191(f); foreign staff recruitment challenges, 127–28; graduates, 38–39, 39(f), 276–77, 277(t), 278(t); Hsu Ai-Chu on, 282; impact at WCUU and beyond, 196–97, 202–3, 226–28, 289–90; and international networks, 289; language of instruction, 10, 16, 36, 130, 158, 193–96, 265; migration of faculty to West China, 176; Nieh's advocacy for faculty, 223–24; Nieh's recruitment as dean, 77–79; Nieh's report on postwar progress, 263–65; Nieh's studies at, 45–47, 47(f); nursing students at WCUU, 227(f); organizational structure at WCUU, 208–9; Pearl Harbor and national exams, 134–37, 163–64; postwar program adjustments and return to Beijing, 246–49, 256; and public health, 14, 42, 51–52, 54–55, 264, 287;

reestablishment under Communists, 279–80; relocation to WCUU, 5, 11, 12, 168, 176–87, 192, 205–7; and Renji School of Nursing, 198; reopening efforts at WCUU, 175–76, 188–89, 193–96, 198–202; senior class practicum, 40(f); staffing issues, 249; student recruitment and promotional materials, 39–41, 42; support for Nieh from Hodgman and Tennant, 218–20; Tennant's defence of, 261–62; uniforms, 201–2, 213–14; vision of nursing, 14, 43–44, 57–58, 80, 260–61, 285; wartime challenges, 196, 200–201; working conditions for staff and nurses, 199; Yuan's recognition of emerging nursing leaders, 245–46

Pen Yen, Victoria, 328n28

Pengxian, 32(t)

Peters, Mary, 233

Planning Committee on Nursing Education, 235–36, 237

Pratt, Miriam I., 154(t), 346n222

Prentice, Margaret May, 135, 136, 137, 138–39, 164, 283, 342n94

Preparatory Committee on Nursing Education, 237

Preston, Clara: departure from China, 173, 283; evacuation to and struggles in West China, 100, 101(t), 103, 104–6, 107, 108, 155, 172(t); in northern China, 102; postwar attempt to return to China, 231, 234–35; on student refugees, 90

Priest, Elsie M., 242, 244–45

public health and public health nursing: crisis in China, 53, 326n150; development of, 43, 70; and Mass Education Movement, 53–54; and PUMC, 14, 42, 51–52, 54–55, 264, 287; and transnational knowledge flows, 285; and wartime, 259. *See also* Beijing Health Station

128; bombing of West China, 94–100, 106, 107, 109–10, 118, 119; end of, 230, 239; impact on China and nursing, 11, 290; internment and restrictions on Westerners, 137, 138–39, 141, 153–55, 154(t), 158–60, 163, 345*n*188; Marco Polo Bridge Incident, 72, 73, 330*n*54; mass migration to West China, 89–90, 100, 102; Nanjing Massacre, 101–2; and Nurses Association of China, 11, 68–69, 246; and nursing, 257–59; occupation and closure of PUMC, 141–46, 146–47, 149–53, 162–63, 163–64; Pearl Harbor and PUMC national exams, 134–37; repatriation of Westerners, 156, 160–61, 192–93; unease in anticipation of, 60–61; waiting for the end, 116, 117–18, 119; wartime conditions, 81

Small, William, 275

Smith, W.E., 81, 95–96, 100

Snapper, Isadore, 139, 154(t), 156

social gospel, 31, 83, 284, 288

South China Mission (SCM), 29, 30(t), 31

Spanish flu, 43

Stanley, Mary Boyd, 102, 155

Stephenson, Gladys, 63–64, 66–67, 69, 158

Stewart, Violet, 268, 271, 272, 274–75

Stockley, Jean Menzies, 103

Streeter, M.E., 224, 225

Struthers, Ernest B., 103–4, 118–19, 181, 357*n*3

Stuart, John Leighton, 139, 156, 159–60, 164, 345*n*195

Sugiman, Pamela, 16

Sun, Helen, 92

Sun Yat-sen, 8, 146–47

Surdain, Jane, 274

Sutherland, Alexander, 29

Sutherland, Harriet, 7

Suzuki, Major, 143, 144

Sze, Sao-ke (Alfred), 222, 239

Taiwan, 279, 290

Tallman, Alma, 101(t), 113, 114, 172(t), 230, 250, 283

Taylor, Lillian, 230, 250, 253, 271–72

Taylor, Mrs. Hugh, 275

Taylor, Ruth, 108

Tennant, Mary Elizabeth, 72–73, 73–74, 130, 133, 218–19, 224, 261–62

Thurmer, Mrs., 144, 149

Tianjin, 8, 138, 146, 158

Tien, Ravenna (Tien Tsai-less), 39(f), 51, 69, 79, 245–46, 261(t)

transnational knowledge flows, 285–86, 290–91

transportation, 118–19, 232

Tsao, Clifford, 268–69

Tsen, Bishop, 232

Tso Han-yeh, 190(t)

Tsur, Y.T.: as China Medical Board trustee, 209; and conflict with Nieh, 208, 210–11, 212, 216, 217, 219, 222–23; and PUMC School of Nursing's departure from WCUU, 239–40, 241; and relocating PUMC to West China, 182

Tung Chi Medical College, 167

Tung Wu University, 248

Turner, Helen, 230–31, 234, 250

uniforms, 201–2, 213–14

United Church of Canada, 29, 287–88. *See also* missionaries and missionary nursing; North China Mission; South China Mission; West China Mission; Women's Missionary Society

United Hospitals of the Associated Universities in Chengdu, 33

United Nations Relief and Rehabilitation Administration (UNRRA), 237, 258, 274

University of Alberta, China Institute, 317*n*7

University of British Columbia, 317*n*7

Printed and bound in Canada by Friesens

Set in Akzidenz and Fournier by Artegraphica Design Co.

Copy editor: Barbara Tessman

Proofreader: Caitlin Gordon-Walker

Indexer: Stephen Ullstrom

Cartographer: Eric Leinberger

Cover designer: Alexa Love

Cover image: WCUU Nurses Dormitory, c. 1946. Courtesy Rockefeller Archive Centre.